MAGNETIC RESONANCE IMAGING TECHNIQUES

MAGNETIC RESONANCE IMAGING TECHNIQUES

Ajay M. Parikh, MBBS, MS

Research Associate
Department of Pharmacology
Medical College of Pennsylvania
Philadelphia, Pennsylvania

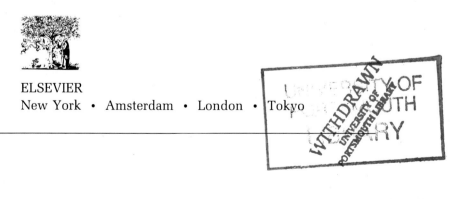

ELSEVIER
New York • Amsterdam • London • Tokyo

Elsevier Science Publishing Co., Inc.
655 Avenue of the Americas, New York, NY 10010

Sole distributors outside the United States and Canada:
Elsevier Science Publishers B.V.
P.O. Box 211, 1000 AE Amsterdam, the Netherlands

Library of Congress Cataloging-in-Publication Data

Parikh, Ajay.
    Magnetic resonance imaging techniques / Ajay Parikh.
      p.   cm.
    Includes index.
    ISBN 0-444-01634-1 (hardcover: acid free paper)
    1. Magnetic resonance imaging—Handbooks, manuals, etc.
  I. Title.
  RC78.7.N83P37   1991
  616.07′548—dc20   91-35160
                                        CIP

Current printing (last digit):
10 9 8 7 6 5 4 3 2 1

Manufactured in the United States of America

To
Reuben Mezrich
and
Rina Mehta

For accepting me when I had nothing to offer them except for the promise of a better future.

Contents

Preface

As an avid reader of various radiological journals and books, I was always a little confused by the variety of acronyms researchers gave to their magnetic resonance imaging (MRI) techniques and pulse sequences. Things got worse when a particular imaging technique would be referred to only by its acronym, and several references had to be read in order to understand it. This experience led me to believe that there was a genuine need for a single reference source which could be consulted whenever a quick description of a particular imaging technique is desired.

During the evolution of this book, I was driven by the urge to include as many different MRI techniques as possible. As a result, I have not included a lot of information about each technique. For example, extensive mathematical treatments are not covered; original references should be reviewed for such in-depth analyses. Furthermore, the following classes of MRI techniques have not been included in the present edition: spectroscopic and chemical shift imaging, perfusion and diffusion imaging, image reconstruction and display algorithms, stereotaxic imaging, and nonhydrogen nuclei imaging. All of these exclusions have helped me to keep the size of the book reasonable.

Each chapter has been divided into three sections. The first section discusses the basic principles of the technique. Pulse sequence diagrams are included for every major technique. In addition to the pulse diagrams, enough illustrations are provided to further explain the technique.[1] Unless stated otherwise, the slice (section) select, the frequency (read) encode, and the phase encode gradients are indicated by the letters Gz, Gx, and Gy, respectively. The second section discusses some of the clinical situations in which the technique has been evaluated. In most cases, a

---

[1] In the illustrations, the rising and falling edges of a gradient pulse are shown as vertical lines only for the convenience of drawing. However, it should not be forgotten that a finite amount of time is required for the attainment of desired amplitude and return to the baseline. Ideally, then, the gradient pulse would look like a trapezoid.

few representative cross-sectional images have been provided. Lastly, an up-to-date listing of journal references, which may be consulted for further reading, is provided.

The chapters have been arranged alphabetically. As a result, the earlier chapters may contain some material for which the reading of the latter chapters may be beneficial. In each chapter, such cross-references have been separately listed under the "*See also*" heading at the end of the first section, so that the reader can more easily locate related information. Indeed, it is understood that this book probably will not be read from the first page straight through to the last page.

Although background knowledge of the basic principles of MRI is assumed, it is my hope that this book will benefit readers who are new to, as well as those who are experienced with, MRI techniques and pulse sequences.

Ajay M. Parikh

Acknowledgments

I would like to express my deepest gratitude to the many distinguished researchers who have responded to my call, from as far away as England, France, Germany, Sweden, Switzerland, and Yugoslavia, and loaned me MR images of their scientific work. Without their support, it would not have been possible for me to produce a book of such high quality.

1

Blipped Echo Planar Imaging (BEPI)

BASIC PRINCIPLES

In echo planar imaging, the echo is evolved while both the phase encoding and frequency encoding gradients are high (Fig. 1.1). As a result, the k-space is traversed in a zig-zag manner (Fig. 1.2). In order to sample the k-space in a more uniform manner, in the "blipped" echo planar version, multiple gradient pulses of very short duration ("blips") are applied in the phase encoding direction in rapid succession. Each successive blip falls between the adjacent frequency encoding pulse and increments the phase-encoding value (in the corresponding k-space, the trajectory of the spins is moved up in the phase direction) until the entire k-space is sampled (Fig. 1.3). After each phase encoding step, data acquisition is carried out by rapid reversal of the frequency encoding gradient.

While the standard EPI consists of two separate pulse applications, the blipped echo planar single-pulse technique (BEST) employs a single RF pulse of angle less than 90° applied in the presence of a slice selective gradient (Fig. 1.4.). Multiple gradient echoes are, then, evolved in the time domain by orthogonal applications of read gradient and phase encoding gradient. Since it scans only half the k-space during a single pass, the collected echoes have to be either temporally rearranged [1] or the entire sequence must be repeated with the starting phase of the phase encoding gradient reversed in order to give the continuous scanning of the spatial frequency domain. Note that time symmetry can be achieved simply by time reversing the alternate echoes (temporal rearrangement), which eliminates the need for the second application of the pulse sequence (as in EPI) [6].

In both the spin echo and gradient echo versions, as the phase encoding

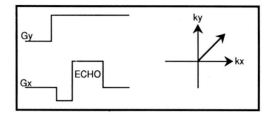

FIG. 1.1 To understand why the echo evolved with both the frequency encode (kx) and phase encode (ky) gradients simultaneously on gives zig-zag k-space sampling, imagine that while Gx is trying to pull the trajectory toward kx, Gy is trying, at the same time, to pull the trajectory toward ky. And, as a result, the trajectory ends up at an angle between the two axes.

gradient is blipped instead of keeping constantly high (as in EPI), the k-space is scanned in a rectilinear manner and is thus more uniformly sampled.

Variants   (A) In BEST, only half of the k-space (spatial frequency domain) is scanned in a one-pass parallel manner; real images based upon the amplitude are obtained by zero-filling the other half of the data set. In the modulus blipped echo planar single-pulse technique (MBEST), a gradient echo version, the entire k-space is scanned, so that both real and imaginary parts of the complex Fourier transform can be used to produce a modulus image that is insensitive to the phase errors [6].

To sample the entire k-space, the spin system is first taken to the negative kx axis by applying a negative gradient prepulse on the readout (Gx) gradient (Fig. 1.5.). The large Gy gradient is then repeatedly switched on

FIG. 1.2

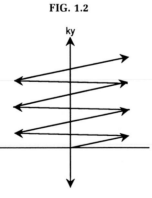

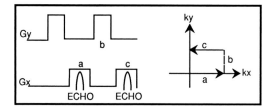

FIG. 1.3 During the time interval a, only Gx is on and, therefore, the trajectory moves only along the kx axis and an echo is collected. During the time interval b, only ky is on and, therefore, the trajectory moves one step forward along the ky axis. During the time interval c, once again, only Gx is on and, therefore, the trajectory moves only along the kx axis. In this way, the entire k-space or its portion is traversed in a rectangular manner.

and off to generate a series of gradient echoes. As it scans the entire k-plane, it takes twice as long as BEST to obtain the same spatial resolution if the gradient strengths are kept identical. A complete image can be obtained in as little as a few milliseconds.

(B) While temporally rearranging the acquired echoes in order to reconstruct an image, any time asymmetry in the gradient creates image artifacts. In order to prevent these artifacts, asymmetric blipped echo planar single-pulse technique (ABEST), a variant of BEST, has been proposed by Feinberg et al [5]. In ABEST, only echoes that have been acquired during the same phase of the gradient (50% of the acquired echoes

FIG. 1.4 Blipped echo planar sequence in which the initial gradient echo is subjected to rapid reversal of the frequency encode gradient. The phase encode gradient is blipped in between the gradient lobes of the frequency encode gradient. The shaded gradient combination is used if it is desired to start k-space sampling at a prescribed location. For example, in MBEST, the k-space is scanned beginning from the negative ky axis (see Fig. 1.5).

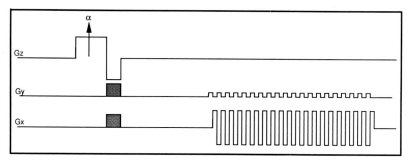

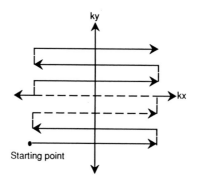

FIG. 1.5 K-space sampling strategy employed in MBEST. The magnetization vector is first moved to the lower left quadrant by prepulsing the phase encode and the frequency encode gradients.

meet this condition) are used to form an image. However, this translates into longer than usual total imaging times. By modifying the readout gradient profile from trapezoidal to asymmetric, it is possible to limit the increase in the acquisition time to about 15%.

(C) In the spin echo version of BEPI (Instascan) [10,11], a 90° slice-selective RF pulse is applied to excite the spins of a given region. This is followed by an 180° RF pulse that refocuses the transverse magnetization. The magnetization vector is, then, shifted from the center of the k-space to its lower left corner by applying an appropriate combination of the phase and frequency encoding gradients [2,4]. The spatial encoding is, then, carried out as described above.

If the principle of conjugate symmetry is used to derive the complete

FIG. 1.6 In mosaicked imaging, the entire k-space is divided into four quadrants and the imaging pulse sequence is repeated in each quadrant. Here, at the cost of increased imaging time, higher resolution is obtained.

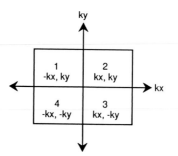

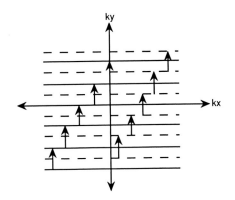

FIG. 1.7 K-space sampling strategy employed in MESH imaging. The left column of arrows indicates odd-numbered phase steps (solid lines) acquired during one application of the pulse sequence; the right column of arrows indicates even-numbered phase encode steps (broken lines) acquired during the second application of the same pulse sequence.

set of image data, the Instascan technique is called the partial k scan Instascan [2]. In another approach, the entire k-space is divided into several blocks, and each block is sampled by repeating the sequence (Fig. 1.6). This approach is called the *mosaic technique*. Although the mosaic technique increases total imaging time, image resolution is considerably improved, especially along the frequency encoding gradient.

In *mosaicked echo scan hybrid* (MESH), two interleaved acquisitions are carried out (Fig. 1.7), one containing odd-numbered phase steps and the other containing even-numbered phase steps. The final image shows an increased signal-to-noise ratio (SNR) with improved resolution along both the kx and ky axes [2].

See also: EPI.

CLINICAL APPLICATIONS
TISSUE CONTRAST

In BEST (and EPI), the zero phase encode step is acquired very early in the experiment. At this time, the echo amplitude is maximum, but is relatively unperturbed by T2 decay. As this phase encode step primarily determines image contrast, the latter is devoid of any T2 weighting.

In MBEST, the zero phase encode step occurs near the echo maximums. Therefore, unlike BEST or EPI images, MBEST images are intrinsically T2 weighted. Although the signal-to-noise ratio is degraded, the contrast-to-noise ratio (CNR) is superior to standard EPI images.

As the RF pulses used in the Instascan technique are similar to those used in SE imaging, the contrast of the images is similar to conventional SE images. If lower than 90° RF pulse is used, for example, to acquire almost instantaneous images, then the contrast becomes at first increasingly T1 weighted, and then proton density weighted [2].

It is possible to introduce any amount of T1 weighting in the images derived from these variants by preceding the initial 90° pulse by a suitable magnetization preparation sequence, such as the inversion recovery [15].

CEREBROSPINAL FLUID

Stehling et al [17] have reported the use of MBEST in analyzing cerebrospinal fluid (CSF) motion. As MBEST can provide both magnitude and phase reconstructed images, their results indicate that it is possible to measure CSF flow velocity in the absence of flow artifacts.

THE HEART

Due to the fast nature of the EPI technique in general, cine-MR studies of the heart may be completed in a few seconds without the need for any motion reduction schemes. As a general class, EPI techniques are useful in clinical settings for imaging organs where the use of more conventional imaging techniques would lead to the creation of motion artifacts in the images. EPI techniques have been used most frequently for real-time cardiac studies (cine-MRI) [3]. A typical cine study using BEST can be completed in as little as one second.

The most challenging task for any fast imaging technique is to depict small vessels accurately without blurring. Using MBEST, it is possible to visualize the coronary arteries of the beating heart [13]. The access to such dynamic information about cardiac functioning is crucial to proper assessment of ischemic disorders. Cardiac cine-studies furnish not only information regarding structural disorders of the valves and septa, but they also shed light on the functional derangements associated with such disorders.

Stehling et al [19] have imaged the motion of the fetal heart using low angle excitation MBEST, without the need for cardiac triggering.

THE ABDOMEN

While conventional T2-weighted SE images provide the best tissue differentiation in the abdomen, such images are grossly spoiled by the presence of motion-induced phase artifacts. In this situation, various versions of BEPI, as described herein, have eliminated motion-related artifacts and provided T2-weighted tissue contrast images of various vascular structures, such as portal, splenic, and mesenteric vessels, and organs, such as the liver, pancreas, adrenal, and kidneys [8,12,14,16,18]. While most of these investigators have employed gradient echo imaging up to the field strength of 0.5 T [8,14], Saini et al [12] have employed the spin echo version at 2.0 T. At higher field strength, magnetic field inhomogeneity effects are exaggerated and the presence of 180° refocusing pulse in the spin echo version partially recovers the signal loss due to spin dephasing. This seems to make implementation of the spin echo EPI feasible at 2.0 T.

PREGNANCY

As noted above, MBEST has been used in MR imaging of the human fetus in utero, and the images produced are free of fetal motion artifacts. Moreover, three-dimensional implementation of MBEST imaging of the fetus has enabled fetal lung volume estimations to be obtained.

ADVANTAGES AND DISADVANTAGES

In contrast to standard EPI, its blipped version traverses the k-space in a more uniform manner. The BEST approach scans only half the k-space and the images are based upon the amplitude of the pixel magnetization. This characteristic makes BEST images susceptible to the field inhomogeneities induced phase artifacts. In the MBEST approach, the entire k-space is traversed. Therefore, image artifacts related to imperfect k-space sampling are mostly removed and the resolution is greatly improved.

Sampling of the entire k-space in MBEST results in an increase in total acquisition time. However, this is outweighed by the fact that the modulus images are insensitive to phase artifacts related to field inhomogeneities and the flowing blood, thus they are technologically more robust than the corresponding EPI or BEST images. For example, MBEST imaging of a zoomed voxel totally avoids image distortion caused by the main magnetic field inhomogeneities seen in unzoomed EP imaging [20]. Ordidge et al [7] have further discussed the relative significance of sampling strategies employed in EPI, BEST, and MBEST imaging.

As the time-reversed (temporally rearranged) echoes are used for image reconstruction, any time-dependent asymmetry in the gradient gives rise to artifacts in the center of the image. This artifact may be removed by nonlinear sampling of the spatial frequency domain or by employing ABEST, a variant of the BEST imaging technique.

The greatest advantage of this technique is its ability to provide real-time MR images of the heart without the need for cardiac triggering. Earlier EPI was unable to function without the triggered mode; this limited the number of images (usually to one) that could be acquired in a single cardiac cycle. With the introduction of BEST, as many as twenty images could be acquired in a single cardiac cycle. Instead of splicing together images from different cardiac cycles, a cine-MR loop consisting of images from the same cardiac cycle provides the essential dynamic information without any phase inconsistencies.

The data in EPI, in general, are acquired in times equivalent to the T2 values for most tissues. Therefore, the influence of the T2 decay is not uniform across the k-space and, as the acquired data are not Hermitian symmetric, this introduces blurring artifacts in Fourier transformed images. Oshio and Singh [9] have proposed an imaging scheme in which data from the entire k-space are acquired. Using the fact that these data are Hermitian symmetric, a correction factor, which is the geometric mean of two symmetric data points, is calculated. The measured point is recalculated using this correction factor before performing the Fourier transform. This method has yielded artifact-free images in computer simulations [9].

As almost all the data acquisition comprising a slice is finished within a single pulse repetition period, the pulse sequence has to be reapplied several times in order to obtain multiple slices. However, this hardly poses a grave difficulty because multiple slices can be acquired in sub-second time periods.

Common to EPI and all its variants, the gradient power supply has to be able to provide enough voltage to achieve very fast rise times (for example 4 G/cm in 150 μsec) [2]. In addition, to collect data very rapidly, a broad receiver bandwidth is required, which decreases the signal-to-noise ratio by a factor of the square root of the applied bandwidth. With appropriate hardware modifications, Cohen and Weisskoff [2] have been able to acquire and display a maximum of five images every second using the Instascan technique.

REFERENCES

1. Chapman B, Turner R, Ordidge RJ, Doyle M, Cawley M, Coxon R, Glover P, Mansfield P (1987): Real-time movie imaging from a single cardiac cycle by NMR. *Magn Reson Med* 5:246–254.
2. Cohen MS and Weisskoff RM (1991): Ultra-fast imaging. *Magn Reson Imag* 9:1–37.

3. Doyle M, Chapman B, Turner R, Ordidge RJ, Cawley M, Coxon R, Glover P, Coupland RE, Morris GK, Worthington BS, Mansfield P (1986): Real-time cardiac imaging of adults at video frame rates by magnetic resonance imaging. *Lancet* 2:682.

4. Farzaneh F, Riederer SJ, Pelo NJ (1990): Analysis of T2 limitations and off-resonance effects on spatial resolution and artifacts in echo-planar imaging. *Magn Reson Med* 14:123–139.

5. Feinberg DA, Turner R, Jakab PD, Von Kienlin M (1990): Echo planar imaging with asymmetric gradient modulation and inner-volume excitation. *Magn Reson Med* 13:162–169.

6. Howseman AM, Stehling MK, Chapman B, Coxon R, Turner R, Ordidge RJ, Cawley MG, Glover P, Mansfield P, Coupland RE (1988): Improvements in snap-shot nuclear magnetic resonance imaging. *Br J Radiol* 61:822–828.

7. Ordidge RJ, Coxon R, Howseman A, Chapman B, Turner R, Stehling M, Mansfield P (1988): Snapshot head imaging at 0.5 T using the echo planar technique. *Magn Reson Med* 8:110–115.

8. Ordidge RJ, Howseman A, Coxon R, Turner R, Chapman B, Glover P, Stehling M, Mansfield P (1989): Snapshot imaging at 0.5 T using echo planar techniques. *Magn Reson Med* 10:227–240.

9. Oshio K, Singh M (1989): A computer simulation of T2 decay effects in echo planar imaging. *Magn Reson Med* 11:389–397.

10. Pykett IL, Rzedzian RR (1987): Instant images of the body by magnetic resonance. *Magn Reson Med* 5:563–571.

11. Rzedzian RR, Pykett IL (1987): Instant images of the human heart using a new, whole-body MR imaging system. *Am J Roentgen* 149:245–250.

12. Saini S, Stark DD, Rzedzian RR, Pykett IL, Rummeny E, Hahn PF, Wittenberg J, Ferrucci JT (1989): Forty-millisecond MR imaging of the abdomen at 2.0 T. *Radiology* 173:111–116.

13. Stehling M, Howseman A, Chapman B, Coxon R, Glover P, Turner R, Ordidge RJ, Jaroszkiewicz G, Mansfield P, Morris GK, Dutka D, Worthington BS, Coupland RE (1987): Real-time NMR imaging of coronary vessels. *Lancet* 2: 964–965.

14. Stehling MK, Howseman AM, Ordidge RJ, Chapman B, Turner R, Coxon R, Glover P, Mansfield P, Coupland RE (1989): Whole body echo-planar MR imaging at 0.5 T. *Radiology* 170:257–263.

15. Stehling MK, Ordidge RJ, Coxon R, Mansfield P (1990): Inversion-recovery echo planar imaging (IR-EPI) at 0.5 T. *Magn Reson Med* 13:514–517.

16. Stehling MK, Charnley RM, Blamire AM, Ordidge RJ, Coxon R, Gibbs P, Hardcastle JD, Mansfield P (1990): Ultrafast magnetic resonance scanning of the liver with echo-planar imaging. *Br J Radiol* 63:430–437.

17. Stehling MK, Firth JL, Worthington BS, Guilfoyle DN, Ordidge RJ, Coxon R, Blamire AM, Gibbs P, Bullock P, Mansfield P (1991): Observation of cerebrospinal fluid flow with echo-planar magnetic resonance imaging. *Br J Radiol* 64:89–97.

18. Stehling MK, Evans DF, Lamont G, Ordidge RJ, Howseman AM, Chapman B, Coxon R, Mansfield P, Hardcastle JD, Coupland RE (1989): Gastrointestinal tract: dynamic MR studies with echo-planar imaging. *Radiology* 171:41–46.

19. Stehling MK, Mansfield P, Ordidge RJ, Coxon R, Chapman B, Blamire AM, Gibbs P, Johnson IR, Symonds EM, Worthington BS, Coupland RE (1990): Echo-planar imaging of the human fetus in utero. *Magn Reson Med* 13: 314–318.

20. Turner R, von Kienlin M, Moonen CTW, van Zijl PCM (1990): Single shot localized echo-planar imaging (STEAM-EPI) at 4.7 Tesla. *Magn Reson Med* 14:401–408.

2

Cardiac Cycle Ordered Phase Encoding (COPE)

BASIC PRINCIPLES

It is widely known that respiratory motion degrades abdominal images and, similarly, cardiac motion causes the intensity of the blood to vary. However, less obvious is the fact that both these physiological motions also make the CSF pulsate [3]; this motion has been documented by various investigators [4,5,7–8]. The CSF pulsations would diminish the signal intensity if flow-induced phase dispersion is not refocused at the imaging time. In certain imaging techniques, this signal loss increases the contrast-to-noise ratio between CSF and the brain/spinal cord. For example, conventional SE images show CSF flowing through the aqueduct as a dark spot due to flow-induced signal loss, and this aids in verifying the patency of the lumen [8]. In most other cases, however, the variable intensity of CSF causes difficulties in the correct interpretation of such images by giving rise to image artifacts [1].

In addition to various general approaches (such as fast imaging), the following specific techniques have been proposed for overcoming CSF motion artifacts.

1. As CSF pulsates in synchrony with the cardiac cycle, it experiences nonconstant flow velocity depending on the status of the cardiac cycle. Therefore, if two separate acquisitions are carried out, one in systole and the other in diastole, an MR myelogram can be obtained by subtracting these two data acquisitions.

2. Similar to the approach described above, two sets of image data are acquired, one with velocity compensation and the other a conventional image. When the latter is subtracted from the former, once again, an MR myelogram is obtained.

In addition to yielding artifact-free myelograms, these two approaches may also permit CSF flow quantification [9]. For example, Quencer et al [6] have used cardiac-triggered gradient echo imaging of the CSF for establishing normal CSF flow patterns and calculating the flow velocity.

Alternatively, if it can be recognized that the cause of the CSF motion artifact is similar to the respiratory motion artifacts, then an approach similar to respiratory ordered phase encoding (ROPE) may be employed for imaging CSF, too. Note that, in ROPE, the acquisition (or positioning) of a phase encoding step is determined by the amplitude of the artifact causing motion. An approach similar to the ROPE technique has been proposed for CSF imaging; it is called cardiac cycle ordered phase encoding, or COPE [2]. The method works as explained below (Fig. 2.1).

A series of RF pulses of identical flip angle are continuously applied at regular intervals. An ECG signal is also being obtained continuously to monitor the phase of the cardiac cycle. The time interval between the R wave and the RF pulse determines which gradient step is next acquired with what strength. Usually, the longer this time interval, the larger is the gradient step to be acquired. The critical point to note is that the total number of phase encode steps is equally distributed over one period of CSF motion. After all the phase encoding values are thus acquired, they are temporally rearranged from k_{min} to k_{max} to reconstruct an MR myelogram.

It is important to distinguish this approach from the more conventional method of cardiac triggering. In both these methods, an ECG signal is

FIG. 2.1 In COPE, the RF pulses are applied in a free-running mode, asynchronous with the ECG wave. The pulse repetition time, TR, is constant regardless of the R-R interval. Therefore, each pulse cycle (shaded areas on the RF axis) is preceded by a variable delay (dotted areas on the RF axis). Depending on this delay value, the amplitude of the phase encode level for that pulse repetition is chosen. Usually, a phase encode step closer to the k_{max} is selected for the pulse cycle triggered by a longer delay, and vice versa. If the selected phase encode step has already been used, the phase encode step next to the selected step is used. The acquired phase encode steps are retrospectively rearranged in the proper order for image reconstruction. Note that the ECG signal is used only for determining the order of the phase encode steps and is *not* used for triggering RF.

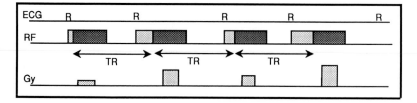

acquired and, in the cardiac-triggered mode, data are acquired only when a particular phase of the cycle is reached. However, in COPE, data are acquired continuously at any phase of the cardiac cycle and they are retrospectively rearranged to yield a final image. This approach simulates the situation as if phase dispersion due to CSF motion is a function of time, varying slowly in concert with the phase encoding function.

See also: DOPE, MAST, RARE.

CLINICAL APPLICATIONS
TISSUE CONTRAST

The CSF appears uniformly bright on both T1- and T2-weighted COPE myelograms. As the flow-related artifacts are essentially eliminated, the contrast-to-noise ratio of COPE images is superior to the CSF images acquired without phase reordering.

CEREBROSPINAL FLUID

Due to the long T2 value of CSF, usually heavily T2-weighted spin echo pulse sequences have been used to obtain CSF myelograms. Such images frequently are marked by severe flow artifacts in the phase encoding direction and the presence of these artifacts sometimes obscures the pathology. As the COPE myelograms are virtually free of flow artifacts, more precise assessment of the pathology is possible.

ADVANTAGES AND DISADVANTAGES

In the past, techniques such as cardiac triggering were used to coordinate the data acquisition from the slowly flowing CSF with the cardiac cycle. Under normal circumstances, this technique provides a powerful way of reducing flow-related artifacts. However, in patients with cardiac rhythm disorder, the image quality is poor. Such abnormal cardiac rhythm may also introduce errors in the time markers used in the COPE technique; but, phantom studies show that these errors would not degrade image quality.

REFERENCES

1. Bock JC, Neumann K, Sander B, Schmidt D, Schorner W (1991): Prepontine artifacts due to cerebrospinal fluid pulsation in the T2 weighted coronal MRT picture: clinical significance, frequency, technique for artifact suppression. ROFO 154:202–205.

2. Cho MH, Kim WS, Cho ZH (1990): CSF flow artifact reduction using cardiac cycle ordered phase-encoding method. *Magn Reson Imag* 8:395–405.

3. Dardenne G, Dereymaeker A, Lacheron JM (1969): Cerebrospinal fluid pressure and pulsatility: an experimental study of circulatory and respiratory influences in normal and hydrocephalic dogs. *Eur Neurol* 2:192–216.

4. Feinberg DA, Mark AS (1987): Human brain motion and cerebrospinal fluid circulation demonstrated with MR velocity imaging. *Radiology* 163:793–799.

5. Lee E, Wang JZ, Mezrich R (1989): Variation of lateral ventricular volume during the cardiac cycle observed by MR imaging. *Am J Neuroradiol* 10:1146–1149.

6. Quencer RM, Post MJ, Hinks RS (1990): Cine MR in the evaluation of normal and abnormal CSF flow: intracranial and intraspinal studies. *Neuroradiology* 32:371–391.

7. Ridgway JP, Turnbull LW, Smith MA (1987): Demonstration of pulsatile cerebrospinal-fluid flow using magnetic resonance phase imaging. *Br J Radiol* 60:423–427.

8. Sherman JL, Citrin CM, Bowen BJ, Gangarosa RE (1986): MR demonstration of altered cerebrospinal fluid flow by obstructive lesions. *Am J Neuroradiol* 7: 571–579.

9. Stahlberg F, Mogelvang J, Thomsen C, Nordell B, Stubgaard M, Ericsson A, Sperber G, Greitz D, Larsson H, Henriksen O, et al (1989): A method for MR quantification of flow velocities in blood and CSF using interleaved gradient-echo pulse sequences. *Magn Reson Imag* 7:655–667.

3

Double Phase Encoding (DOPE)

BASIC PRINCIPLES

Numerous approaches have been implemented in MR imaging for examining the morphological and quantitative characteristics of CSF. Even on conventional T2-weighted spin echo imaging, CSF shows up as a highly intense structure without the need for any special maneuvers. However, much like blood, the CSF pulsates, albeit slowly, in phase with the cardiac cycle [8] and flow-related artifacts degrade the contrast-to-noise ratio between the CSF and adjacent tissues. To avoid these artifacts, one of the earliest approaches has been to link the CSF data acquisition to a particular phase of the cardiac cycle [1,2,7,9,10]. For still better performance, two acquisitions, one sampled in systole and the other in diastole, may be subtracted to achieve only CSF visualization [8]. Recently, motion compensating gradients have been employed to obtain artifact-free CSF images (GMN or MAST). With the availability of gradient echo based, low flip angle rapid imaging techniques, such as GRASS, and flow-encoding gradient waveforms, phase-contrast imaging of the CSF also has been possible [3].

An alternative to the approaches mentioned above is a spin echo based rapid pulse sequence proposed by Hennig and Friedburg [5], called double phase encoding (DOPE). DOPE uses the principle of interferography. Based on the Fourier shift theorem, DOPE simultaneously generates two signals with different phase encoding information from the same tissue parameter, such as flow. Thus, two superimposed data sets are generated; when they are displayed simultaneously in the gray scale format, a pattern of parallel bands of alternating intensities appears across the display.

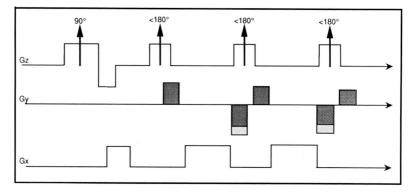

FIG. 3.1 The DOPE pulse sequence is a modified RARE sequence. The striking feature of the pulse sequence is that the phase compensating lobe differs from the phase encoding lobe by some constant amount (dotted areas). (Modified, with permission, from Hennig et al [6]).

The DOPE pulse sequence is shown in Fig. 3.1. In fact, DOPE is a modified RARE sequence. As in the standard RARE sequence, variable phase encoding between the RF pulses exists. However, unlike in RARE, the refocusing pulses in DOPE are slightly lower than 180°. The effect of such low angle refocusing pulses on transverse magnetization established by 90° pulse has been studied by Hahn in his original paper on spin echoes [4]. In short, it has been shown that transverse magnetization is parted into two components with different phases [5]. Moreover, the phase encoding (Ge) and phase encoding compensating (Gc) gradient pulses have differing amplitudes (A). In other words,

$$A(Gc) = A(Ge) + C$$

where C is constant for the entire pulse sequence. Note that, in RARE, C = 0. With these modifications, two series of echoes are produced simultaneously, but with different phase encoding; the difference, $\Delta\phi$, between them, at position p is equivalent to $(\gamma C\tau)p$, where γ is the gyromagnetic ratio and τ is the time for which the gradient is switched on [6].

As these two echo series are phase shifted from each other, they encode the flow information differently. Therefore, using the Fourier shift theorem, desired interferograms can be obtained from these two simultaneously acquired, but phase shifted, data sets (see NIMAT).

See also: COPE, FISP, MAST, RARE.

CLINICAL APPLICATIONS
TISSUE CONTRAST

The images show alternating horizontal bright/dark bands in the regions where flow is present, and the areas corresponding to the stationary tissues are not visualized at all.

CEREBROSPINAL FLUID

The significance of the shape and integrity of the stripes is as follows:

1. Spacing between adjacent stripes is proportional to the flow velocity. As the minimum spacing between stripes can be one pixel wide, the

FIG. 3.2 (a) T2-weighted RARE myelogram showing a subarachnoid cyst (C) fails to indicate whether a communication exists between the cyst and the spinal canal. **(b)** The DOPE myelogram shows the flow pattern inside the cyst similar to the flow pattern in the spinal canal, which is suggestive of the possibility that the CSF in the spinal canal may communicate with the cystic contents. (Courtesy of J. Hennig; reproduced, with permission, from Hennig et al [6]).

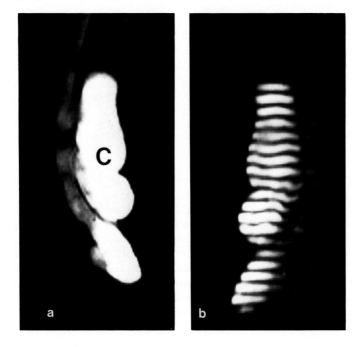

minimum flow velocity (per pixel, mm/sec) that can be resolved is (2 × FOV)/(Echo spacing × Total number of pixels) [6]. For a typical image of 128 phase encodings and 40 cm FOV, this becomes 1.3 mm/sec/pixel. As the stripes bulge in the direction of the flow, the flow direction also can be readily determined by looking at the curvature of the stripes.

2. Clinically, it may be important to determine whether the intracranial shunt installed to bypass an obstructive pathology is patent. In this situation, any discontinuity in the stripes may suggest that the flow is absent in that region, eg, around a blocked shunt.

3. Alignment of the stripes may suggest whether multiple aqueous spaces lying in close proximity communicate with one another. For example, the standard T2-weighted RARE myelogram often fails to demonstrate whether a communication exists between a neural cyst and the spinal canal (Fig. 3.2a). In such a situation, if a DOPE myelogram shows stripes overlying the cyst running parallel to those overlying the spinal canal, it strongly indicates the presence of a communication between them (Fig. 3.2b).

ADVANTAGES AND DISADVANTAGES

The DOPE sequence is inherently sensitive only to flow. In other words, the phase information in DOPE is not corrupted by localized field inhomogeneities or any other nonvelocity-dependent phase changes. This feature is a distinct advantage over other phase-based myelographic techniques.

In contrast to ECG-gated MR myelography, the examination time for a DOPE myelogram is only about a few seconds. This may prove advantageous in small children and hyperirritable or terminally ill patients.

MR myelograms with similar stripes have been obtained by others [2,10]; however, unlike these approaches, no postprocessing of the data is necessary in the DOPE experiment.

The DOPE technique gives only the time averaged flow velocity. Thus, dynamic information about the pulsatility is lost. As long as the flow profile is laminar, time averaged flow velocity equals the mean velocity over the period of data acquisition. However, if the flow profile becomes turbulent during some part of the data acquisition, experimental results have shown that the quantitative assessment of flow is weighted toward that part of the period in which the laminar flow is more prominent [6].

This technique has been implemented on a Bruker 2 T whole body superconductive system (S200).

REFERENCES

1. Bergstrand G, Bergstrom M, Nordell B, Stahlberg F, Ericsson A, Hemmingson A, Sperber G, Thomas KA, Jung B (1985): Cardiac gated MR imaging of cerebrospinal fluid flow. *J Comput Assist Tomogr* 9:1003–1006.

2. Edelman RR, Wedeen VJ, Davis KR, Widder D, Hahn P, Shoukimas G, Brady TJ (1986): Multiphasic MR imaging: a new method for direct imaging of pulsatile CSF flow. *Radiology* 161:779–783.

3. Enzmann DR, Pecl NJ (1991): Normal flow patterns of intracranial and spinal cerebrospinal fluid defined with phase-contrast cine MR imaging. *Radiology* 178:467–474.

4. Hahn EL (1950): Spin echoes. *Phys Rev* 80:580–594.

5. Hennig J, Friedburg H (1988): Clinical applications and methodological developments of the RARE technique. *Magn Reson Imag* 6:391–395.

6. Hennig J, Ott D, Adam TH, Friedburg H (1990): Measurement of CSF flow using an interferographic MR technique based on the RARE-fast imaging sequence. *Magn Reson Imag* 8:543–556.

7. Mascalchi M, Ciraolo L, Tanfani G, Taverni N, Inzitari D, Siracusa GF, DalPozzo GC (1988): Cardiac-gated phase MR imaging of aqueductal CSF flow. *J Comput Assist Tomogr* 12:923–926.

8. Njemanze PC, Beck OJ (1989): MR-gated intracranial CSF dynamics: evaluation of CSF pulsatile flow. *Am J Neuroradiol* 10:77–80.

9. Quencer RM, Post MJ, Hinks RS (1990): Cine MR in the evaluation of normal and abnormal CSF flow: intracranial and intraspinal studies. *Neuroradiology* 32:371–391.

10. Wedeen VJ, Rosen BR, Chesler D, Brady TJ (1985): MR velocity imaging by phase display. *J Comput Assist Tomogr* 9:530–536.

4

Echo Planar Imaging (EPI)

BASIC PRINCIPLES

The echo planar imaging technique, as proposed by Mansfield in 1977 [14], is one of the earliest fast NMR imaging techniques. Although many other spin mapping techniques were proposed before EPI, their performances were suboptimal for a number of reasons, primarily the lengthy image acquisition times, which were undesirable in clinical applications. Therefore, one of the intentions of EPI was to achieve good quality images in clinically acceptable time periods. While the earliest techniques collected NMR signals from a single point or, at best, a single line of the two-dimensional plane after each excitation, the revolutionary echo planar imaging method could collect all the data points comprising a selected plane following the application of a single excitation pulse.

A simple illustrative EPI pulse sequence is given in Fig. 4.1. The 90° RF pulse excites the spins in a plane selected by the slice selection gradient. After spin excitation, both the frequency and phase encoding gradients are turned on simultaneously. The decaying FID is transformed into a gradient echo by rapidly reversing the frequency encode gradient. This echo contributes a line along the kx axis. Most conventional gradient echo techniques abandon the echo here and repeat the pulse sequence with different phase encoding steps. However, in EPI, the first echo is repeatedly dephased and rephased by rapidly oscillating the frequency encode gradient. Each successive echo is phase encoded differently, due to the time interval that exists between the echoes. Thus, a series of differently phase encoded echoes is obtained by only a single RF excitation of the plane.

The resultant k-space trajectories are shown in Fig. 4.2a. In order to

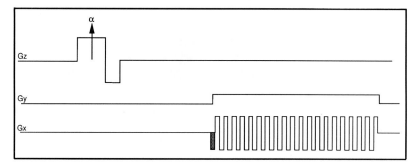

FIG. 4.1 An illustrative echo planar sequence. The initial echo is further phase encoded by the constant phase encoding gradient and a series of gradient echoes is obtained by rapidly reversing the frequency encode gradient. An RF refocused spin echo may be used initially to decrease the harmful effects of field inhomogeneities. As the single application of the pulse sequence scans the k-space in a zig-zag manner, it is repeated with the starting polarity of the frequency encode gradient reversed (shaded area). Also see Fig. 4.2.

perform the Fourier transform on the data, it is necessary for all the echoes to evolve in the same direction along the frequency axis (Fig. 4.2b). Therefore, the pulse sequence of Fig. 4.1 is reapplied, but now with the starting phase of the frequency encode gradient reversed (the dashed part in the figure). This second pulse application scans the k-space as shown in Fig. 4.2c. If alternate lines from Figs. 4.2a and 4.2c are concatenated, two sets

Fig. 4.2 (a) K-space sampling if the pulse sequence of Fig. 4.1 is used. However, in order to perform artifact-free Fourier transform, the echoes have to evolve either only along the solid lines or only along the broken lines **(b)**. Therefore, the pulse sequence of Fig. 4.1 is reapplied with the starting phase of the oscillating gradient in the opposite direction, which gives the k-space sampling as shown in **(c)**. If the alternate lines from (a) and (c) are spliced together, two data sets corresponding to the solid lines and the broken lines are obtained.

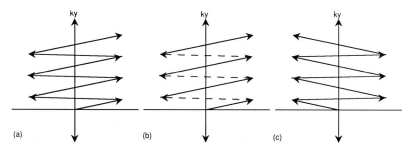

of data are obtained with the k-space traversal as shown in Fig. 4.2b. Before performing the Fourier transform, the individual data sets are zero-filled. Alternatively, the half-Fourier approach may be used [6]. The resultant two images may be summed (after one of the images is reversed) to achieve an improvement in the signal-to-noise ratio by a factor of 1.4 [2].

Two alternative algorithms for reconstructing an image from a zig-zag trajectory have been proposed. Sekihara and Kohno [20] have proposed using odd- and even-numbered echoes to create two individual images. However, as the sampling interval is doubled for each image, aliasing artifacts appear. Sekihara and Kohno have demonstrated that when these two images are combined, the artifacts disappear. Yan and Braun [23] have proposed using the generalized Fourier transform theory to reconstruct an image directly, using the data of even–odd zig-zag trajectory without any artifacts.

The following points should be noted from the above discussion:

1. As each echo evolves at a different time, TE is not the same for all the phase encoded lines. In addition, the amplitude of the successive echoes decreases by a factor of $e^{\tau/T2}$ (Fig. 4.3). This is analogous to the echo attenuation that occurs in a multiecho series. The maximum number of echoes that can be obtained is limited by T2/(2 × Echo decay time). Obviously, the image contrast is not uniform everywhere.
2. The RF pulse angles of the two pulse applications are 45° and 90°, to keep the signal amplitude the same in two echo series (tan a = sin b, where a and b are excitation flip angles of two RF pulses) [2]. These rather large pulse angles increase the TR, especially for the tissues with long T1. Thus, the latter may not be imaged rapidly.
3. The k-space trajectories of Fig. 4.2 are zig-zag shaped, which results in nonuniform sampling of the k-space.

FIG. 4.3 The amplitude of the successive echoes diminishes as a result of concomitant T2 decay.

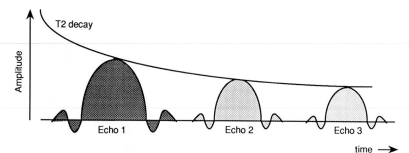

4. As only half the k-space is explicitly sampled and the other half is derived by zero-filling the data set, only the real (R) part of the Fourier transformed data set may be used (the imaginary (I) part is cosine convoluted). The real image is prone to the field inhomogeneity effects. The modulus image is less sensitive to the phase inconsistencies but, for reconstructing a modulus image (M), both the real and imaginary parts are required [12].

$$M = \sqrt{(R^2 + I^2)}.$$

The difficulties mentioned in points 2 through 4 now have been largely overcome by modifying the original EPI as described below.

Variants   (A) In order to enhance the time efficiency of EPI (particularly for tissues with long T1), the large excitation pulses may be replaced by low flip angle pulses. In a low angle version of EPI, fast low angle excitation echo planar technique (FLEET), both the RF pulse angles are maintained at about 20° [2].

(B) In order to scan the k-space uniformly, the k trajectories need to be made rectilinear. The reason for zig-zag trajectories in the original EPI is that the echo is collected while both the frequency encode and the phase encode gradients are on. Therefore, in blipped echo planar imaging, the phase encode gradient is switched off at the time of the echo collection. This results in a rectilinear trajectory parallel to the kx axis (see BEPI).

(C) If the entire k-space is sampled (from ky_{min} to ky_{max}), the data do not have to be zero filled, and both the real and imaginary terms can be used for calculating the modulus image (see BEPI) [12]. Field inhomogeneity artifacts are less conspicuous on a modulus image.

(D) The other alternative for reducing field inhomogeneity artifacts is to use 180° refocusing pulses to generate the echoes (π-EPI or double π-EPI) [11].

The following three variants of EPI have been used for chemical shift imaging.

(E) *Echo planar shift imaging (EPSM):* This is a three-dimensional version of EPI in which the third dimension is filled by the chemical shift information, in addition to the two spatial dimensions. The resolution of EPSM is poor because a large amount of data have to be collected in a relatively short period of time (about 100 msec) [9,15].

(F) *Projection-reconstruction echo planar (PREP):* As the name suggests, this technique combines the echo sampling strategy of echo planar imaging with image reconstruction by the projection method (Fig. 4.4). By rotating the axis of the oscillating gradient, the object is scanned with respect to the chemical shift dimension [7]. In comparison to EPSM, ex-

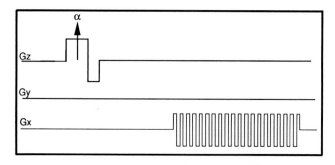

FIG. 4.4 The PREP pulse sequence for chemical shift imaging. It is similar to Fig. 4.1, except that no explicit phase encoding is used. Note that the presence of chemical shifts provides a constant phase encoding for the evolving series of echoes. (Modified, with permission, from Doyle and Mansfield [7]).

cellent resolution is obtained; however, the improved resolution is received at the cost of increased time (about four minutes for 64 images) [7]. Therefore, unlike EPSM, PREP has no real-time capabilities.

(G) *Phase encoded echo planar (PEEP):* This is a two-dimensional Fourier transform version of PREP in which a standard phase encode gradient has been incorporated (Fig. 4.5) [10]. At each RF excitation, a full plane defined by the chemical shift and frequency axis is sampled. To sample the next plane, the phase encode gradient is increased in the spatial direction. Thus, a full set of three-dimensional data is obtained. Compared to EPSM, PEEP takes about 64 seconds; however, the resolution ($64 \times 64 \times 128$) is much higher than EPSM.

See also: BEPI, MR fluoroscopy, RARE, SFI.

FIG. 4.5 The PEEP pulse sequence for chemical shift imaging. The 180° pulse is used to refocus magnetic field inhomogeneity effects. (Modified, with permission, from Guilfoyle et al [10]).

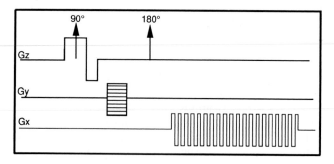

CLINICAL APPLICATIONS
TISSUE CONTRAST

As commonly no refocusing pulses are used, T2-dependent contrast is compromised and the decay of transverse magnetization is dominated by T2* rather than T2. As the main magnetic field inhomogeneity determines T2* decay, it also influences image resolution. Generally, the signal-to-noise ratio is low and the in-plane spatial resolution is limited to only a couple of millimeters.

To introduce T1-dependent image contrast in EPI images, an approach analogous to the IR-FLASH experiment can be employed simply by preceding the EPI pulse sequence by a nonselective 180° inverting pulse [22]. After a variable time interval (TI) following the inverting pulse, the actual imaging sequence is begun. The resultant images are, then, T1 weighted (see IR-FLASH).

THE BRAIN

In diffusion studies of organs such as the brain, it is of the utmost importance to prevent any type of inadvertent macromotion from creating image artifacts, otherwise the precise assessment of diffusion (micromotion) will be jeopardized. This requires fairly rapid imaging times. EPI has been used successfully in brain diffusion studies.

An article by Worthington and Mansfield [24] briefly discusses the role of echo planar imaging in the examination of the nervous system.

THE HEART

Earlier EPI was unable to provide instant cardiac images without cardiac triggering. However, with more recent technological improvements (see BEST and MBEST), it is possible to obtain a series of real-time echo planar images of the heart and coronary arteries during a single cardiac cycle. A single such image may be obtained in about 60 msec. Such cine-MRI of cardiac motion using EPI may be clinically useful in studying blood flow abnormalities associated with various valvular disorders, such as regurgitation or stenosis, and other congenital diseases of the heart [4,5].

Blackband et al [1] have characterized the rat heart as a model for echo planar imaging. The smaller size of the organ requires field homogeneity on a relatively smaller spatial volume, which may be achieved with less stringent hardware specifications. They have implemented EPI at 4.7T and have obtained images free from inhomogeneity artifacts. Probably, for the same reason, the initial experiments of the EPI technique were done on infants, who could be accommodated by a smaller size magnet.

Even today, considerable effort seems to be targeted at the pediatric age group [3,17,18].

THE ABDOMEN

MR evaluation of motions such as swallowing and peristalsis was made possible with the advent of EPI. Due to its real-time imaging abilities, respiratory or other random-motion related artifacts are virtually absent. Recently, 128 × 128 images of the normal and pathologic liver have been obtained, each in approximately 100 msec.

PREGNANCY

Intrauterine assessment of fetal structures is critical for determining the normal growth and wellbeing of the fetus. Besides ultrasonography, MRI is the only other noninvasive imaging technique available for use during pregnancy. The early results of EPI in normal and abnormal pregnancies are encouraging [13,16,21]. However, the effects of rapidly switching magnetic fields on a developing fetus are not completely known; this fact demands cautious use of EPI during pregnancy.

T1 CALCULATION

Ordidge et al [19] have used echo planar imaging for creating calculated T1 images of the brain using the same pulse sequence used for the IR-EPI experiment [22].
    See also: MORT.

ADVANTAGES AND DISADVANTAGES

Echo planar imaging is one of the fastest MR imaging methods in existence. As the image acquisition times are in the range of 30 to 130 msec (as the rule of thumb, each phase encode step takes approximately 1 msec), image degradation due to motion-induced artifacts is virtually eliminated. This makes EPI particularly appropriate for imaging moving organs (such as the heart) and studying organs surrounded by various kinds of motion (such as the liver).

    The main advantage of FLEET is its ability to provide real-time MR images of the whole body without the need for cardiac triggering. Earlier EPI was unable to function without the triggered mode; this limited the number of images (usually to one) that could be acquired in a single cardiac cycle. With the introduction of FLEET, as many as 20 images can be acquired in a single cardiac cycle. Instead of splicing together images from different cardiac cycles, a cine-MR loop consisting of images from the same cardiac cycle provides the essential dynamic information without any phase inconsistencies.

Despite the fact that, in both EPI and RARE, a series of echoes is generated in an analogous fashion, the minimum spacing between echoes is much less in EPI than in RARE, as there are no refocusing pulses in EPI. Unfortunately, if the entire data acquisition is not finished in the time comparable to the tissue T2 value (see above), blurring artifacts appear in the images. To reduce these artifacts, the data sampling rate has to be decreased, which ultimately results in a poor signal-to-noise ratio.

The image resolution of EPI is poorer when compared to snapshot FLASH. As refocusing pulses commonly are not used, the tissue contrast in EPI is inferior to that achieved using spin echo based rapid imaging techniques such as RARE. To increase the image signal-to-noise ratio, usually multiple images are averaged.

At higher field strengths, chemical shift artifacts have been reported, which may further degrade image quality. Farzaneh et al [8] have discussed the effect of the sampling rate and the off resonance artifacts that occur due to chemical shift and local susceptibility effects in echo planar imaging.

The other (and more troublesome) disadvantage of EPI is that it places stringent requirements on the imaging hardware. Its implementation requires the highest achievable main magnetic field homogeneity and gradients with sufficient speed and strength.

The evolution of echo planar imaging, since its first report in 1977, has been as fascinating and rapid as the parent technology of magnetic resonance imaging. With numerous recent modifications in its armament, EPI is well set to be one of the most promising imaging techniques of the future.

At present, EPI is not available on any commercial MR scanner. However, this situation is likely to change very soon with the introduction of ultrafast gradients and other necessary hardware.

REFERENCES

1. Blackband SJ, Chatham JC, O'dell W, Day S (1990): Echo planar imaging of isolated perfused rat hearts at 4.7 T: a comparison of Langendorff and working heart preparations. *Magn Reson Med* 15:240–245.

2. Chapman B, Turner R, Ordidge RJ, Doyle M, Cawley M, Coxon R, Glover P, Mansfield P (1987): Real-time movie imaging from a single cardiac cycle by NMR. *Magn Reson Med* 5:246–254.

3. Chapman B, O'Callaghan C, Coxon R, Glover P, Jaroszkewicz G, Howseman A, Mansfield P, Small P, Milner AD, Coupland RE (1990): Estimation of lung volume in infants by echo planar imaging and total body plethysmography. *Arch Diseases in Childhood* 65:168–170.

4. Chrispin A, Small P, Rutter N, Coupland RE, Doyle M, Chapman B, Coxon R, Guilfoyle D, Cawley M, Mansfield P (1986): Echo planar imaging of normal and abnormal connections of the heart and great arteries. *Pediatric Radiol* 16:289–292.

5. Chrispin A, Small P, Rutter N, Coupland RE, Doyle M, Chapman B, Coxon R, Guilfoyle D, Cawley M, Mansfield P (1986): Transectional echo planar imaging of the heart in cyanotic congenital heart disease. *Pediatric Radiol* 16:292–297.

6. Crooks LE, Arakawa M, Hylton NM, Avram H, Hoenninger JC, Watts JC, Hale JD, Kaufman L (1988): Echo-planar pediatric imagery. *Radiology* 166:157–163.

7. Doyle M, Mansfield P (1987): Chemical-shift imaging: a hybrid approach. *Magn Reson Med* 5:255–261.

8. Farzaneh F, Riederer SJ, Pelc NJ (1990): Analysis of T2 limitations and off-resonance effects on spatial resolution and artifacts in echo-planar imaging. *Magn Reson Med* 14:123–139.

9. Guilfoyle DN, Mansfield P (1985): Chemical-shift imaging. *Magn Reson Med* 2:479–489.

10. Guilfoyle DN, Blamire A, Chapman B, Ordidge RJ, Mansfield P (1989): PEEP—a rapid chemical-shift imaging method. *Magn Reson Med* 10:282–287.

11. Hennel F, Jasinski A, Tomanek B (1990): Double EPI sequence with 180° RF pulses. *Magn Reson Med* 16:161–165.

12. Howseman AM, Stehling MK, Chapman B, Coxon R, Turner R, Ordidge RJ, Cawley MG, Glover P, Mansfield P, Coupland RE (1988): Improvements in snap-shot nuclear magnetic resonance imaging. *Br J Radiol* 61:822–828.

13. Johnson IR, Stehling MK, Blamire AM, Coxon RJ, Howseman AM, Chapman B, Ordidge RJ, Mansfield P, Symonds EM, Worthington BS, et al (1990): Study of internal structures of the human fetus in utero by echo-planar magnetic resonance imaging. *Am J Obst Gynec* 163:601–607.

14. Mansfield P (1977): Multi-planar image formation using NMR spin echoes. *J Phys C: Solid State Physics* 10:L55–L58.

15. Mansfield P (1984): Spatial mapping of the chemical shift in NMR. *Magn Reson Med* 1:370–386.

16. Mansfield P, Stehling MK, Ordidge RJ, Coxon R, Chapman B, Blamire A, Gibbs P, Johnson IR, Symonds EM, Worthington BS, et al (1990): Echo planar imaging of the human fetus in utero at 0.5 T. *Br J Radiol* 63:833–841.

17. O'Callaghan C, Chapman B, Coxon R, Howseman A, Jaroszkiewicz G, Stehling M, Mansfield P, Milner AD, Swarbrick A, Small P, et al (1988): Evaluation of infants by echo planar imaging after repair of diaphragmatic hernia. *Arch Disease in Childhood* 63:186–189.

18. O'Callaghan C, Chapman B, Howseman A, Stehling M, Coxon R, Mansfield P (1990): Echo planar imaging of an infant with pectus excavatum. *Eur J Pediatrics* 149:698–699.

19. Ordidge RJ, Gibbs P, Chapman B, Stehling MK, Mansfield P (1990): High-speed multislice T1 mapping using inversion-recovery echo-planar imaging. *Magn Reson Med* 16:238–245.

20. Sekihara K, Kohno H (1987): New reconstruction technique for echo-planar imaging to allow combined use of odd- and even-numbered echoes. *Magn Reson Med* 5:485–491.

21. Stehling MK, Mansfield P, Ordidge RJ, Coxon R, Chapman B, Blamire A, Gibbs P, Johnson IR, Symonds EM, Worthington BS, et al (1989): Echo-planar magnetic resonance imaging in abnormal pregnancies. *Lancet* 2:157.

22. Stehling MK, Ordidge RJ, Coxon R, Mansfield P (1990): Inversion-recovery echo-planar imaging (IR-EPI) at 0.5T. *Magn Reson Med* 13:514–517.

23. Yan H, Braun M (1991): Image reconstruction from Fourier domain data sampled along a zig-zag trajectory. *Magn Reson Med* 18:405–410.

24. Worthington BS, Mansfield P (1990): The clinical applications of echo planar imaging in neuroradiology. *Neuroradiology* 32:367–370.

5

Fast Acquisition Double Echo (FADE)

BASIC PRINCIPLES

In an SSFP experiment, a bicomponent steady state signal is produced during each pulse repetition period, TR (see SSFP). The first component of this signal is analogous to an FID in that it arises due to the RF pulse preceding the TR, and it disappears fairly rapidly. The second component of this signal is analogous to a time reversed FID, in that it gradually increases to attain a peak at the echo time (which occurs just as the following RF pulse is being applied).

Most of the current two-dimensional Fourier transform SSFP pulse sequences generate only one echo, corresponding to either component, during each TR. However, two different echoes can be acquired during each TR by properly modifying the frequency encoding gradient (Gx) of the pulse sequence. And there is a strong clinical motivation for obtaining two echoes because each component of the signal signifies different relaxation mechanisms. While the initial decaying part is influenced by T1 relaxation, the terminal rising part is influenced by T2 relaxation. Therefore, if these signal components are acquired separately after each RF application, two images with varying contrast properties can be reconstructed.

It is important to examine how the other SSFP sequences acquire only one echo in order to understand how two echoes may be generated during each TR. The FLASH type sequences use readout (Gx) reversal (an unbalanced bipolar gradient pulse) to generate the first echo and then dephase the second signal by applying only a monopolar gradient pulse (Fig. 5.1a). The CE-FAST-type sequences use Gx reversal toward the end of the TR to generate an echo and dephase the first component of the

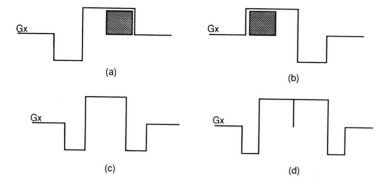

FIG. 5.1 (a) The frequency encoding gradient profile of FLASH-type sequence; only FID is collected. (b) The frequency encoding gradient profile of CE-FAST-type sequence; only the echo is collected. In both cases, the shaded gradient area destroys the unwanted signals. If these two gradient profiles are added together with differential time shift, the gradient profiles as shown in (c) and (d) are obtained. (c) The balanced FAST frequency encoding gradient profile in which both SSFP signals are superimposed. (d) The unbalanced frequency encoding gradient of FADE keeps the FID and the echo signal components separate.

FIG. 5.2 Unlike FISP, the frequency encode gradient is not balanced (shaded gradient lobes) in FADE sequence, which prevents the superimposition of the two SSFP signal components; they are acquired separately by gradient reversal.

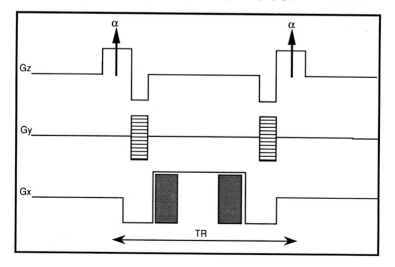

signal by applying a monopolar gradient pulse during the initial part of the TR (Fig. 5.1b). Sequences such as FISP use balanced Gx, so that both components are superimposed onto each other (Fig. 5.1c).

It is obvious from Fig. 5.1 that the combination of the first and second read gradients will give two different echoes. The combined Gx is shown in Fig. 5.1d [1–3]. Note that the phase encoding gradient is identical (and balanced) in all the SSFP sequences (except for the spoiled FLASH). Incidentally, this makes it similar to the FISP Gx, with the exception that the Gx is now made unbalanced (Fig. 5.2). Enough time should be allowed between echoes in order to keep them temporally separate, otherwise contrast interference may be generated.

See also: SSFP.

CLINICAL APPLICATIONS
TISSUE CONTRAST

As the relaxation processes underlying each signal component are different, the images derived from individual echoes display distinct tissue contrast. While the image reconstructed from the first echo exhibits strong T1 weighting, the second image exhibits heavy T2 weighting. As with other SSFP sequences, the contrast of the individual images may be altered by varying the excitation flip angle.

THE BRAIN

It is interesting to note that three different groups have presented the identical approach for separately acquiring the SSFP signal components [1–3]. All three groups reported their initial results using this pulse sequence in the brain.

While the first echo image is more like FISP (brighter tissue intensity), the second echo image is more like FLASH (darker tissue intensity). As expected, the second echo image shows strong T2 weighting and, as expected, the CSF (with its long T2 value) appears bright (Fig. 5.3). In contrast to the first echo images reported by Redpath and Jones [3] and Lee and Cho [2], the first echo images reported by Bruder et al [1] also seem to register a bright CSF signal.

Another noticeable feature of the images is that the flow perpendicular to the image section appears bright on the first echo images because the spins that do not reach the steady state, due to flow, yield a higher intensity signal. In contrast, the second echo images show such flow consistently as signal void because the second component of the SSFP signal grows more slowly with the number of RF pulses than the first component [2].

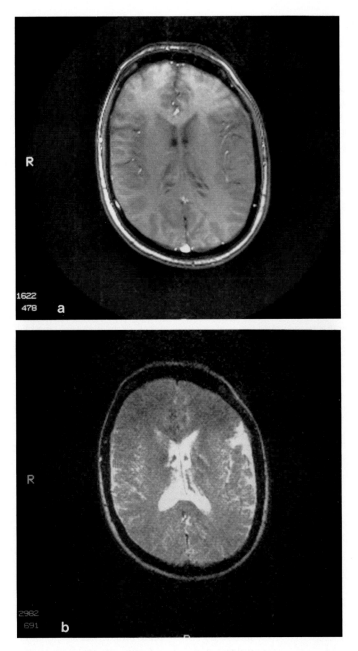

FIG. 5.3 First **(a)** and second **(b)** component images obtained at the level of the ventricles through the head of a normal volunteer (60° excitation; TR = 50 msec; slice thickness = 10 mm; 8 averages; total time 102 sec). (Courtesy of T. Redpath; reproduced, with permission, from T.W. Redpath and R.A. Jones [3].)

ADVANTAGES AND DISADVANTAGES

The FADE sequence has a twofold advantage over other FFE-SSFP techniques. First, it provides two images with different contrast characteristics in the same time interval as other SSFP techniques, such as FISP and FLASH, which provide only one image. Second, even though two signals are read during each TR, the imaging time is only slightly increased when compared to a single echo SSFP sequence. This time superiority is greatly enhanced when compared to the T2-weighted SE images. For example, two images (256 × 256) with TR/TE of 40/11 msec and EFA of 30° can be produced in about ten seconds [2]. Clearly, this acquisition time is much less than the conventional long TR/long TE SE data acquisition.

Similar to gradient recalled echo techniques in general, susceptibility artifacts appear near the bone/air interface in these images.

REFERENCES

1. Bruder H, Fischer H, Grumman, Deimling M (1988): A new steady state imaging sequence for simultaneous acquisition of two MR images with clearly different contrasts. *Magn Reson Med* 7:35–42.

2. Lee SY, Cho ZH (1988): Fast SSFP gradient echo sequences for simultaneous acquisitions of FID and echo signals. *Magn Reson Med* 8:142–150.

3. Redpath TW, Jones RA (1988): FADE—a new fast imaging sequence. *Magn Reson Med* 6:224–234.

6

Fourier Angiography (FANG)

BASIC PRINCIPLES

The net phase shift experienced by a spin flowing in the direction of a
bipolar gradient is given by the relationship

$$\delta\phi = \gamma \times A_G \times T \times V$$

where γ is the gyromagnetic ratio, v is the velocity, and the other symbols
are as explained in Fig. 6.1. From the above equation, it is evident that,
on increasing the gradient amplitude of a bipolar gradient pulse, the velocity-dependent phase shift increases linearly with the amplitude.
Therefore, if a stepwise increasing bipolar gradient is used, a direct relationship between the spin phase and the velocity can be obtained,
which, after the Fourier transform, yields a relationship between the spin
density and the velocity [4]. Fourier transform based angiographic methods exploit this fact by incorporating stepwise increasing bipolar gradients in the direction of the velocity encoding. Note that the more conventional phase based flow imaging techniques usually use gradient
pulses of constant amplitude and an image is derived from the subtraction
of two data sets obtained using different permutations of the bipolar pulse
(see PBANG).

In this Fourier transform angiographic technique, N images corresponding to N different gradient amplitude levels are obtained. Therefore, each
original image represents a distinct phase shift corresponding to the gradient amplitude. Based upon the final display format, N point one (or
two-dimensional) Fourier transform is performed using N different points
given by P(q,r,n) where q and r specify the pixel position in the image
indexed by n (n $\leq$ N).

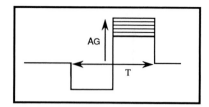

FIG. 6.1 A simple bipolar pulse with varying amplitude.

Once the velocity data are obtained, several options exist for displaying the velocity information, as described below.

1. In a conventional two-dimensional Fourier transform MR imaging experiment, an image is created by performing two-dimensional Fourier transform of the data acquired in the presence of the phase and frequency encoding gradients, where the encoded phase and frequency constitute two necessary spatial dimensions. Unless the three-dimensional Fourier technique is used, there is no room for directly displaying any additional dimension, such as the chemical shift, magnetic field inhomogeneities, or flow velocity. Note that the total imaging time is directly proportional to the total number of the phase encoding steps in the spatial direction(s) (Np) and in the velocity encode direction (Nv). Therefore, the implementation of three-dimensional Fourier transform increases the total imaging time by a factor directly proportional to the number of encoding steps in the new dimension.

2. If it is desired to keep the imaging time the same as in the case of two-dimensional Fourier transform nonvelocity encoding imaging, Np has to be decreased to accommodate Nv. The result is that image resolution degrades. For example, Redpath et al [8] have obtained 64 × 64 images of a flow phantom with eight velocity phase encoding steps in about eight minutes. As expected, the image quality of this reduced data set is poor.

3. Sacrifice the spatial information along one dimension (usually the phase encoding) and substitute velocity encoding in lieu of the sacrificed dimension. Hennig et al [4,5] have successfully employed this approach (Fig. 6.2), together with very fast data acquisition (FLASH type sequence) and selectively saturating the stationary spins (to optimize the signal-to-noise ratio), for obtaining angiograms in about seven minutes (64 separate flow images, each taking 6.5 seconds, TR 44 msec, 128 velocity encoding steps, 20 presaturating cycles).

4. Use the projective format of display in which the third imaging gradient is used for neither spatial encoding nor spatial selection (pro-

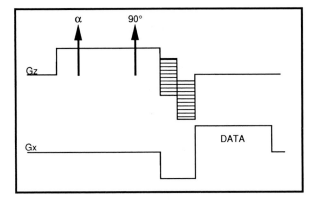

FIG. 6.2 The amplitude of the bipolar pulse is varied for different pulse applications to encode different flow velocities. This is similar to the conventional phase encoding achieved via varying the gradient amplitude. The angle of the first RF pulse may be varied to optimize the suppression of the stationary tissue. (Modified, with permission, from Hennig et al [5].)

jective Fourier angiography, PFA). Using this approach, Norris et al [7] have obtained arterial and venous angiograms of the neck vessels in about 8.5 minutes (TR 500 msec, 128 phase encoding steps, eight velocity encoding steps). Even though the time taken is similar to that of the technique of Redpath et al (see above), resolution in the phase encoding direction is considerably improved.

FIG. 6.3 The flow encoding step is incremented after each cardiac trigger until the desired resolution is reached in the flow encoding direction. Note that, in both Figs. 6.2 and 6.3, a dephasing gradient may be used after the excitation pulse to disperse any unwanted magnetization. (Modified, with permission, from Cho et al [1].)

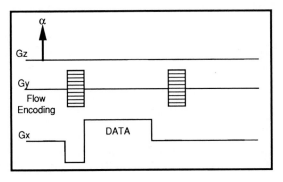

Variants   (A) The signal intensity of the arteries is determined by the flow velocity, which affects both the phase shift induced by the gradient magnetic fields and the inflow of unsaturated spins. At each point in the cardiac cycle, arterial blood flow velocity is different (pulsatile flow) and, therefore, the signal intensity is different.

The Fourier transform arteriography as proposed by Cho et al [1] is based upon the following principle: if, during a cardiac cycle, N data acquisitions are carried out using a suitable pulse sequence with stepwise increasing bipolar gradient pulses (Fig. 6.3), one-dimensional Fourier transformation of these data sets results in the formation of N spectral

FIG. 6.4 Each coronal projection image of the human legs represents a spectrally decomposed Fourier transformed magnitude image acquired with TR = 45 msec and TE = 12 msec. (Courtesy of K-J. Jung; reproduced, with permission, from Cho et al [1].)

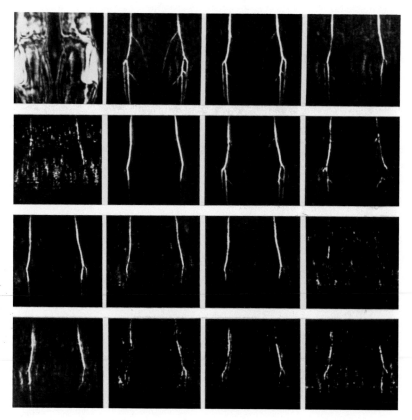

images (Fig. 6.4), each one representing a different spatial and temporal location due to the pulsatile nature of the arterial blood flow. If these spectral images are added together after taking magnitude of the images, an arteriogram is obtained (Fig. 6.5). While doing the summation, the spectral image corresponding to the zero harmonic is conveniently left out, as it contains information about the static tissue and the veins (non-pulsatile flow) (the spectral image lying at the intersection of the top row and the left column in Fig. 6.4) [1,7].

(B) In the method proposed by Hou et al (Fig 6.6) [6], the flow encoding bipolar pulses are applied in the direction of the slice selection. The phase encoding gradient is the same as in other conventional pulse sequences. However, two gradient echoes are obtained following an RF pulse. The first gradient echo gives an anatomic map of the vessel in the direction of the slice select gradient and the second echo is flow encoded so that it provides a velocity profile.

See also: LISA, PBANG, TOF.

FIG. 6.5 An arteriogram obtained by adding together the second and third images of the first two rows from Fig. 6.4. (Courtesy of K-J. Jung; reproduced, with permission, from Cho et al [1].)

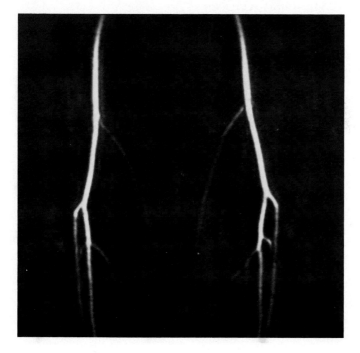

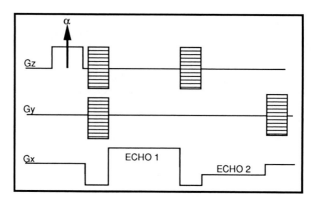

FIG. 6.6 Conventional phase encoding pulses are applied in the direction of the slice selection and flow encoding pulses are applied along the Gy gradient. ECHO 1 is the standard phase encoded echo for image construction; ECHO 2 is the velocity encoded echo for velocity measurement. (Modified with permission, from Hou et al [6].)

CLINICAL APPLICATIONS

Feinberg and Mark [3] have implemented the Fourier flow imaging principle for analyzing CSF motion and have demonstrated that the pulsatile blood-induced motion of the brain principally pushes the CSF through the ventricles.

Dousset et al [2] have evaluated the accuracy of the velocity values obtained using the Fourier angiography technique with the corresponding values obtained using Doppler ultrasound. Their MR data in the popliteal artery show significant correlation with the Doppler data.

As a side note, while comparing the MR velocity data with the Doppler, it is critical to remember that these different experiments usually are performed sequentially to avoid RF interference. As the pattern of rapidly

FIG. 6.7 Generic pulse timing diagram showing only the frequency encoding gradient **(a)**. As shown in **(b)**, ultrasound is disabled only when echo sampling is being performed. At all other times (shaded areas), ultrasound measurements are continuously being acquired.

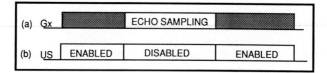

flowing blood flow may change from time to time, spurious results may be obtained, which may undermine the significance of the MR examination. Therefore, to make a fair comparison between the MR and Doppler data, both examinations should be carried out near simultaneously. Sebok et al [9] have proposed an approach for interleaving the data acquisitions from the Doppler and MR. As shown in Fig. 6.7, Doppler data acquisition is disabled whenever MR data acquisition is performed.

ADVANTAGES AND DISADVANTAGES

In general, the ability to resolve the maximum velocity is determined by the gradient integral (Amplitude × Time) [4]:

$$V_{max} = 8\pi N/(\gamma \times A_G \times T),$$

where N is the total number of the phase encoding steps in the velocity direction and the denominator is as explained previously. It is important to design the pulse sequence so that the range of phase shift, as given by the denominator term, falls between ±180°; otherwise, velocity aliasing may occur. Obviously, this puts a restriction on the range of the velocity values that may be resolved.

Fourier flow imaging has the advantage of directly displaying the velocity values. In addition, projective Fourier angiography has the capability of obtaining velocity information from a large volume of tissue and the course of tortuous vessels can be visualized more precisely.

In addition to saving considerable imaging time, the omission of the phase encoding gradient [4,5] also means that proper anatomic localization of the vessel may be problematic.

REFERENCES

1. Cho ZH, Jung KJ, Ro YM (1990): MR Fourier transform arteriography using spectral decomposition. *Magn Reson Med* 16:226–237.
2. Dousset V, Wehrli FW, Louie A, Listerud J (1991): Popliteal artery hemodynamics: MR imaging—US correlation. *Radiology* 179:437–441.
3. Feinberg DA, Mark AS (1987): Human brain motion and cerebrospinal fluid collection demonstrated with MR velocity imaging. *Radiology* 163:793–799.
4. Hennig J, Muri M, Brunner P, Friedburg H (1988): Quantitative flow measurement with the fast Fourier flow technique. *Radiology* 166:237–240.
5. Hennig J, Muri M, Brunner P, Friedburg H (1988): Fast and exact flow measurements with the fast Fourier flow technique. *Magn Reson Imag* 6:369–372.
6. Hou P, Parker DL, Blatter DD, Robinson RO (1991): Hybrid MR angiography and Fourier velocity imaging using two echo 3D acquisition. *Magn Reson Med* 19:203–208.

7. Norris DG, Jones RA, Hutchison JMS (1988): Projective Fourier angiography. *Magn Reson Med* 7:1–10.

8. Redpath TW, Norris DG, Jones RA, Hutchison JMS (1984): A new method of NMR flow imaging. *Phys Med Biol* 29:891–898.

9. Sebok DA, Wilkerson D, Schroder W, Mezrich R, Zatina M (1991): Interleaved magnetic resonance and ultrasound by electronic synchronization. *Invest Radiol* 26:353–357.

7

Fast Acquisition in Steady State (FAST)[1]

BASIC PRINCIPLES

When steady state magnetization is achieved by applying low angle RF pulses in very rapid succession, at least two separate signals can be acquired during each interpulse interval (see SSFP). Either of these signals may be transformed into a gradient echo by reversing the readout gradient. If the slice select and the frequency encode gradients are balanced before the echo is acquired, then the gradient reversal refocuses the first signal. Here, a dephasing gradient following the echo collection destroys the second signal. If all the gradients are balanced after the echo is acquired, then the gradient reversal refocuses the second signal. Here, a dephasing gradient preceding the echo collection destroys the first signal. This has been shown schematically in Fig. 38.3.

A variety of fast imaging techniques have been proposed to acquire these SSFP signals. While the original FLASH uses an unbalanced phase encoding gradient to destroy residual transverse magnetization, in FAST, the latter is made balanced to preserve the transverse magnetization and thus achieve the steady state in both (longitudinal and transverse) directions in (Fig. 7.1). Both FLASH and FAST collect the first component (FID) of the steady state signal. Thus, while FAST is similar to FLASH with a bipolar phase encoding gradient (refocused FLASH), it is also similar to FISP with an unbalanced slice and frequency encoding gradients (ROAST).

Variants The second SSFP signal is much like a spin echo in a classic SE sequence (Fig. 38.2). Therefore, if the first signal is dephased by gra-

---

[1] Also called Fourier acquired steady state [1].

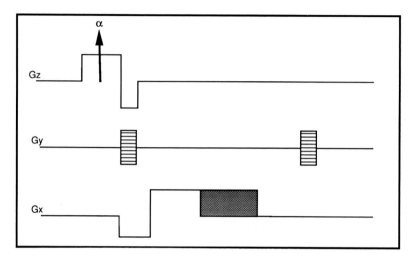

FIG. 7.1 The FAST SSFP sequence. Note the balanced phase encoding gradient. The shaded gradient lobe destroys the second (echo) component of the SSFP signal.

FIG. 7.2 The CE FAST SSFP sequence. The RF pulse shown above refocuses the FID following the previous RF pulse. Note that the slice rephasing gradient lobe is delayed until after the data acquisition (or just preceding the next RF pulse).

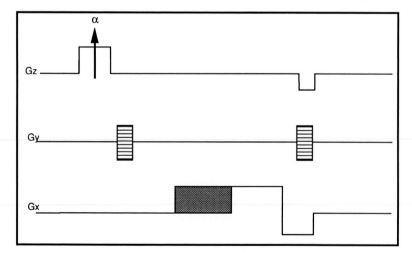

dient pulses and only the second signal is acquired by the gradient reversal, a strongly T2-weighted image is obtained. This modified pulse sequence is known as contrast enhanced-FAST (CE-FAST, Fig. 7.2).

As we shall see below, the CE-FAST pulse sequence has been used to visualize the intravoxel incoherent motion (IVIM), which includes such diverse dynamic phenomena as molecular diffusion and perfusion. The common goal of any IVIM technique is to be able to depict signal attenuation due to IVIM without contamination from any other sources of motion.

See also: FISP, FLASH, ROAST, SSFP.

CLINICAL APPLICATIONS
TISSUE CONTRAST

The FAST images show T1-weighted image contrast, which is dependent on the excitation pulse angle and the pulse repetition time (TR). The CE-FAST images are heavily T2 weighted, and the intensity of the contrast is determined by the ratio T2/TR.

THE BRAIN

In general, brain images obtained by FAST have poor contrast-to-noise ratios because the ratio T1/T2 for white and gray matter are quite similar (even though they have distinct T1 and T2) [2]. However, CE-FAST images provide excellent white/gray matter differentiation due to the T2 contrast capability [1] of CE-FAST.

DIFFUSION STUDIES

As perfusion and diffusion take place at the molecular level, it is very likely that deviation from their normal character would result in some type of organ dysfunction. For example, a poorly perfused area eventually becomes an infarct. Therefore, it may be clinically rewarding to monitor perfusion/diffusion noninvasively before any gross changes occur.

Recently, the CE-FAST sequence has been used for studying diffusion and perfusion in the brain (Figs. 7.3 and 7.4) [3–5].

ADVANTAGES AND DISADVANTAGES

An article by Gyngell [1] discusses, at length, the relative features of the FAST and CE-FAST sequences.

In the past, spin echo based techniques have been used for diffusion

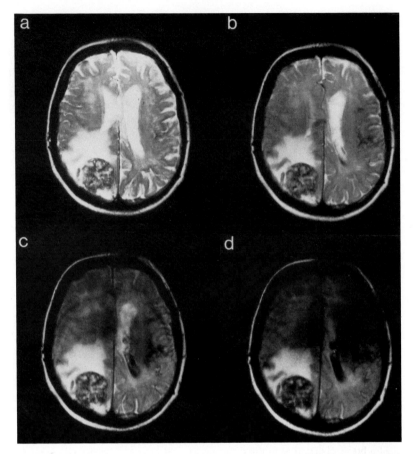

FIG. 7.3 Series of four axial sections of the human brain, obtained using the diffusion weighted CE-FAST sequence. For all images, the image matrix is 256 × 256; TR = 25 msec **(a)** and **(b)**, 29 msec **(c)** and **(d)**; 8 averages; 10 mm slice thickness; and total imaging time about 1 min. The diffusion gradient duration was 5 msec **(a)** and **(b)** and 9 msec **(c)** and **(d)**. The diffusion gradient strength (mTm^{-1}) was 1 **(a)**, 7**(b)** and **(c)** and 9.8 **(d)**. All images show right cerebral metastasis with associated edema. However, as the diffusion weighting is increased **(c)** and **(d)**, CSF becomes less visualized. (Courtesy of K-D. Merboldt; reproduced, with permission, from Merboldt et al [4].)

studies [6]. Usually, the diffusion encoding gradient pulses are made very long, so that the IVIM accumulates enough phase shift. However, extra long gradients signify greater signal loss due to T2 decay. Moreover, it is difficult to control the artifacts from other sources of motion. The use of the CE-FAST sequence for studying diffusion has the advantage that

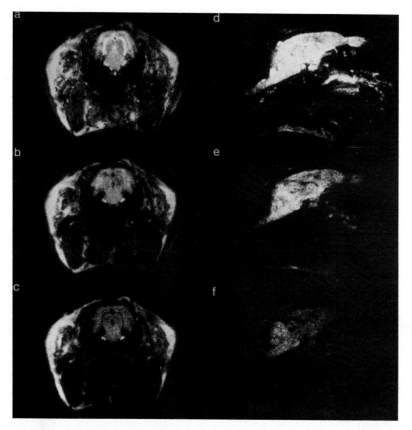

FIG. 7.4 Series of axial **(a)**, **(b)**, and **(c)** and sagittal **(d)**, **(e)**, and **(f)** images of a rabbit brain, obtained with the diffusion weighted CE-FAST pulse sequence. For all images, the image matrix is 256×256; TR = 45 msec; 8 averages; 4 mm slice thickness; total imaging time about 1.5 min, and the diffusion gradient duration was 15 msec. The diffusion gradient strength (mTm^{-1}) was 0 **(a)** and **(d)**; 7.5 **(b)** and **(e)**, and 13.2 **(c)** and **(f)**. Note that the CSF signal disappears with increased diffusion weighting. Images **(c)** and **(f)** show signal attenuation probably due to widespread diffusional processes. On the axial images, the signal from the sub-cutaneous fat is not diminished because of the lower diffusional coefficient of lipids [5]. (Courtesy of K-D. Merboldt; reproduced, with permission, from Merboldt et al [5].)

it is not necessary to use extra long (or large) gradients because of the slow flow sensitivity of the SSFP experiment. However, motion artifacts persist despite the use of gating or motion refocused gradient waveforms [5]. Merboldt et al [4,5] have averaged the data in order to make these artifacts less conspicuous.

This pulse sequence is available on Picker MR scanners.

REFERENCES

1. Gyngell ML (1988): The application of steady-state free precession in rapid 2DFT NMR imaging: FAST and CE-FAST sequences. *Magn Reson Imag* 6:415–419.

2. Just M, Higer HP, Schwarz M, Bohl J, Fries G, Pfannensteil P, Thelen M (1988): Tissue characterization of benign brain tumors: use of NMR-tissue parameters. *Magn Reson Imag* 6:463–472.

3. Le Bihan D (1988): Intravoxel incoherent motion imaging using steady-state free precession. *Magn Reson Med* 7:346–351.

4. Merboldt KD, Bruhn H, Frahm J, Gyngell ML, Hanicke W, Deimling M (1989): MRI of "diffusion" in the human brain: new results using a modified CE-FAST sequence. *Magn Reson Med* 9:423–429.

5. Merboldt KD, Hanicke W, Gyngell ML, Frahm J, Bruhn H (1989): The influence of flow and motion in MRI of diffusion using a modified CE-FAST sequence. *Magn Reson Med* 12:198–208.

6. Taylor DG, Bushell MC (1985): The spatial mapping of translational diffusion coefficient by the NMR imaging technique. *Phys Med Biol* 30:345–349.

7. van der Muelen P, Groen JP, Tinus AMC, Bruntink G (1988): Fast field echo imaging: an overview and contrast calculations. *Magn Reson Imag* 6:355–368.

8

Field Even Echo Rephasing (FEER)

BASIC PRINCIPLES

Phase shifts occur in the presence of a bipolar gradient modulation. During the first half of a bipolar gradient pulse, all the spins, stationary as well as moving, experience gradient field dependent phase changes. During the second half of the gradient modulation, the sign of the gradient field is reversed. This results in the complete phase restoration of the spins only if they have not moved during the entire duration of the modulation. Otherwise, they will gain a net phase shift. Thus, at the end of a bipolar gradient, the flowing spins accumulate a net phase shift ϕ, proportional to the velocity and the gradient integral, which contributes to signal loss.

However, if the first bipolar gradient modulation (which gives a phase shift of $+\phi$) is followed by a second antisymmetric (of the same duration, but of opposite polarity) bipolar gradient modulation in the same direction (which gives a phase shift of $-\phi$), the net phase of the flowing spins is restored (or rephased). This rephasing occurs for any odd derivative of the position if the refocusing gradient is an even function of time (Fig. 8.1) [11]. This is equivalent to the process of even echo rephasing seen with the SE sequence briefly reviewed below.

The stationary spins in the presence of a linear gradient rephase completely at the initial echo time (TE), and at any multiple of TE thereafter. However, the flowing spins, in the presence of a linear field gradient (the gradient may be pulsed as long as it is switched on simultaneously with the 90° pulse), do not rephase completely after the first 180° refocusing pulse, and some signal loss occurs proportional to the flow velocity and the gradient strength. When a second 180° refocusing pulse is applied,

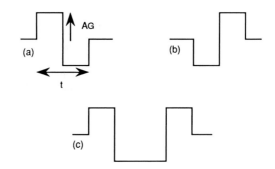

FIG. 8.1 **(a)** Shows a bipolar gradient pulse that refocuses the magnetization for the stationary spins and the following spins acquire a phase shift (ϕ), which is proportional to the flow velocity, the gradient amplitude, AG, and the time, t. **(b)** The stationary spins are again refocused; however, the flowing spins acquire an opposite phase shift ($-\phi$). Therefore, it is evident that if the bipolar pulse is followed by its antisymmetric (in the time domain) pulse, the net phase shift will become zero and a maximum signal will be obtained from the flowing spins. This is shown in **(c)**.

FIG. 8.2 The FEER sequence. The slice select and the frequency encode gradients are balanced (shaded areas). In fact, the shaded areas represent a pair of bipolar pulses joined in an antisymmetric manner as shown in Fig. 8.1. This effectively refocuses the flowing spins. To encode the velocity information, the gradient profile is altered as shown by the dotted gradient lobes in inset. (Modified, with permission, from Nayler et al [11].)

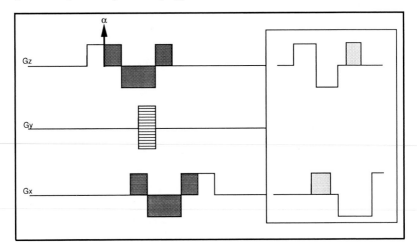

complete rephasing of the flowing spins is achieved, and a higher intensity echo is obtained. Thus, after every 360° rotation, the voxel magnetization of the spins flowing with constant velocity is stronger than at any other time. This is the principle of even echo rephasing [1,7,13,14]. As the flow velocity increases, the signal difference between the first and second echoes, at first, decreases, and then both become equivalent. At still higher velocities, the second signal further diminishes and eventually disappears.

To encode the velocity, the terminal portion of a refocusing gradient is time-shifted (Fig. 8.2), thus making the phase shift a known function of time. The pulse sequence is run twice (with and without time shifting the gradient), in an interleaved manner. The data acquisition is carried out gated to the cardiac cycle; a subtraction of two data sets leaves only the flow-induced phase shifts in the direction of the flow-encoding gradient. By changing the orientation of this gradient, flow can be encoded in any direction.

See also: FLAG, PBANG.

CLINICAL APPLICATIONS
TISSUE CONTRAST

Magnitude-based FEER images show the flowing blood as a high intensity area due to the even echo refocusing effect of the flowing spins. On the phase maps, however, the flowing blood may appear dark if it is flowing away from the direction of the refocusing gradient.

Under normal nonturbulent conditions, velocity quantification of the aortic [2], mitral, and pulmonary [4,10] blood flow with FEER pulse sequence has provided very good correlation with other flow-calculating techniques, such as multislice imaging or Doppler sonography [3,5,11]. Fig. 8.3 shows a representative FEER cross-section (magnitude as well as phase reconstructed) of the heart.

In numerous cardiovascular anomalies, such as intracardiac septal defects, aortic coarctation, valvular disorders (including poststenotic evaluation of the blood flow), femoral vein thrombosis, and coronary bypass grafts, FEER has aided in the correct diagnosis and quantitative assessment of the underlying pathology. Although the diagnosis of many of these defects may be apparent on the standard MR image, the degree of functional deficit is not readily evident. Moreover, in certain clinical situations (eg, tetralogy of Fallot; multiple intracardiac shunts), more than one structural defect may coexist, and then it becomes important to determine the relative contributions of the defects to the overall clinical

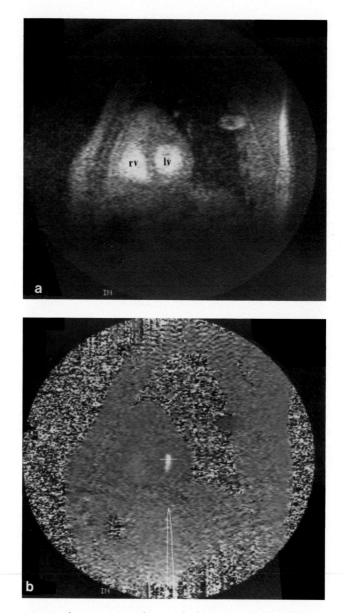

FIG. 8.3 Magnitude reconstructed **(a)** and phase reconstructed **(b)** maps of the human heart along the short axis of the left ventricle (lv) in a patient with mitral stenosis. The images (TE = 3.6 msec; 128 × 128; 2 averages) were acquired triggered by the R wave. The stenotic jet is seen in (b) as a bright region and its velocity profile (mm/sec) is also shown. (Courtesy of R. Mohiaddin; reproduced, with permission, from Mohiaddin et al [10].)

problem. In such conditions, FEER has successfully identified the defect through which the majority of abnormal blood flow occurs [12].

NONLAMINAR FLOW

Poststenotic flow and flow near an atherosclerotic plaque represent turbulent flow characteristics. The presence of higher-order terms (eg, acceleration) in the turbulent conditions lead to rapid phase incoherence and, despite the presence of gradient rephasing, result in signal loss (Fig. 8.4). This signal loss can be minimized by decreasing TE, which allows accurate mapping of the turbulent flow velocities of up to 6 m/sec [6,11]. Clinical studies of various stenotic disorders, such as aortic stenosis, have shown agreement with the velocity values obtained using Doppler sonography [8]. Moreover, Mitchell et al [9] have demonstrated that it is possible to grade the stenosis by measuring the extent of poststenotic signal loss.

As the signal from the flowing blood is recovered, it is possible to

FIG. 8.4 View along the horizontal long axis of the left ventricle in a patient with mitral stenosis (TE = 14 msec). The arrow indicates turbulence near the stenotic jet as an area of signal loss. (Courtesy of R. Mohiaddin; reproduced, with permission, from Mohiaddin et al [10].)

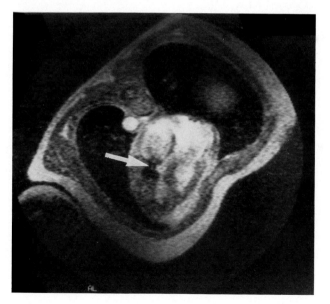

distinguish a thrombus (area of signal loss) from the flowing blood (area of bright intensity) [2].

ADVANTAGES AND DISADVANTAGES

Unlike the magnitude-based angiographic methods (see TOF), FEER uses the phase information. The phase shifts provide velocity information independent of the spin density. Therefore, FEER images provide a more precise determination of the flow velocity. Moreover, the process of image subtraction eliminates the phase shifts caused by local field inhomogeneities or susceptibility effects. Therefore, in addition to a magnitude image, a phase map is obtained that directly maps the velocity to the pixel intensity.

As two pulse repetitions are required for every phase encoding step, the total imaging time for a single slice may be 5 to 8 minutes, depending on the heart rate. Even though it is possible to measure turbulent flow velocities by decreasing TE (to about 3 to 4 msec), the complete study is time-consuming and takes about 1 to 2 hours.

Most often, the FEER sequence has been implemented on Picker MR scanners.

REFERENCES

1. Axel L (1984): Blood flow effects in magnetic resonance imaging. *Am J Radiol* 143:1157–1166.
2. Bogren HG, Underwood SR, Firmin DN, Mohiaddin RH, Klipstein RH, Rees RSO, Longmore DB (1988): Magnetic resonance velocity mapping in aortic dissection. *Br J Radiol* 61:456–462.
3. Bogren HG, Klipstein RH, Firmin DN, Mohiaddin RH, Underwood SR, Rees RSO, Longmore DB (1989): Quantitation of antegrade and retrograde blood flow in the human aorta by magnetic resonance velocity mapping. *Am Heart J* 117:1214–1222.
4. Bogren HG, Klipstein RH, Mohiaddin RH, Firmin DN, Underwood SR, Rees RSO, Longmore DB (1989): Pulmonary artery distensibility and blood flow patterns: a magnetic resonance study of normal subjects and of patients with pulmonary arterial hypertension. *Am Heart J* 118:990–999.
5. Firmin DN, Nayler GL, Klipstein RH, Underwood SR, Rees RSO, Longmore DB (1987): In vivo validation of MR velocity imaging. *J Comput Assist Tomogr* 11:751–756.
6. Firmin DN, Nayler GL, Pennell D, Kilner P, Longmore DB (1990): Short (TE 3.5 msec) field even echo rephasing sequences for improved blood flow measurement. *Magn Reson Imag* 8:S14.
7. Katz J, Peshock RM, Malloy CR, Schaefer S, Parkey RW (1987): Even-echo rephasing and constant velocity flow. *Magn Reson Med* 4:422–430.

8. Kilner PJ, Firmin DN, Rees RSO, Martinez J, Pennell DJ, Mohiaddin RH, Underwood SR, Longmore DB (1991): Valve and great vessel stenosis: assessment with MR jet velocity mapping. *Radiology* 178:229–235.

9. Mitchell L, Jenkins JPR, Watson Y, Rowlands DJ, Isherwood I (1989): Diagnosis and assessment of mitral and aortic valve disease by cine-flow magnetic resonance imaging. *Magn Reson Med* 12:181–197.

10. Mohiaddin RH, Amanuma M, Kilner PJ, Pennell DJ, Manzara C, Longmore DB (1991): MR phase-shift mapping of mitral and pulmonary venous flow. *J Comput Assist Tomogr* 15:237–243.

11. Nayler GL, Firmin DN, Longmore DB (1986): Blood flow imaging by cine magnetic resonance. *J Comput Assist Tomogr* 10:715–722.

12. Underwood SR, Firmin DN, Klipstein RH, Rees RSO, Longmore DB (1987): Magnetic resonance velocity mapping: clinical application of a new technique. *Br Heart J* 57:404–412.

13. von Schulthess GK, Higgins CB (1985): Blood flow imaging with MR: spin-phase phenomena. *Radiology* 157:687–695.

14. Waluch V, Bradley WG (1984): NMR even echo rephasing in slow laminar flow. *J Comput Assist Tomogr* 8:594–598.

9

Fast Imaging with Steady State Precession (FISP)

BASIC PRINCIPLES

Originally proposed in 1986 [8], FISP is one of several fast field echo (FFE) techniques based on the principle of steady state free precession.

As in all FFE techniques, FISP employs a small flip angle (less than 90°) RF excitation pulse without any refocusing pulses. After several such cycles with short TR, a coherent steady state magnetization is achieved (see SSFP). In this steady state, a bicomponent signal is produced. While either component of the signal may be used to generate a gradient echo, in FISP, the components are superimposed onto each other due to the balanced frequency encode gradient (Fig. 9.1) [18]. The overall balanced gradient structure of FISP makes the sequence insensitive to motion. Moreover, the balanced phase encoding gradient restores transverse magnetization for stationary spins, which increases sensitivity to T2*. Note that in contrast to the FISP approach, in FLASH (another variety of FFE), transverse magnetization is destroyed by a spoiler gradient pulse before the next RF excitation pulse is applied.

Variants As shown in Fig. 9.1, in FISP, all three imaging gradients are balanced. While a balanced (bipolar) phase encoding gradient is essential for the rephasing of stationary spins, balanced readout and slice select gradients ensure velocity insensitivity at the time of the echo readout. This approach of implementing FISP, however, does not correct for field inhomogeneity phase artifacts, which become more prominent with increasing RF flip angle. Such artifacts occur due to a wide variety of resonant offsets coexisting within a single voxel. To eliminate these artifacts, the readout and slice select gradients of the FISP sequence may be made

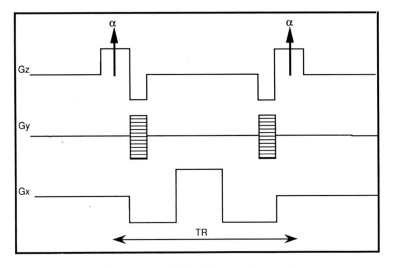

FIG. 9.1 Note that in FISP, all the gradients are balanced.

unbalanced. This unbalancing of the gradients systemically averages out the range of phase values for a particular voxel (resonant offset averaging in the steady state, see ROAST).[1] However, this also disperses coherent transverse magnetization, especially for fast flowing spins.

   See also: FADE, ROAST, SSFP.

CLINICAL APPLICATIONS
TISSUE CONTRAST

The T1 contrast in FISP is dependent on such factors as the excitation flip angle (EFA) and TR, and the ratio T1/T2* determines the ultimate contrast observed on FISP images [11,14]. However, if T1 and T2* of the diseased tissue change such that the ratio T1/T2* remains unaltered (or becomes the same as the surrounding tissue), FISP may fail to differentiate abnormal tissue from normal tissue.

CONTRAST ENHANCEMENT AND FISP

As Gd-DTPA decreases T1 of blood, the incoming blood is even more relaxed and, therefore, the vessels appear brighter on the angiograms [2].

---

[1] Just to confuse things a little bit more, ROAST has been referred to as conventional FISP and FISP, as outlined here, as true FISP!

For similar reasons, Gd-enhanced FISP also has been used in breast examinations [6]. The newer experimental contrast agent ^{17}O (in the form of $H_2^{17}O$) decreases T2 but has no effect on T1. Therefore, instead of lengthy T2-weighted SE images, FISP images provide comparable image contrast in a very short period of time [5].

CEREBROSPINAL FLUID

Usually, the larger the excitation flip angle, the brighter the CSF signal, because of increased T2 weighting. Moreover, refocusing of the motion further enhances the CSF signal.

THE ABDOMEN

Being very fast due to extremely short repetition times, FISP allows the entire data acquisition to be finished in a very short period of time, eg, a single breath holding. Thus, the degradation in signal-to-noise ratio due to respiratory motion is minimized. Complete MR studies of the abdomen can be carried out within a few seconds. As T2* contrast is more dominant than T1 contrast in FISP, hepatic tumors (long T2) usually appear brighter than normal liver tissue. However, as the blood appears bright, flow-related artifacts may be enhanced and, particularly in case of the left of the lobe, lesions may be disguised by these artifacts [16].

THE JOINTS

FISP has been employed in the morphological examination of the normal and abnormal hip and knee joints [1,9,12,15]. The differentiation of various internal structures is determined by image contrast, which, in turn, is determined by the EFA. For example, it has been found that while a 10° EFA outlines the knee cartilages very well, a 90° EFA shows the best fat–muscle differentiation [15]. In the case of the hip joint, FISP, using a 70° RF excitation pulse with TR (33 msec) and TE (12 msec), provides the best arthrographic images (Fig. 9.2) [1]. Tyrrell et al [15] have found the diagnostic merit of FISP images comparable to that of the arthroscopy, but Solomon et al [12] have found FISP images no better than spin echo images in identifying meniscal lesions.

THE BLOOD

The fact that FISP is more sensitive to magnetic susceptibility effects than spin echo techniques has been cleverly used in the detection of acute hemorrhage. Areas of acute hemorrhage may contain deoxyhemoglobin,

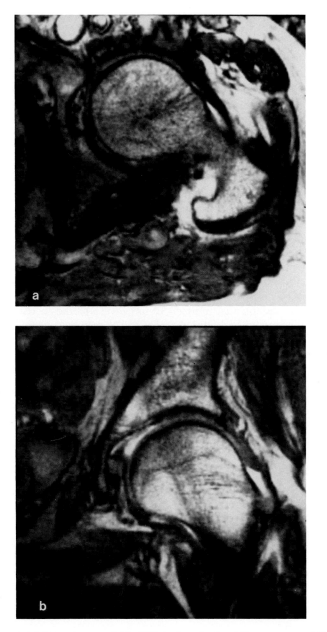

FIG. 9.2 Axial **(a)** and coronal **(b)** FISP (70° excitation; TR = 30 msec; TE = 12 msec) images of the hip joint of a normal volunteer. Note the high intensity of the synovial fluid and bone marrow on the coronal section. (Courtesy of G. Bongartz; reproduced, with permission, from Bongartz et al [1].)

which is paramagnetic. In a region where there is an accumulation of deoxyhemoglobin, magnetic susceptibility is very high and, as a result, T2* is greatly reduced. Being very sensitive to this reduction in T2*, FISP shows areas of acute hemorrhage as dark spots [17]. However, FLASH provides better delineation of subacute and chronic clots (see FLASH). In addition, as the flowing blood also appears bright, the definitive diagnosis of a hyperintense thrombus may be difficult.

THE ANGIOGRAPHY

FISP is the only FFE technique in which all the gradients are balanced. This balanced gradient structure makes FISP velocity insensitive. In other words, the flowing spins are refocused at the echo time. Therefore, the flowing blood appears bright, with the surrounding tissues appearing dark. However, lowering the excitation flip angle may increase the signal intensity of the surrounding tissue, which may then increase the background signal. This counteracts the benefit of the increased blood signal. In the three-dimensional form, FISP has been utilized to obtain angiograms of the carotids and intracranial vessels in time periods ranging from 6 to 13 minutes, without the need for cardiac gating [7,10].[2] Fig 9.3 shows a three-dimensional FISP angiogram of the forearm vessels. TR 50 msec and 15° RF flip angle seems to provide the best contrast between the flowing blood and the surrounding brain tissue/CSF.

ADVANTAGES AND DISADVANTAGES

FISP has the ability of delivering T1-weighted MR scans in a short period of time. The rapidity of the sequence permits contrast-enhanced studies of the heart, breast, and other structures to be performed.

As FISP and FLASH belong to the same general class of fast imaging techniques, there has been a considerable effort to evaluate their respective roles in clinical MRI. Overall, FISP has been rated, in terms of speed and the ability to suppress motion-induced artifacts, at par with FLASH [14].

Like most other gradient echo techniques, FISP does not have a 180° refocusing pulse. So, in general, it is more sensitive to magnetic inhomogeneities than conventional spin echo techniques, and the decay of

---

[2] Three-dimensional FISP also has been used successfully to study the inner ear structures [13].

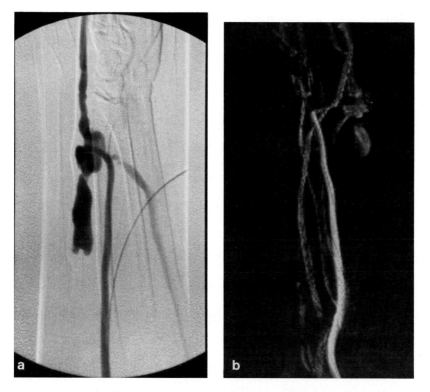

FIG. 9.3 Digital subtraction angiogram **(a)** and the corresponding three-dimensional FISP (20° excitation; TR = 40 msec; TE = 14 msec) angiogram **(b)** of the forearm in a patient with hemodialysis fistula. The feeding artery is clearly seen on both images. However, the size of the venous convolution and the aneurysmic venous sac are underestimated on the FISP angiogram. (Courtesy of H-B. Gehl; reproduced, with permission, from H-B. Gehl [3].)

transverse magnetization is described by T2* rather than T2. However, the degree of this sensitivity to field inhomogeneities is somewhat more pronounced in FISP than in other FFE sequences [18], the reason being the image intensity fluctuates with inhomogeneity-induced changing phase rotations. The latter makes the FISP sequence very sensitive to local magnetic field inhomogeneity artifacts and, not so uncommon, such artifacts may degrade image quality beyond its usefulness. In addition, as the flowing spins are refocused, they register a higher signal, which may further enhance flow-related artifacts. ROAST, a modified FISP sequence, is designed to decrease FISP image sensitivity to local inhomogeneities [4].

FISP is available on Siemens MR scanners.

REFERENCES

1. Bongartz G, Bock E, Horbach T, Requard H (1989): Degenerative cartilage lesions of the hip—magnetic resonance evaluation. *Magn Reson Imag* 7: 179–186.

2. Creasy JL, Price RR, Presbrey T, Goins D, Partain CL, Kessler RM (1990): Gadolinium-enhanced MR angiography. *Radiology* 175:280–283.

3. Gehl HB (1991): Imaging of hemodialysis fistulas: limitations of MR angiography. *J Comput Assist Tomogr* 15:271–275.

4. Haacke EM, Wielopolski PA, Tkach JA, Modic MT (1990): Steady-state free precession imaging in the presence of motion: application for improved visualization of the cerebrospinal fluid. *Radiology* 175:545–552.

5. Hopkins AL, Haacke EM, Barr RG, Tkach J (1988): Oxygen-17 contrast agents: fast imaging techniques. *Invest Radiol* 23:S240–S242.

6. Kaiser WA, Zeitler E (1989): MR imaging of the breast: fast imaging sequences with and without Gd-DTPA. Preliminary observations. *Radiology* 170: 681–686.

7. Masaryk TJ, Modic MT, Ross JS, Ruggieri PM, Laub GA, Lenz GW, Haacke EM, Selman WR, Wiznitzer M, Harik SI (1989): Intracranial circulation: preliminary clinical results with three-dimensional (volume) MR angiography. *Radiology* 171:793–799.

8. Oppelt A, Graumann R, Barfuss H, Fischer H, Hartl W, Schajor W (1986): FISP—a new imaging sequence with rapid pulses for magnetic resonance tomography. *Electromedica* 54:15–18.

9. Reiser MF, Bongartz G, Erlemann R, Strobel M, Pauly T, Gaebert K, Stoeber U, Peters PE (1988): Magnetic resonance in cartilaginous lesions of the knee joint with three-dimensional gradient-echo imaging. *Skeletal Radiology* 17:465–471.

10. Ruggieri PM, Laub GA, Masaryk TJ, Modic MT (1989): Intracranial circulation: pulse-sequence considerations in three-dimensional (volume) MR angiography. *Radiology* 171:785–791.

11. Runge VM, Wood ML (1988): Fast imaging and other motion artifact reduction schemes: a pictorial overview. *Magn Reson Imag* 6:595–608.

12. Solomon SL, Totty WG, Lee JK (1989): MR imaging of the knee: comparison of three-dimensional FISP and two-dimensional spin-echo pulse sequences. *Radiology* 173:739–742.

13. Tanioka H, Shirakawa T, Machida T, Sasaki Y (1991): Three-dimensional reconstructed MR imaging of the inner ear. *Radiology* 178:141–144.

14. Tkach JA, Haacke EM (1988): A comparison of fast spin echo and gradient field echo sequences. *Magn Reson Imag* 6:373–389.

15. Tyrrell RL, Gluckert K, Pathria M, Modic MT (1988): Fast three-dimensional MR imaging of the knee: comparison with arthroscopy. *Radiology* 166:865–872.

16. Unger EC, Cohen MS, Gatenby RA, Clair MR, Brown TR, Nelson SJ, McGlone JS (1988): Single breath-holding scans of the abdomen using FISP and FLASH at 1.5 T. *J Comput Assist Tomogr* 12:575–583.

17. Unger EC, Cohen MS, Brown TR (1989): Gradient echo imaging of hemorrhage at 1.5 Tesla. *Magn Reson Imag* 7:163–172.

18. van der Meulen P, Groen JP, Tinus AMC, Bruntink G (1988): Fast field echo imaging: an overview and contrast calculations. *Magn Reson Imag* 6:355–368.

10

Flow Adjustable Gradient Echo (FLAG)

BASIC PRINCIPLES

Flow adjustable gradient echo (FLAG) angiography [2,7] is based on the phase-sensitive projection method of MR angiography [1], in which two data acquisitions are carried out, each containing distinct flow velocity dependent phase information. An angiogram is obtained by a subtraction of these two data sets, as explained below.

As the excited spins move within the selected plane, they experience phase changes along the direction of a field gradient. Gradients can be designed such that these changes in the spin phase can be registered (flow sensitive or *uncompensated*). Gradients can also be designed such that they do not encode these changes (flow insensitive or *compensated*). If such gradients are alternated during the image acquisition, two separate data sets are obtained, one with velocity-induced phase shifts, and the other with rephased flowing spins (no phase shifts). A complex subtraction of these data sets yields an angiogram (Fig. 10.1).

The FLAG pulse sequence consists of a low flip angle (usually 20°) RF excitation pulse to establish steady state magnetization, followed by the acquisition of gradient echoes. The standard sequence contains both flow-compensated and flow-uncompensated bipolar gradients (Fig. 10.2). By varying the amplitude of the bipolar gradient pulses, velocity sensitivity and compensation may be adjusted [5].

The sequence may be applied in either cardiac-triggered mode (where the phase shift at each phase encoding step in both images corresponds to the distinct flow components, thus temporally resolved) or the non-triggered mode (where the phase shift at each phase encoding step in both images is not time-related to the distinct flow components; thus temporally averaged).

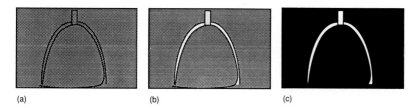

(a)   (b)   (c)

FIG. 10.1 (a) The vessel is barely seen as a result of signal loss due to random phase shifts. **(b)** The flowing spins are refocused and the signal from the vessel is brighter. To achieve a better contrast-to-noise ratio, the stationary surround has to be eliminated. This is achieved by subtracting image (a) from image (b). The resultant flow image is shown in **(c)**. (This illustration represents an ideal situation, in which complete elimination of the stationary surround is achieved. In reality, residual phase errors do not easily permit us to obtain the excellent contrast-to-noise ratio shown in **(c)**).

Variants   In the standard cardiac-triggering approach, flow-compensated and flow-sensitive components of the sequence are acquired in two successive cardiac cycles, while maintaining their temporal relationship to the triggering signal (Fig. 10.3a). The underlying assumption is that flow remains identical at the same time point in two different cardiac cycles.

FIG. 10.2 FLAG pulse sequence with a velocity-compensated balanced gradient profile. The dotted areas represent the gradient lobes whose amplitude is changed for achieving the desired velocity sensitivity. Two applications of the sequence are used: velocity compensated and velocity sensitive. A complex subtraction of the signals then yields a flow image. The shaded gradient lobe may be used to destroy any residual transverse magnetization at the end of the repetition period. (Modified, with permission, from Lanzer et al [5].)

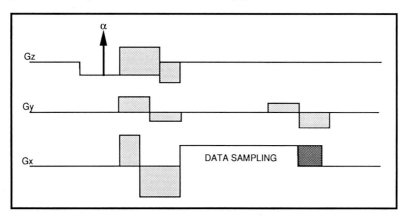

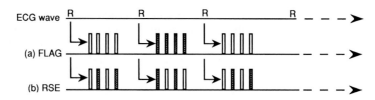

FIG. 10.3 Depending on the length of the cardiac cycle and the pulse timing parameters, a variable number of pulse applications may be performed during each R-R interval. In this illustration, four such pulse applications are shown by the vertical columns. **(a)** In FLAG, during each R-R interval, either only velocity-compensated data acquisitions (clear columns) or only velocity-sensitive data acquisitions are performed (shaded columns). In contrast, in RSE, the applications of velocity-compensated and velocity-sensitive sequences are interleaved during each R-R interval **(b)**, and their order is alternated during every other R-R interval.

However, this is not true and, in reality, some phase errors may be introduced on the subtraction of the data sets. To avoid this problem, a novel triggering scheme, rapid sequential excitation (RSE), has been proposed. Under this scheme, flow-compensated and flow-sensitive acquisitions are undertaken, one immediately following the other, in the same cardiac cycle (Fig. 10.3b) [3].

See also: FEER, PBANG.

CLINICAL APPLICATIONS
TISSUE CONTRAST

On the magnitude images, the flowing blood appears uniformly bright, the intensity being determined by the flow velocity, and the timing of the data acquisition with respect to the cardiac cycle. For example, the best diagnostic quality angiograms are obtained when the data are acquired 30 to 60 msec *before* the peak flow velocity [4].

So far, clinical studies of the carotids, aortoiliac, and femoropopliteal junctions of normal subjects using this sequence have been reported [3–8]. Experience shows that the triggered mode of data acquisition gives a higher percentage of diagnostic aortograms than the nontriggered mode [6]. FLAG MR aortograms acquired in the nontriggered mode suffer from the presence of unwanted venous structures and greater background noise.

Even in the triggered mode, the best image quality is obtained when systolic blood flow is near its peak value, probably because higher velocity gives better contrast due to the flow-sensitive nature of this pulse. This leaves a window of about 60 to 90 msec for data acquisition. Typically, a time resolved FLAG MR angiographic study (128 × 128 × 2 pulse repetitions) of the aortoiliac or femoropopliteal junction can be completed in approximately 15 minutes. In addition to this time, a considerable amount of time is needed to process the acquired image data.

Some quantitative information regarding blood flow velocity in the carotid arteries also has been obtained using this pulse sequence [6]. To accomplish this, a phase map is created by subtracting two images with different phase information. By selecting a region of interest (ROI) over the vessel, the average velocity in that region is derived, which, together with the area of ROI, may be used to calculate vessel flow. Such quantitative analysis of the circulatory system is quite helpful in the evaluation of peripheral vascular disorders.

ADVANTAGES AND DISADVANTAGES

As FLAG provides time-averaged flow quantification, nontriggered data acquisition can be carried out, which may reduce the total study time. For example, a typical study comprising 16 images with 30° RF pulse excitation, TR 200 msec, TE 30 msec and eight averages takes about 14 minutes. However, this amount of time is still considerably higher than other fast angiographic methods (see SFI), which provide imaging time of a few seconds.

In the study reported by Tarnawski et al [7], the carotid blood flow quantification by the FLAG pulse sequence was found to be highly correlated with the Doppler ultrasound examination. This may be clinically significant in cases where ultrasound examination of the vessels is not feasible, for example, if the vessels are deeply buried beneath the tissue layers.

The RSE approach increases the flow-related signal. Together with the fact that near complete static tissue subtraction is achieved with the RSE approach, the increased signal from the blood increases the diagnostic quality of the FLAG angiograms.

FLAG pulse sequence is available on Philips MR imaging scanners.

REFERENCES

1. Dumoulin CL, Hart HR (1986): Magnetic resonance angiography. *Radiology* 161:717–720.

2. Groen JP, van Dijk P (1987): Design of flow adjustable gradient waveforms. *Magn Reson Med* 6:S868.

3. Lanzer P, Bohning J, Groen J, Gross G, Nanda N, Pohost G (1990): Aortoiliac and femoropopliteal phase-based NMR angiography: a comparison between FLAG and RSE. *Magn Reson Med* 15:372–385.

4. Lanzer P, Gross G, Nanda N, Pohost G (1990): Timing of data acquisition de-

termines image quality in femoropopliteal phase-sensitive MR angiography. *Angiology* 41:817–823.

5. Lanzer P, McKibbin W, Bohning D, Thorn B, Gross G, Cranney G, Nanda N, Pohost G (1990): Aortoiliac imaging by projective phase sensitive MR angiography: effects of triggering and timing of data acquisition on image quality. *Magn Reson Imag* 8:107–116.

6. Smith MA, Tarnawski M, Padayachee TS, West DJ, Graves M, Taylor MG (1988): Measurement of time-averaged flow in the carotid arteries. *Magn Reson Med* 7:S179.

7. Tarnawski M, Padayachee TS, West DJ, Graves MJ, Ayton VT, Taylor MG, Smith MA (1990): The measurement of time-averaged flow by magnetic resonance imaging using continuous acquisition in the carotid arteries and its comparison with Doppler ultrasound. *Clin Phys Physio Measurement* 11:27–36.

8. van Dijk P, Groen JP, de Graaf RG (1987): Three applications of a flow adjustable gradient echo sequence. *Radiology* 165:S130.

11

Fast Low Angle Spin Echo (FLASE)

BASIC PRINCIPLES

In an NMR experiment, the signal amplitude is directly determined by the magnitude of the longitudinal magnetization (Mz). After the first RF excitation, the amount of Mz available for the next pulse cycle is dependent on the recovery of Mz from the previous excitation; the time required for the latter is directly related to the degree of flipping experienced by the Mz. The Mz recovery time can become prohibitively longer, especially if the tissue T1 is longer (eg, various bodily fluids), which, in turn, increases the pulse repetition time (TR). However, if Mz is flipped by a lower angle, less time is required for its complete recovery; thus, the data acquisition can be completed in a relatively short period of time. This is the principle of partial flip angle imaging [6,7] (Fig. 11.1).

While partial flip angle imaging has been popularly associated with gradient echo imaging [1,12], it is important to note that the principle of partial flip angle imaging is general and is applicable to almost any type of pulse sequence. When this principle is applied to spin echo sequences, it may be called partial flip angle spin echo imaging (PFA SE) or fast low angle spin echo (FLASE).

The standard SE sequence uses a 90° RF pulse to flip the Mz into the transverse xy plane. The resulting FID is refocused by a 180° RF pulse to form a spin echo. By properly adjusting the echo time (TE) and TR, either T1 or T2 weighted images are obtained. As the spin dephasing due to field inhomogeneities is almost completely recovered by using 180° refocusing pulses, the decay in transverse magnetization is described by T2 rather than by T2*. The diagnostic significance of T2-weighted SE images is very well known and, in practice, such images are usually ob-

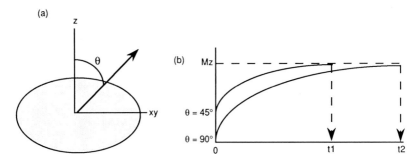

FIG. 11.1 (a) The magnetization vector is flipped by an angle θ, which is less than 90°. As a result, the steady state longitudinal magnetization is reached very rapidly **(b)**.

tained by setting TR to 2000 msec and TE to 80 msec. Long TR is necessary to allow near complete recovery of the longitudinal magnetization. This makes T2-weighted study very time-consuming (the imaging time increases linearly with TR). However, a considerable reduction in the imaging time can be obtained by flipping only a part of the available Mz every time the sequence is repeated (thereby, reducing the TR).

Various spin echo based fast imaging approaches have been proposed, sometimes with different acronyms, such as *fast low angle multiecho* (FLAME) [5] or *fast optimal angle spin echo sequence with a short TE* (FATE) [11]. All of these approaches are essentially low angle versions of the SE sequence (except for RARE). It will be helpful to review the FATE pulse sequence as a representative example.

As shown in Fig. 11.2, FATE is essentially a double spin echo sequence with a low angle excitatory RF pulse. While the reduced angle of the excitation pulse helps to decrease the overall TR, the presence of the 180° refocusing pulses ensures that field inhomogeneity effects are accurately refocused at the echo time. However, some signal loss may still occur due to imperfections in the 180° pulse profile. This signal loss may be minimized by using nonselective 180° pulses [11]. Alternatively, the pulse sequence of Fig. 11.2 may be modified as described below.

Variants In yet another approach to achieve faster imaging times without the disadvantages of using gradient echo sequences, *rapid spin echo excitation* (RASEE), a variant of the FATE sequence, has been proposed [2]. It consists of a nonselective 180° pulse applied just before the selective excitation pulse of angle less than 90°. After a time interval TE/2, another nonselective 180° RF pulse is applied to invert the longitudinal magnetization, and a spin echo is obtained (Fig. 11.3). The time interval

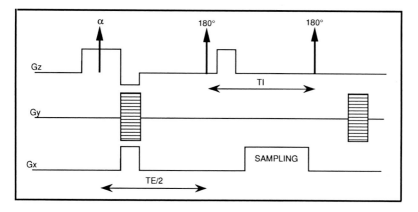

FIG. 11.2 FATE pulse sequence. It is similar to a double spin echo sequence but the 90° excitation pulse is replaced by a pulse of angle less than 90°. (Modified, with permission, from Bogdan and Joseph [2].)

between two 180° pulses is known as the interpulse time (TI). Note that, in RASEE, the sampling of the data occurs outside the time interval TI. In FATE, the sampling of data occurs during the time interval TI. This has a profound effect on the signal-to-noise ratio, as discussed later.

The pairing of the selective low angle RF pulse with a nonselective 180° RF pulse is similar to a spatially selective RF pulse whose angle is close to 180° [2]. Therefore, RASEE also may be called large angle spin

FIG. 11.3 RASEE pulse sequence. Note that the second 180° pulse of Fig. 11.2 has been moved just before the 90° excitation pulse. As a result, the data sampling occurs outside the interpulse time TI, which has a significant influence on the signal-to-noise ratio. See text for details. (Modified, with permission, from Bogdan and Joseph [2].)

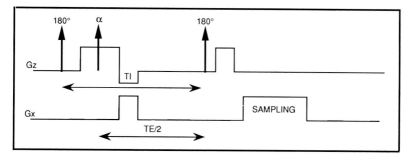

echo (LASE). However, the disadvantages of nonlinearity and poor pulse profile associated with a large angle selective pulse are eliminated.

See also: FLASH, GREASE, RASE.

CLINICAL APPLICATIONS
TISSUE CONTRAST

By retaining 180° refocusing pulses, FLASE is made insensitive to field inhomogeneities, and it does not suffer from the signal loss due to T2* decay (Fig. 11.4). Improved contrast-to-noise ratio is thus achieved, leading to better detection of the pathology via T2-weighted FLASE images in less time than long TR/long TE spin echo images. In general, T2-weighted image contrast can be obtained by using only half as long TR as the standard SE sequence. As the TR is decreased, the T1 weighting may be increased, which is offset by the lower excitation flip angle in an even echo spin echo sequence. Note that the same condition may be met by increasing the RF flip angle beyond 90° in case of an odd echo spin echo sequence [8]. As a result, the signal intensity of the images is diminished when compared to the standard SE images (see below) [5]. However, the resolution of the FATE images is similar to that of the conventional T2-weighted SE images.

THE BRAIN

While gradient echo techniques provide very rapid scan times, their clinical utility is limited by local inhomogeneity artifacts, especially near the bone/air or brain tissue/bone interfaces (eg, paranasal sinuses and the cranial fossa) [10]. In such situations, better quality images have been obtained by using partial RF flip angle sequences, which retain 180° refocusing pulses [4,5,8]. The CSF flow void sign is preserved and fewer CSF flow-related artifacts are present than the 90° SE images [3].

THE SPINE

Unlike FLASH, there is no signal loss from the vertebral body and the vertebra appears bright, almost isointense with the intervertebral discs, on the FATE images. However, the presence of the cortical bone, which appears as a dark border, defines the disc margins very well [11]. This may facilitate the visualization of diseases afflicting the bone marrow.

THE BLOOD

Unlike FLASH, the signal from the flowing material is not registered in FATE; the flowing blood, thus, appears dark (signal void). This results in elimination of flow-related artifacts [11].

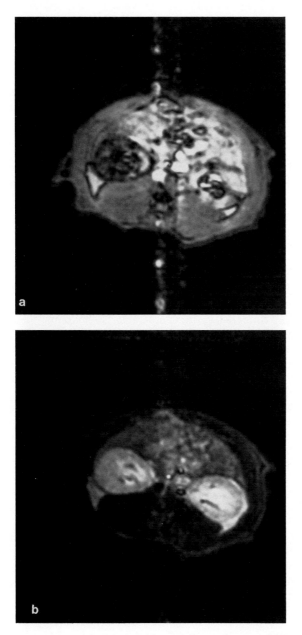

FIG. 11.4 A comparison between the fast gradient echo **(a)** and RASEE **(b)** post-gadolinium images of the rat kidney. Both images were obtained with 40° excitation, TR = 50 msec, and TE = 13.5 msec. Note the image degradation in (a) due to field inhomogeneities and flow effects. (Courtesy of Peter Joseph; reproduced, with permission, from Bogdan and Joseph [2].)

MUSCLE

Fat appears almost as bright as on T1-weighted SE images because the spin dephasing of fat is effectively rephased by the 180° pulses. Thus, unlike FLASH, there is better contrast between muscle mass and subcutaneous fat [11].

THE PELVIS

The contrast-to-noise ratio of urine (long T1) and pelvic fat (short T1) is increased at below 90° RF flip angles. Similarly, the internal structure of the prostate and the uterus appears more clearly demarcated than the corresponding 90° SE images [8].

ADVANTAGES AND DISADVANTAGES

The lower flip angle RF excitation helps to reduce the TR. However, the presence of 180° refocusing pulses prolongs the minimum achievable echo time (TE). Nonetheless, for comparable TE, image matrix, and number of averages, a two- to threefold reduction in imaging time is possible.

As only a part of the Mz is transformed into transverse magnetization, the amplitude of the resultant echo is diminished, and so is the signal intensity. Moreover, the shorter TR may permit only a limited number of slices to be obtained in a time-multiplexed multiecho series.

Even though FATE sequence is not as fast as some other gradient echo techniques such as FLASH (TR is longer due to the presence of 180° pulses), the spatial resolution of FATE images is far greater than that of the corresponding gradient echo images [11].

The time interval between the two 180° pulses (TI) determines the loss of signal due to recovery of longitudinal magnetization. The lesser the time interval TI, the lesser is the signal loss due to the recovery of longitudinal magnetization. In FATE, TI is directly proportional to the TE and the sampling time (Fig. 11.2). In RASEE, a variant of FATE, TI does not depend on the sampling time, as the latter is done outside the TI (Fig. 11.3). So, for the same value of TE, more sampling can be done with RASEE without increasing the interpulse time TI (and the resultant signal loss), and, therefore, a signal-to-noise ratio higher than that of the FATE images may be achieved [2].

REFERENCES

1. Bendel P (1987): T2-weighted contrasts in rapid low flip-angle imaging. *Magn Reson Med* 5:366–370.
2. Bogdan AR, Joseph PM (1990): RASEE: a rapid spin-echo pulse sequence. *Magn Reson Imag* 8:13–19.

3. Chang KH, Yi JG, Han MH, Cho MH, Han MC, Cho ZH, Kim CW (1990): Clinical utility of partial flip angle T2 weighted spin-echo imaging of the brain. Neuroradiology 32:255–260.

4. Chisin R, Buxton RB, Ragozzino MW, Beaulieu PA, Fabian RL, Brady TJ (1989): Preliminary results with low flip angle spin-echo MR imaging of the head and neck. Am J Neuroradiol 10:719–724.

5. Hackney DB, Lenkinski RE, Grossman RI, Zimmerman RA, Goldberg HI, Bilaniuk LT, Young SC, Nowell MA, Kemp SS (1988): Initial experience with fast low-angle multiecho (FLAME) imaging of the central nervous system. J Comput Assist Tomogr 12:171–174.

6. Mills TC, Ortendahl DA, Hylton NM (1986): Investigation of partial flip angle magnetic resonance imaging. IEEE Trans Nucl Sci 33:496–500.

7. Mills TC, Ortendahl DA, Hylton NM, Crooks LE, Carlson JW, Kaufman L (1987): Partial flip angle MR imaging. Radiology 162:531–539.

8. Mitchell DG, Vinitski S, Burk DL, Levy D, Rifkin MD (1989): Variable-flip-angle spin-echo MR imaging of the pelvis: more versatile T2-weighted images. Radiology 171:525–529.

9. Laissy JP, Hugonet P (1989): Partial flip-angle spin-echo imaging: clinical applications. (letter) Am J Roentgen 153:883–884.

10. Ludeke KM, Roschmann P, Tischler R (1985): Susceptibility artifacts in NMR imaging. Magn Reson Imag 3:329–343.

11. Tkach JA, Haacke EM (1988): A comparison of fast spin echo and gradient field echo sequences. Magn Reson Imag 6:373–389.

12. Winkler ML, Ortendahl DA, Mills TC, Crooks LE, Sheldon PE, Kaufman L, Kramer DM (1988): Characteristics of partial flip angle and gradient reversal MR imaging. Radiology 166:17–26.

12

Fast Low Angle Shot (FLASH)

BASIC PRINCIPLES

Fast low angle shot (FLASH) [9] sequence is one of the earliest fast field echo (FFE) techniques in magnetic resonance imaging. As in all other FFE techniques, FLASH consists of a reduced angle slice selective RF excitation pulse and, after establishment of the steady state (longitudinal) magnetization, a gradient recalled echo acquisition is carried out (Fig. 12.1). As in any other two-dimensional Fourier transform technique, a single line of k-space is sampled for each RF pulse. Note that, unlike the spin echo techniques, 180° refocusing pulses are conspicuously absent from the pulse sequence. The absence of 180° pulse allows the echo train to be moved closer to the excitation pulse for a shorter effective echo time (TE). As the excitation pulse angle is less than 90°, TR also can be made very short (usually less than 10 msec); the net result is very fast data acquisition.

For three-dimensional implementation of FLASH, an extra phase encoding gradient is introduced, as shown in Fig. 12.2 [8,24]. As a result of this gradient, the motion sensitivity of the sequence is increased. Alternatively, multiple two-dimensional FLASH images can be acquired and then stacked on top of one another. Runge et al [23] have used this approach for volume imaging of the brain.

In the FLASH sequence, the phase encoding gradient is not symmetric around the data acquisition. And as the amplitude of the phase encoding gradient is varied for every pulse repetition (as in any spin warp method), but without the unwarping lobe of the gradient, image artifacts may arise due to a constantly changing precession angle of the spins located away from the center of the gradient, if any transverse coherence is allowed to

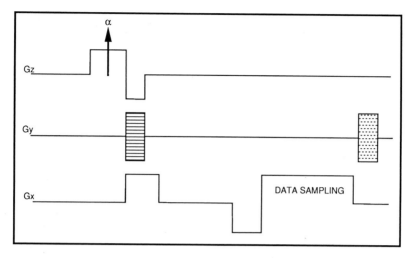

FIG. 12.1 Original ("spoiled") FLASH pulse sequence in which the phase encoding gradient is not balanced. In the refocused FLASH version, a second gradient pulse is applied after the data sampling (the dashed gradient lobe) to restore the phase of the stationary spins.

persist [7]. This artifact manifests itself near the region where the phase encoding gradient is zero [10], and it lies parallel to the direction of the frequency encoding gradient [7]. A variety of approaches have been proposed to eliminate this artifact, as described below:

1. Simply follow the data acquisition with a gradient lobe of the opposite polarity but equal amplitude. This preserves the transverse magnetization. Now the T2 relaxation process competes with the T1 relaxation process for determining image contrast, and the latter is much altered. In fact, the use of refocused FLASH (see below) effectively broadens the artifact band and spreads it over the entire image [7]. The image as a whole appears brighter, which increases the signal-to-noise ratio; but, the contrast-to-noise ratio is deteriorated.

2. Alternatively, disperse the transverse magnetization by adding a spoiler gradient pulse. Most commonly, such a spoiler pulse is applied in the slice select direction [33,34]. In the approach by Wood ėt al [34], the amplitude of the spoiler gradient steadily decreases from the highest in the first repetition cycle to the lowest in the last such cycle. The benefit of this approach is that it minimizes the transverse magnetization without altering image contrast. In the approach proposed by Wang and Riederer [33], the gradient amplitude (A_G) increases in a geometric manner (A_G, $2A_G$, $4A_G$, $8A_G$, ...). Alternatively, an arith-

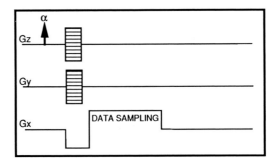

FIG. 12.2 In three-dimensional FLASH implementation, the phase encoding is performed in two perpendicular directions. Each phase encoding step takes about 10 msec, depending on the gradient hardware. For 128 phase encode steps in each direction, the total acquisition time is about 3 min.

metic series is used, in which a large gradient pulse (nA$_G$) is followed by a series of gradient pulses of increasing amplitudes (A$_G$ + k, A$_G$ + 2k, A$_G$ + 3k, . . ., A$_G$ + nk; where k = constant and n is less than the total number of phase encoding steps). The entire series repeats itself after the nth phase encode step, until the last cycle is reached.

3. The above approach of adding spoiler gradient pulses of variable amplitudes has not been found effective for three-dimensional FLASH imaging [35]. In this situation, Wood and Runge [35] have found that the addition of a spoiler pulse of constant amplitude in the refocused FLASH sequence reduces the overall image intensity by a factor of 50%. Thus, it can be readily seen that the disadvantage of the first approach has been attenuated by combining it with the second approach.

4. Crawley et al [7] have shown that if the RF pulses are increasingly frequency shifted, then results similar to the application of a spoiler gradient pulse are achieved. However, this approach has been found technically more demanding for RF electronics.

Variants   Following are variations of the original FLASH sequence that have been proposed.

(A) In the original FLASH sequence, the phase encoding gradient is not made balanced by rewinding it after the echo acquisition (the spoiled FLASH, because the transverse magnetization is destroyed). In what is known as the refocused FLASH, the phase encoding gradient is reversed (and thus made balanced) after the echo readout (Fig. 12.1), as in other FFE-SSFP varieties. This simple modification restores the steady state transverse magnetization response.

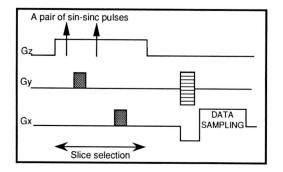

FIG. 12.3 RAPID pulse sequence. The shaded gradient lobe dephases any incidental transverse magnetization. (Modified, with permission, from Brooks et al [3].)

(B) The FLASH sequence may be preceded by either a 180° RF pulse (to achieve variable T1 contrast; see IR-FLASH) or a 90°–180°–90° (DISE) pulse triplet (to achieve variable T2 contrast; see IR).

(C) By improving gradient switching times, various faster versions of the original FLASH sequence have been proposed (see snapshot FLASH imaging, SFI).

(D) In FLASH, the slice select gradient is switched on every time an RF pulse is applied, and is then reversed to rephase the magnetization of the stationary spins. For an acquisition comprised of 128 phase encode steps, this process is repeated as many times. Surely, this involves a lot of gradient switching on and off. Brooks et al [3] have proposed a technique in which the slice selection is achieved by a pair of sin-sinc pulses (Fig. 12.3). This eliminates the need for continuously switching the gradient on and off for slice selection. This method, called RAPID (rapid acquisition of proton images using DIGGER) has been found as fast as the FLASH sequence [3].

See also: FLASE, RARE, SFI, SSFP.

CLINICAL APPLICATIONS
TISSUE CONTRAST

For large EFA (close to 90°), the contrast is primarily T1 weighted. However, the contrast-enhanced 90° FLASH has been found inferior to the T1-weighted SE images in brain studies [4]. As the EFA is lowered to 30°, T2* weighting increases [30], which may decrease the contrast-to-noise ratio [28]. For EFAs below 20°, only proton density weighted contrast is available. FLASH images usually show the paradoxical enhancement of the flow perpendicular to the selected slice. The muscle mass and sub-cutaneous fat have almost identical signal intensity.

CONTRAST ENHANCEMENT AND FLASH

As FLASH is sensitive to paramagnetism, perfusion studies using contrast agents, such as Gd-DTPA, may be completed within a very short period of time [13]. FLASH has already shown superior contrast of various hepatic lesions when used along with Gd-DOTA [16]. In the brain, the Gd-DTPA–enhanced FLASH shows similar contrast characteristics (in terms of the pathology demarcation from the normal brain tissue) to the Gd-DTPA–enhanced SE images [25]. However, a report by Tovi et al [29] suggests that, in the case of gliomas, postgadolinium FLASH images provide less information than T1-weighted SE images. Ross et al [22] have compared two- and three-dimensional postgadolinium FLASH images and concluded that the three-dimensional images provide more information regarding intradural and parenchymal diseases.

THE BRAIN

For any pulse sequence, the ultimate test for providing excellent tissue contrast should be its ability to differentiate the white matter from the gray matter in normal as well as pathologic conditions. In this regard, the performance of FLASH is variable in that it provides variable contrast (see above) depending on the pulse parameters. For example, according to Stadnik et al [26], FLASH sequence with 70°–120°/150–300/10 provides T1-weighted contrast. If the EFA is lowered to less than 30°, the contrast is decreased mainly because at such lower flip angles, the signal is primarily dependent on the proton density; the water content of the gray and white matter is very similar.

THE SPINE

The extradural pathologies are better highlighted on FLASH images. In particular, a 10° FLASH has been found to be the most useful for identifying the extradural pathologies, as the vertebral bodies appear dark and the CSF appears very bright. In contrast, the intradural lesions are better highlighted with T1-weighted SE images [32].

CEREBROSPINAL FLUID

Using ECG-gated FLASH, it has been possible to demonstrate the direction and velocity of CSF flow through the aqueduct [27]. Commonly, two acquisitions with different phase encodings are subtracted to derive an image of the flow.

THE HEART

Dynamic examinations of the heart have been possible with FLASH. Usually, several cardiac cycles are needed in order to construct a single image of the beating heart; several such images are needed to construct a loop for the standard cine-FLASH MR imaging. This means that at least several minutes are required for a complete dynamic study of the heart. However, by using 10° RF pulses, 64 phase encode × 128 spatial resolution and extremely short TR (4.8 msec) and TE (2.8 msec), it is possible to acquire an image of the beating heart, without cardiac triggering or the need for breath holding, in about 300 msec, which closely equals the duration of a single cardiac cycle [12]. In the cine mode, the myocardium appears bright and the blood shows velocity-dependent variable intensity. By using several presaturating 90° pulses before the imaging sequence, the contrast between the flowing blood and the myocardium can be optimized. Such cine-FLASH studies offer the facility for examining the blood flow through structural defects in the heart [20].

THE ABDOMEN

T1-weighted and T2-weighted SE images provide excellent tissue contrast in abdominal images. However, motion-induced phase shifts may create annoying image artifacts. When T2-weighted SE images are considerably degraded due to these artifacts, FLASH may be used because of its speed advantage. A single artifact-free image may be acquired in as little as a few seconds. T1-weighted FLASH (50° to 60°) shows hepatic tumors darker than the surrounding liver tissue. Ohtomo et al [19] have found FLASH very effective in differentiating the hepatic hemangiomas from the hepatocellular carcinoma. Similarly, various hepatic metastases have been correctly identified by using FLASH sequence [1].

The distinction between the hepatic and portal venous systems is not readily obvious, more so peripherally, on standard MR images, as both of them appear isointense. By selectively presaturating spins of one of the venous systems, we can make their appearances unequivocal. To this end, FLASH, with 90° pulses to presaturate spins of the portal system, has been able to show only the hepatic veins [21].

THE BLOOD

Areas of acute hemorrhage may contain deoxyhemoglobin, which is paramagnetic and reduces the $T2^*$ by increasing local magnetic field inhomogeneities. Being very sensitive to $T2^*$, FLASH shows acute hemorrhage as a dark spot (T1-weighted SE fails to identify such clots altogether, and T2-weighted SE has inferior contrast compared to FLASH or FISP). Areas of chronic hemorrhage may contain methemoglobin, which shortens T1 considerably. On FLASH, such areas appear bright because of increased signal intensity [31].

ANGIOGRAPHY

The flowing blood appears bright on the FLASH images because it is less saturated at the low excitation flip angle and the stationary tissue remains fully saturated because it receives multiple RF pulses at very short time intervals [11]. Masaryk et al [15] have found three-dimensional FLASH as effective as conventional contrast-enhanced digital subtraction angiography in identifying aneurysms and stenotic lesions of the carotid bifurcation. Matthaei et al [17] have measured blood flow with gated FLASH acquisition and found fairly accurate velocity measurements.

THE JOINTS

FLASH with 20° RF pulse, long TR and long TE brightens both the synovial fluid and the hyaline cartilage. The structural details of wrist joints inflicted with rheumatoid arthritis show contrast characteristics comparable to T2-weighted SE images. However, in hip joint assessment, FISP has been found superior to FLASH in providing a higher contrast-to-noise ratio (Fig. 12.4) [2]. In temporomandibular joint studies, the pseudodynamic cine-FLASH has provided information regarding disc displacement that previously was unavailable using the gradient echo or spin echo techniques [5,6]. The short imaging time also eliminates joint motion related artifacts. Meske et al [18] have compared the performance of FLASH images with T1/T2-weighted spin echo images in the wrist joints, and have found that FLASH provides adequate anatomic details and visualization of the synovial infiltration in rheumatoid arthritis of the wrist joints.

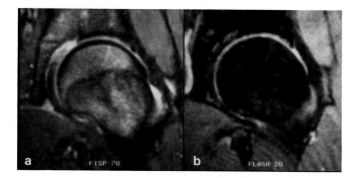

FIG. 12.4 Comparison between FISP (70° excitation; TR = 33 msec; TE = 12 msec), left **(a)** and FLASH (20° excitation; TR = 200 msec; TE = 24 msec), right **(b)** coronal images of a normal hip joint. The FISP image shows excellent separation between the hyaline cartilages and the synovial fluid. Also note that the bone marrow is brighter on the FISP image than on the FLASH image. (Courtesy of G. Bongartz; reproduced, with permission, from Bongartz et al [2].)

ADVANTAGES AND DISADVANTAGES

FLASH is utilized frequently because it has a time advantage over conventional SE imaging schemes. A typical FLASH examination may be completed in about 20 to 30 sec. While the standard cine-FLASH may take several minutes, the segmented turbo FLASH approach results in reduced data acquisition time and performs the cardiac cine studies in about 10 sec. In three-dimensional implementation of FLASH, 128 × 128 × 128 data sets of the extremities have been obtained within four minutes using 15° RF pulses, TR 10 to 20 msec and TE 9 msec.

Several different artifacts, as described below, may appear on the FLASH images.

1. The standard cine-FLASH MR has respiratory ghost artifacts, which may disappear with the use of multiple excitation FLASH imaging or retrospective gating and respiratory ordering of the phase encoding steps (ROPE).
2. As the flowing blood appears bright, it may result in flow-related artifacts in the phase encoding direction. These artifacts may be removed using appropriate flow-suppression techniques (eg, presaturation pulses).
3. If transverse magnetization is not completely destroyed by spoiler gradients before a new excitation pulse is applied, band artifacts in the

direction of the frequency encode axis appear (see Basic Principles) [7].

Recently, a spectroscopic version of three-dimensional FLASH has been proposed for ^{31}P imaging. In the future, such spectroscopic studies may provide in vivo information regarding, among many other things, ATP generation and utilization [14].

REFERENCES

1. Andersson T, Nyman R, Ericsson A, Hemmingsson A (1989): Field-echo pulse sequences used under suspended respiration for detection of liver metastases. Acta Radiologica 30:285–289.

2. Bongartz G, Bock E, Horbach T, Requard H (1989): Degenerative cartilage lesions of the hip-magnetic resonance evaluation. Magn Reson Imag 7:179–186.

3. Brooks WM, Brereton IM, Doddrell DM (1987): RAPID—a new method for fast imaging using a single slice of z-magnetization. Magn Reson Med 5:191–195.

4. Cherryman G, Golfieri R (1990): Comparison of spin echo T1-weighted and FLASH 90 degrees gadolinium-enhanced magnetic resonance imaging in the detection of cerebral metastases. Br J Radiol 63:712–715.

5. Conway WF, Hayes CW, Campbell RF (1988): Dynamic magnetic resonance imaging of the temporomandibular joint using FLASH sequences. J Oral Maxillofac Surg 46:930–938.

6. Conway WF, Hayes CW, Campbell RL, Laskin DM (1989): Temporomandibular joint motion: efficacy of fast low-angle shot MR imaging. Radiology 172: 821–826.

7. Crawley AP, Wood ML, Henkelman RM (1988): Elimination of transverse coherences in FLASH MRI. Magn Reson Med 8:248–260.

8. Frahm J, Haase A, Matthaei D (1986): Rapid three-dimensional MR imaging using the FLASH technique. J Comput Assist Tomogr 10:363–368.

9. Frahm J, Haase A, Matthaei D (1986): Rapid NMR imaging of dynamic processes using the FLASH technique. Magn Reson Med 3:321–327.

10. Frahm J, Hanicke W, Merboldt KD (1987): Transverse coherence in rapid FLASH NMR imaging. J Magn Reson 72:307–314.

11. Frahm J, Merboldt KD, Hanicke W, Haase A (1987): Flow-suppression in rapid FLASH NMR imaging. Magn Reson Med 4:372–377.

12. Frahm J, Merboldt KD, Bruhn H, Gyngell ML, Hanicke W, Chien D (1990): 0.3-second FLASH MRI of the human heart. Magn Reson Med 13:150–157.

13. Haase A, Matthaei D, Hanicke W, Frahm J (1986): Dynamic digital subtraction imaging using fast low-angle shot MR movie sequences. Radiology 160: 537–541.

14. Haase A, Leibfritz D, Werk W (1988): ^{31}P FLASH MR imaging. Magn Reson Med 7:358–363.

15. Masaryk TJ, Modic MT, Ruggieri PM, Ross JS, Laub G, Lenz GW, Tkach JA, Haacke EM, Selman WR, Harik SI (1989): Three-dimensional (volume) gradient-echo imaging of the carotid bifurcation: preliminary clinical experience. Radiology 171:801–806.

16. Marchal G, Decrop DE, Hecke PY, Baert AL (1990): Gadolinium-DOTA enhanced fast imaging of liver tumors at 1.5 T. *J Comput Assist Tomogr* 14: 217–222.

17. Matthaei D, Haase A, Merboldt KD, Hanicke W, Deimling M (1987): ECG-triggered arterial FLASH-MR flow measurement using an external standard. *Magn Reson Imag* 5:325–330.

18. Meske S, Friedburg H, Hennig J, Reinbold W, Stappert K, Schumichen C (1990): Rheumatoid arthritis lesions of the wrist examined by rapid gradient-echo magnetic resonance imaging. *Scand J Rheumatol* 19:235–238.

19. Ohtomo K, Itai Y, Yoshida H, Kokubo T, Yoshikawa K, Ilo M (1989): MR differentiation of hepatocellular carcinoma from cavernous hemangioma: complementary roles of FLASH and T2 values. *Am J Roentgen* 152:505–507.

20. Onishi S, Fukui S, Atsumi C, Morita R, Fuji K, Kusuoka H, Kitabatake A, Kamada T, Takizawa O (1989): Clinical evaluation of regurgitant blood flow by rapid cine magnetic resonance imaging in patients with valvular heart disease. *J Cardiol* 19:571–582.

21. Otake S, Matsuo M, Kuroda Y (1990): Distinction of hepatic vein from portal vein by MR imaging. *J Comput Assist Tomogr* 14:201–204.

22. Ross JS, Masaryk TJ, Modic MT (1989): Three-dimensional FLASH imaging: applications with gadolinium-DTPA. *J Comput Assist Tomogr* 13:547–552.

23. Runge YM, Wood ML, Kaufman DM, Nelson KL, Trail MR (1988): FLASH: clinical three-dimensional magnetic resonance imaging. *Radiographics* 8: 947–965.

24. Runge YM, Gelblum DY, Wood ML (1990): 3-D imaging of the CNS. *Neuroradiology* 32:356–366.

25. Schomer W, Sander B, Henkes H, Heim T, Lanksch W, Felix R (1990): Multiple slice FLASH imaging: an improved pulse sequence of contrast enhanced MR brain studies. *Neuroradiology* 32:474–480.

26. Stadnik TW, Luypaert RR, Neirynck EC, Osteaux M (1989): Optimization of sequence parameters in fast MR imaging of the brain with FLASH. *Am J Neuroradiol* 10:357–362.

27. Thomsen C, Stahlberg F, Stubgaard M, Nordell B (1990): Fourier analysis of cerebrospinal fluid velocities: MR imaging study. The Scandinavian Flow Group. *Radiology* 177:659–665.

28. Tkach JA, Haacke EM (1988): A comparison of fast spin echo and gradient field echo sequences. *Magn Reson Imag* 6:373–389.

29. Tovi M, Lilja A, Bergstrom M, Ericsson A, Bergstrom K, Hartman M (1990): Delineation of gliomas with magnetic resonance imaging using Gd-DTPA in comparison with computed tomography and positron emission tomography. *Acta Radiologica* 31:417–429.

30. Unger EC, Cohen MS, Gatenby RA, Clair MR, Brown TR, Nelson SJ, McGlone JS (1988): Single breath-holding scans of the abdomen using FISP and FLASH at 1.5 T. *J Comput Assist Tomogr* 12:575–583.

31. Unger EC, Cohen MS, Brown TR (1989): Gradient-echo imaging of hemorrhage at 1.5 tesla. *Magn Reson Imag* 7:163–172.

32. VanDyke C, Ross JS, Tkach J, Masaryk TJ, Modic MT (1989): Gradient-echo MR imaging of the cervical spine: evaluation of extradural disease. *Am J Neuroradiol* 10:627–632.

33. Wang HZ, Riederer SJ (1990): A spoiling sequence for suppression of residual transverse magnetization. *Magn Reson Med* 15:175–191.

34. Wood ML, Silver M, Runge YM (1987): Optimization of spoiler gradients in FLASH-MRI. *Magn Reson Imag* 5:455–463.

35. Wood ML, Runge YM (1988): Artifacts due to residual magnetization in three-dimensional magnetic resonance imaging. *Med Phys* 15:825–831.

13

Fluoroscopy in Magnetic Resonance Imaging

BASIC PRINCIPLES

The reasons for developing very fast MR imaging techniques are numerous. The most important reasons are the need to improve image quality by eliminating motion artifacts; to analyze the motion of a moving structure, such as the valvular cusps; and to increase the total number of scans per unit time. To this end, various fast imaging techniques have been proposed. Fast field echo techniques such as FLASH and GRASS provide image acquisition times on the order of a few seconds; imaging techniques based on the principle of planar data acquisition (EPI) further reduce data acquisition times to about 100 to 200 msec. Taking the time required for reconstructing an image from the acquired data, total imaging times may be higher.

It should be recognized that fast imaging mainly decreases only data acquisition times (eg, by decreasing the number of excitations or the pulse repetition time (TR) and the number of phase encoding steps per image). But this is only a first step toward achieving real-time imaging capabilities. In order to achieve real-time interactive manipulation of MR images, it is equally important to decrease image reconstruction time (eg, by adopting new and faster image reconstruction strategies). Finally, image display rate also has to be increased to keep up with image flow. By a combination of these factors, a type of MR fluoroscopy has been proposed by Riederer et al [1,2,7].

In the scheme, proposed by Riederer et al, image data are acquired using a fast sequence such as FLASH or GRASS (conceptually, spin echo based pulse sequence, such as RARE, also may be used). The TR is reduced to about 10 msec by decreasing the phase encoding steps to 48 or 64, reducing the readout points to 128, and decreasing the RF pulse width.

To achieve faster image reconstruction, a "sliding window" approach is used [1] in which, for each successive image, only a small number (usually one or two) of new temporally displaced phase encoding steps are recruited, and an equal number of corresponding phase encoding steps are eliminated (Fig. 13.1). As the number of phase encoding steps for every image remains same, the image resolution is constant throughout the image series. To achieve the maximum image output, the image window is moved only one TR interval forward.

Conventionally, the images are displayed on the monitor only after the complete data set is collected and reconstructed. However, by modifying the imaging hardware, it is possible to display the image within a time span of about 120 msec after the signal is acquired [8]. Wright et al [8] have elaborately discussed the hardware requirements for such an instant-display device.

See also: BEPI, EPI, LISA, SFI.

FIG. 13.1 The sliding window concept. An image (rectangular box) is comprised of four phase encoding steps and is laterally shifted as soon as data acquisition is completed. Here, lateral displacement is one phase encode step. In this manner, only one new phase encode step has to be acquired to reconstruct each subsequent image frame. As a result, the image reconstruction rate is greatly enhanced and, if matched by proper hardware, the image display rate is correspondingly increased.

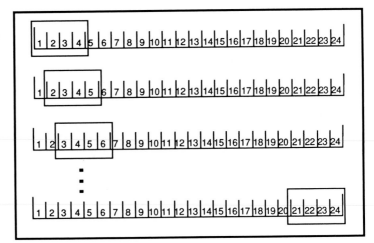

CLINICAL APPLICATIONS
TISSUE CONTRAST

The penalty that is paid to achieve very fast imaging times is in the form of poor contrast-to-noise ratio. However, a recent modification of the method allows some manipulation of the image contrast by inserting a 180° slice selective refocusing pulse during ongoing data acquisition, and waiting for a time period TI to allow T1 contrast to develop [2]. Subsequent images, then, are T1 weighted. In theory, any type of contrast can be achieved by preceding the data acquisition sequence by a suitable magnetization preparation sequence.

ADVANTAGES AND DISADVANTAGES

The fluoroscopic examination may allow the operator to change the imaging protocol (eg, field of view, patient position, view angle) by looking at the region of interest in real-time. It also offers the choice of carrying out the complete radiographic study only if the suspected pathology is found on the initial images.

Such fluoroscopic techniques also offer the potential for interventional MR procedures in the future [5]. For example, Jolesz et al [3] have imaged in near real time thermal changes due to laser–tissue interaction. Pearlman et al [6] have proposed an imaging scheme that displays in real time the vascular blood flow and the valvular cusp motion in a manner analogous to M mode ultrasonography.

Even though inadvertent subject motion may occur during the acquisition of the image series, each individual image is free from motion artifacts because it is acquired in a very short period of time (300 to 600 msec per image). Nonetheless, Korin et al [4] have proposed a compensation scheme for motion occurring at a known velocity (such as that which may occur during the operation of the gantry). They have derived the following formula for the signal $S_n'(t)$, which occurs in the presence of a known velocity in the y direction (Vy) and the x direction (Vx):

$$S_n'(t) = S_n(t) \times P1(Vy) \times P2(Vx),$$

where $S_n(t)$ is the signal that would have been obtained in the absence of the motion, and

$$P1(Vy) = e^{(-i2\pi(n-(N-1)/2)Vy \times tn/FOV)}$$

and

$$P2(Vx) = e^{(-i2\pi(m-(M-1)/2)Vx \times tn/FOV)},$$

where n = the index of the phase encoding step, N = the total number of phase encoding steps, m = the index of the echo sample, M = the total number of echo samples, and t_n = the time of the motion. It is apparent from the above formula that in order to derive the motion-free signal value from the acquired signal, the acquired signal simply has to be multiplied by $P1^{-1}P2^{-1}$ in order to correct for motion.

As noted above, the image contrast is inferior to that achieved using more conventional imaging techniques. But, then, obtaining well-contrasted images has been the lowest priority objective of fluoroscopic examination. After the pathology has been located, a detailed examination of the region always can be carried out to obtain good diagnostic quality images.

REFERENCES

1. Farzaneh F, Riederer SJ, Lee JN, Tasciyan T, Wright RC, Spritzer CE (1989): MR fluoroscopy: initial clinical studies. *Radiology* 171:545–549.

2. Holsinger AE, Wright RC, Riederer SJ, Farzaneh F, Grimm RC, Maier JK (1990): Real-time interactive magnetic resonance imaging. *Magn Reson Med* 14: 547–553.

3. Jolesz FA, Bleier AR, Jakab P, Ruenzel PW, Huttl K, Jako GJ (1988): MR imaging of laser-tissue interactions. *Radiology* 168:249–253.

4. Korin HW, Farzaneh F, Wright RC, Riederer SJ (1989): Compensation for effects of linear motion in MR imaging. *Magn Reson Med* 12:99–113.

5. Lufkin RB, Robinson JD, Castro DJ, Jabour BA, Duckwiler G, Layfield LJ, Hanafee WN (1990): Interventional magnetic resonance imaging in the head and neck. *Topics in Magn Reson Imag* 2:76–80.

6. Pearlman JD, Hardy CJ, Cline HE (1990): Continual NMR cardiography without gating. *Radiology* 175:369–373.

7. Riederer SJ, Tasciyan T, Farzaneh F, Lee JN, Wright RC, Herfkens RJ (1988): MR fluoroscopy: technical feasibility. *Magn Reson Med* 8:1–15.

8. Wright RC, Riederer SJ, Farzaneh F, Rossman PJ, Liu Y (1989): Real-time MR fluoroscopic data acquisition and image reconstruction. *Magn Reson Med* 12:407–415.

14

Gating

BASIC PRINCIPLES

Very early in the development of MRI, the potential harmful effects of subject motion, such as respiration, became obvious. Motion-related artifacts appear on MR images because there is asynchrony between the motion and the data acquisition, specifically the phase encoding steps. To achieve the optimum contrast-to-noise ratio, it is highly desirable that these artifacts be eliminated from the final image. This can be accomplished in a variety of the ways (see ROPE).[1] An alternative approach to those described in ROPE is to establish temporal synchrony (gating) be-

---

[1] The following are general approaches not discussed in ROPE.

1. *Data averaging:* When multiple NMR signals (FID or echo) are obtained from the same spatial location, the signal-to-noise ratio of the detected NMR signal increases by the square root of the number of signals acquired. This translates directly into an increase in the signal-to-noise ratio of the image because with each successive data addition, the signal accumulates and the random noise cancels out. However, this is true only if the image noise is random (white noise). Once the noise becomes organized due to imperfections in the system, the linear relationship between signal averaging and the signal-to-noise ratio of the signal no longer exists; acquiring multiple averages beyond this point does not increase the signal-to-noise ratio of the image [27]. For most systems, this cut-off point is well above the number of averages employed in clinical practice and, therefore, the above anomaly is not readily apparent.

   To obtain an improved signal-to-noise ratio, a penalty is paid in the form of increased total data acquisition time (which equals the number of averages × the number of phase values × TR). If, however, only a limited number of phase values are averaged (selective averaging of phase encoding lines, SAPEL), then the degree of increased imaging time may be somewhat diminished. Recently, it has been reported that the signal-to-noise ratio also decreases when selective averaging is employed [26]. In addition, the texture of the image changes considerably, which may interfere with the identification of small lesions.

tween different phases of the motion and the phase encoding process. Such gating techniques already have been used in x-ray computer tomography.

Though the terms *gating* and *triggering* seem similar, their underlying mechanisms for data acquisition are different (Fig. 14.1) [23]. The purpose of gated data acquisition is to enable pulse application only when motion amplitude is considerably low (eg, the end expiratory stage of respiration). On the other hand, the purpose of triggered data acquisition is to enable pulse application whenever a predetermined stage of motion is reached (eg, halfway between the baseline and the peak of the inspiration or the late diastolic stage of the cardiac cycle). However, in the literature, gating and triggering are used interchangeably, especially in case of the heart. We shall use the term cardiac triggering instead of cardiac gating.

CARDIAC TRIGGERING

Unlike respiratory motion, "silent" periods (periods with minimal or no motion) do not occur during cardiac motion. Moreover, the appearance of the heart and fluid such as the blood and the CSF alter distinctly during the cardiac cycle. Therefore, it is important to determine the phase of the cardiac cycle at the beginning of the data acquisition.

In the literature, usually the term cardiac-triggered MRI implies the electrocardiographic- (ECG) triggered MRI. In ECG-triggered MRI, data acquisition is possible only when the heart is at a specific phase along the ECG. Most commonly, the peak or the juxta peak region of the R wave (diastole) is used to trigger data acquisition, and the R-R interval (or the heart rate) determines the effective pulse repetition time (TR). Alternatively, T waves may be used to obtain images during the cardiac systole.

The above technique may be called central (or direct) cardiac triggering. However, in addition to ECG, there are many other avenues for obtaining information regarding cardiac motion. In peripheral (or indirect) cardiac triggering, usually a plethysmograph [31] is used to establish a direct relationship between the cardiac cycle induced pulsatile blood flow and the size of a peripheral part such as a finger. Alternatively, a laser or Doppler ultrasound device may also be used to monitor the cardiac phase.

---

2. *Restrain:* To limit abdominal motion during data acquisition, a tight nonmagnetic band may be placed around it. This diminishes considerably the intensity of the artifacts; however, some patients may find it uncomfortable.

3. *Breath holding:* Here, the goal is to finish the entire data acquisition in a single breath hold interval, which typically lasts for 15 to 30 sec [40]. Obviously, this approach can be implemented only with fast imaging techniques such as RARE-, EPI-, or SSFP-based sequences. However, a multiple breath hold approach has been designed which may be useful for conventional data acquiring sequences (see Pause).

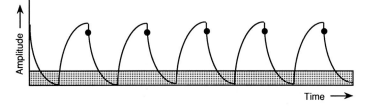

FIG. 14.1 Hypothetical waveform illustrating the distinction between gating and triggering. In gating, data acquisition is enabled whenever motion amplitude is less than a preset threshold value (dotted area). For example, in respiratory gating, data are acquired usually during the end-expiratory stage, when the respiratory amplitude is approximately 20% of maximum. In contrast, in triggered data acquisition, data are acquired only when the motion cycle is at a particular phase (indicated by the black dots). For example, cardiac data are usually triggered by the R wave.

In what is called multiphasic cardiac triggering, images are acquired at many points (many phases) during the cardiac cycle [16]. When using gradient echo techniques, typically 12 to 16 RF pulses are delivered in one R-R interval. While the temporal resolution of such cine-MR is on the order of 40 to 50 msec, total data acquisition and image display times are fairly long (60 to 90 min). These time estimates become still longer if multiplanar multiphasic spin echo techniques are used. Alternatively, total time can be decreased by limiting the number of cardiac phases that are sampled during each R-R interval. For example, only the end diastolic (peak of the R wave) and the end systolic (downslope of the T wave) cardiac phases are important for determining the left ventricular blood volume. Therefore, greater time efficiency can be obtained by implementing biphasic imaging techniques (Figs. 14.2 and 14.3) [6,29].

RESPIRATORY GATING

What makes respiratory motion different from cardiac motion is the fact that the former contains at least two stages during which there is minimal or absolutely no motion (the end expiratory and end inspiratory stages). In respiratory gating, usually data acquisition is limited to the end expiratory stage. In contrast, in respiratory triggering, any phase along the respiratory cycle may be used for data acquisition. The two modes for data acquisition [12] are as follows:

1. *Spin conditioning:* Data are acquired only when the desired stage of motion is reached; RF excitation is halted during other stages.

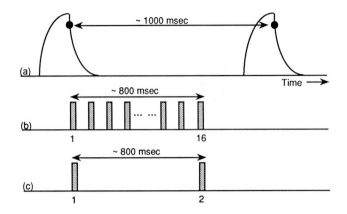

FIG. 14.2 **(a)** The repetition period of the wave is varying, but is approximately 1000 msec. The data are triggered just after the peak of the wave. **(b)** In gradient recalled multiphasic imaging, typically 12 to 16 time frames are acquired at 50 msec intervals during one such wave cycle. Due to unpredictability of the occurrence of the next trigger, data acquisition cannot be prolonged to the very end of the cycle period. **(c)** In biphasic imaging, data are sampled only at the two phases of most interest. Even though the effective repetition time of data acquisition may be identical to the multiphasic case, a considerable amount of time is saved, as fewer data frames have to be reconstructed.

2. *Without spin conditioning:* Data are continuously acquired, but only those pieces of data that occurred during the desired stage of motion are retained.

Because most people, especially men, are abdominal breathers, usually movement of the anterior abdominal wall is monitored by a suitable sensor and data acquisition is possible only when the desired respiratory stage is reached. Amoore and Ridgway [2] and Ehman et al [12] have discussed a variety of sensors for monitoring respiratory motion.

Variants (A) *Pseudo gating:* Gating or triggering, as employed above, uses some type of physiological measurement for motion synchronization (physiological gating), and requires additional hardware and/or software. In an approach advocated by Haacke et al [19], gating is accomplished by properly modifying the pulse parameters such as the TR and the number of averages (n). Before knowing how this technique works, it should be recognized that the purpose of implementing gated MRI is to achieve motion synchronization in order to eliminate motion-related artifacts. Therefore, if the TR (or the spacing between the adjacent phase encode

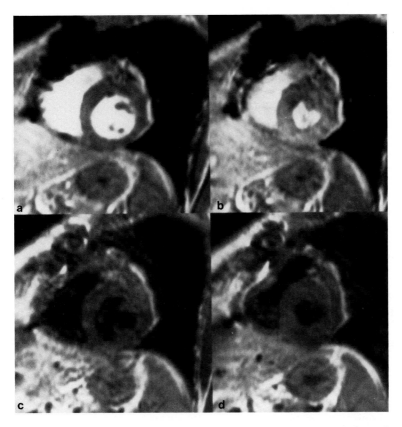

FIG. 14.3 A pair of cine-MR images obtained at end diastole **(a)** and end systole **(b)**. Corresponding biphasic images are shown in **(c)** and **(d)**. (Courtesy of G. Caputo; modified, with permission, from Caputo et al [6].)

steps) is made the same as the motion period 1/f (where f is the frequency of motion), then data acquisition would always begin at the same phase of the motion. This could be accomplished simply by making TR just as long as the motion period, TR = 1/f. Under this condition, the artifacts would be minimally separated from the image plane, and the image as well as the artifacts appear superimposed. To achieve a simultaneous increase in the signal-to-noise ratio, multiple averages (n) of the phase encode steps may be obtained, now maintaining the equality TR × n = 1/f. As no explicit gating is used to obtain artifact-free images, this has been called "pseudo-gating" (see ROPE for alternative methods of artifact separation).

Note that if the entire image acquisition is completed in a time span equivalent to or less than a single period of motion ($N \times TR = 1/f$, where N is the number of phase encoding steps), then no gating is required. Such rapid image acquisition is possible with EPI, SFI, or similar ultrafast imaging techniques. However, it may still be necessary to use gated data acquisition in rapid imaging to achieve phase specificity for a series of images taken at varying temporal positions—for example, to monitor an ischemic region of the myocardial wall.

(B) *Retrospective gating:* Cardiac triggering employed concomitantly with data acquisition is called prospective cardiac triggering. The disadvantage of prospective (ECG) triggering is that the performance of the technique is highly dependent on the ECG signal, and data acquisition is unable to self-adjust to the conditions of normal variations in R-R interval or abnormal impulse conduction such as ectopic beats. Moreover, it is not possible to acquire data in the late diastole (just before the R wave) [35]. In addition, uneven longitudinal magnetization recovery during data idling causes the first few images to be very bright—the "lightening" effect [28].

In what is called retrospective cardiac triggering, data are continuously acquired in a nontriggered mode. In the wireless retrospective mode, any information regarding cardiac motion is derived from the raw data acquired using specially designed pulse sequences [18,35]. In general, these pulse sequences obtain two echoes during one pulse repetition: a phase encoded echo for imaging data, and a nonphase encoded echo for timing the motion (such as Hinks' monitored echo gating (MEGA) [20]) or tagging the data caused by motion (see NAVEC). Such nonimaging data then properly direct the reconstruction of an image at a particular phase of the cardiac cycle or, alternatively, they may be used to reject the motion causing data (see SLO-MOTION).

COMBINED CARDIAC AND RESPIRATORY GATING

The advantages of cardiac triggering and respiratory gating may be combined if both are employed simultaneously. For example, in abdominal examinations, cardiac triggering may eliminate intense blood flow related artifacts and respiratory gating may eliminate abdominal motion artifacts. Similarly, this approach may be used for cardiac studies. While Ehman et al [12] have found only slightly more cardiac detail using this combined approach than using cardiac triggering alone, a study by Thickman et al [36] indicates that the best image quality is obtained with the combined approach.

See also: COPE, DOPE, GMN, MAST, NAVEC, Pause, ROPE, SLO-MOTION.

CLINICAL APPLICATIONS
TISSUE CONTRAST

The image contrast-to-noise ratio is considerably increased by using time synchronized gating techniques as described above. In addition, flowing spins are depicted with consistent signal intensity on successive images of a multislice acquisition.

CEREBROSPINAL FLUID

Just as the blood pulsates with the cardiac cycle, so does the cerebrospinal fluid [8,15]. Therefore, when CSF data are acquired without cardiac triggering, flow-related artifacts and signal loss decrease the clinical utility of such myelograms. Considerable improvement in the image contrast-to-noise ratio has been achieved by implementing cardiac triggering in CSF studies [13,14,32]. For example, the nerves entering and leaving the spinal cord can be visualized adequately on the triggered myelograms.

THE HEART

Currently, almost all cardiac MR studies are carried out with triggering. In addition to eliminating artifacts, the clinical interpretation of a series of time-multiplexed triggered images is simplified. Using cardiac-triggered MRI, various congenital disorders [10,17], myocardial infarction [24,25,33], and ventricular hypertrophy have been correctly diagnosed. Numerous investigators have discussed the technical aspects of implementing cardiac triggering in various clinical situations [1,9,21,22]. For example, Buckwalter et al [4] and Edelman et al [11] have implemented cardiac triggering to determine ventricular volume and blood outflow. Burbank et al [5] have attempted to find cardiac-triggered MRI views similar to echocardiographic angles. Such interdisciplinary analysis would further strengthen the role of clinical cardiac MRI.

   Although generally it is believed that nontriggered cardiac images are useless because of artifacts, Choyke et al [7] have shown that by using short TR/TE (10 to 20 msec), values, good quality cardiac images can be obtained without triggering. This was later confirmed with the introduction of fast imaging techniques such as turboFLASH and echo planar imaging.

THE ABDOMEN

One of the reasons MRI did not achieve early success in abdominal studies is that respiratory motion quite often rendered nongated T2-weighted (long TR/long TE) SE abdominal scans clinically almost incompetent.[2] With the advent of respiratory gating and various other artifact-reducing techniques such as MAST and ROPE, the quality of abdominal images has improved a great deal. Intraabdominal organs such as the liver, pancreas, kidneys, and abdominal aorta can be routinely identified on abdominal images properly acquired with motion-reduction schemes.

Abdominal images obtained without gating have a considerable number of artifacts, and it has been thought that these artifacts alter the measurement of true T1 or T2 values by altering image contrast. However, Thomsen et al [37] have shown that this is true only if the pathology is focal. In cases of diffuse pathology or normal tissue, relaxation curves are not influenced by respiratory gating.

ANGIOGRAPHY

As the blood pulsates in synchrony with the cardiac cycle, it exhibits different flow velocities during the systole and diastole. The intensity of the flowing blood depends on, among other factors, flow velocity (other factors are the excitation status of the spins, amount of flowing blood, local inhomogeneity and susceptibility influences, and strength of the gradients). Therefore, the pulsatile nature of the flowing blood gives off variable intensity signals when the data are acquired without paying attention to the phase of the cardiac cycle. Moreover, the "accidental" velocity encoding that occurs in most MR pulse sequences gives rise to disc-shaped artifacts extending from the vessel to the image periphery on either side in the phase encoding direction [30]. These artifacts make correct interpretation of the images difficult. Therefore, cardiac-triggered MRI is needed in order to provide angiograms with predictable intensity. In fact, the very first MR angiograms were produced by cardiac-triggered data acquisition. Since then, cardiac triggering has been used extensively for obtaining a wide variety of angiograms based on both TOF effects and phase manipulations.

---

[2] The other reason for MRI's lack of early success was the absence of a reliable intraluminal contrast agent such as barium sulfate, which is widely used in x-ray radiography. In spite of recent developments in oral MRI contrast agents (such as various superparamagnetic and ferromagnetic compounds) and very fast imaging techniques such as EPI, the x-ray barium examination still is clinically the most useful procedure for demonstrating various intraluminal, endothelial, and intraabdominal lesions.

ADVANTAGES AND DISADVANTAGES

Gated or triggered data acquisition eliminates the appropriate physiological motion-related artifacts (Fig. 14.4). In addition to spatial domain,
the images are stabilized along the temporal axis, too. The latter aids
considerably in evaluating various cardiac functional disorders such as
blood flow abnormalities through septal or valvular defects.

As the TR is fixed by the period of motion, it is difficult to achieve
flexible T1 weighting in gated acquisitions. However, TR may be increased by gating data acquisition to every other motion cycle. This yields
highly T2-weighted images [21,22].

Although triggering does not increase imaging time, gating invariably
increases total image acquisition time. Wood and Henkelman [41] have
proposed the concept of fractional respiratory gating to balance this increased imaging time. In fractional respiratory gating, only a fraction of
the total number of phase encoding steps is acquired in the gated mode

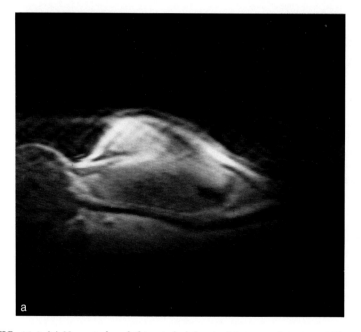

FIG. 14.4 (a) Nongated and **(b)** gated abdominal images of a mouse. Notice the
absence of artifacts and image blurring in the gated image. The arrow shows the
area of hemorrhage from a subcutaneous tumor that was not identifiable in the
nongated image. (Courtesy of N. V. Bruggen; reproduced, with permission, from
Bruggen et al [3].)

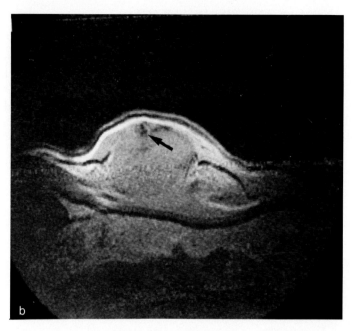

FIG. 14.4 (*Continued*)

(Fig. 14.5). Depending on the region of the k-space chosen for gated acquisition, some artifacts are eliminated. As the increase in acquisition time is determined by the size of the fraction, this approach gives a means for offsetting the increase in time (if one can tolerate the remaining artifacts).

FIG. 14.5 In fractional respiratory gating, only those phase encoding steps that may be degraded the most by motion are gated. Depending on the particular clinical situation, the region of the k-space that is gated differs. For example, in the accompanying illustration, only those phase steps near the zero phase encoding are gated. Therefore, a considerable amount of time may be saved by performing the nongated data acquisition elsewhere.

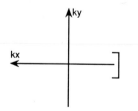

Both triggering or gating require special hardware for monitoring motion. The leads used for cardiac triggering may sometimes give rise to image artifacts. Wendt et al [39] and van Genderingen et al [38] have discussed various possibilities for minimizing these artifacts. Conversely, the RF and gradient magnetic fields may induce spurious voltages in the ECG leads and, thus, trigger excitation at inappropriate times. Shetty [34] has proposed a filtering and preamplifier blanking device for eliminating premature RF excitation.

REFERENCES

1. Alfidi RJ, Haaga JR, El Yousef SJ, Bryan PJ, Fletcher BD, LiPuma JP, Morrison SC, Kaufman B, Richey JB, Hinshaw WS, et al (1982): Preliminary experimental results in humans and animals with a superconducting, whole-body, nuclear magnetic resonance scanner. *Radiology* 143:175–181.

2. Amoore JN, Ridgway JP (1989): A system for cardiac and respiratory gating of a magnetic resonance imager. *Clin Phys Physio Measurement* 10:283–286.

3. Bruggen NV, Syha J, Busza AL, King MD, Stamp GWH, Williams SR, Gadian DG (1990): Identification of tumor hemorrhage in an animal model using spin echoes and gradient echoes. *Magn Reson Med* 15:121–127.

4. Buckwalter KA, Aisen AM, Dilworth LR, Mancini GBJ, Buda AJ (1986): Gated cardiac MRI: ejection-fraction determination using the right anterior oblique view. *Am J Roentgen* 147:33–37.

5. Burbank F, Parish D, Wexler L (1988): Echocardiographic-like angled views of the heart by MR imaging. *J Comput Assist Tomogr* 12:181–195.

6. Caputo GR, Suzuki JI, Kondo C, Cho H, Quaife RA, Higgins CB, Parker DL (1990): Determination of left ventricular volume and mass with use of biphasic spin-echo MR imaging: comparison with cine MR. *Radiology* 177:773–777.

7. Choyke PL, Kressel HY, Reichek N, Axel L, Gefter W, Mamourian AC, Thickman D (1984): Nongated cardiac magnetic resonance imaging: preliminary experience at 0.12 T. *Am J Roentgen* 143:1143–1150.

8. Citrin CM, Sherman JL, Gangarosa RE, Scanlon D (1987): Physiology of the CSF flow-void sign: modification by cardiac gating. *Am J Roentgen* 148:205–208.

9. Crooks LE, Barker B, Chang H, Feinberg D, Hoenninger JC, Watts JC, Arakawa M, Kaufman L, Sheldon PE, Botvinick E, et al (1984): Magnetic resonance imaging strategies for heart studies. *Radiology* 153:459–465.

10. Didier D, Higgins CB, Fisher MR, Osaki L, Silverman NH, Cheitlin MD (1986): Congenital heart disease: gated MR imaging in 72 patients. *Radiology* 158:227–235.

11. Edelman RR, Thompson R, Kantor H, Brady TJ, Leavitt M, Dinsmore R (1987): Cardiac function: evaluation with fast-echo MR imaging. *Radiology* 162:611–615.

12. Ehman RL, McNamara MT, Pallack M, Hricak H, Higgins CB (1984): Magnetic resonance imaging with respiratory gating: techniques and advantages. *Am J Roentgen* 143:1175–1182.

13. Enzmann DR, Rubin JB, O'Donohue J, Griffin C, Drace J, Wright A (1987): Use

of cerebrospinal fluid gating to improve T2-weighted images: part II—temporal lobes, basal ganglia, and brain stem. *Radiology* 162:768–773.

14. Enzmann DR, Rubin JB, Wright A (1987): Use of cerebrospinal fluid gating to improve T2-weighted images: part I—the spinal cord. *Radiology* 162:763–767.

15. Enzmann DR, Pelc NJ (1991): Normal flow patterns of intracranial and spinal cerebrospinal fluid defined with phase-contrast cine MR imaging. *Radiology* 178:467–474.

16. Fisher MR, von Schulthess GK, Higgins CB (1985): Multiphasic cardiac magnetic resonance imaging: normal regional left ventricular wall thickening. *Am J Roentgen* 145:27–30.

17. Fletcher BD, Jacobstein MD, Nelson AD, Riemenschneider TA (1984): Gated magnetic resonance imaging of congenital cardiac malformations. *Radiology* 150:137–140.

18. Glover GH, Pelc NJ: A rapid-gated cine MRI technique, in Kressel HY (ed): *Magnetic Resonance Annual.* New York, Raven Press, 1988, pp. 288–333.

19. Haacke EM, Lenz GW, Nelson AD (1987): Pseudo-gating: elimination of periodic motion artifacts in magnetic resonance imaging without gating. *Magn Reson Med* 4:162–174.

20. Hinks RS (1988): Monitored echo gating (MEGA) for the reduction of motion artifacts. *Magn Reson Imag* 6:S48.

21. Lanzer P, Botvinick EH, Schiller NB, Crooks LE, Arakawa M, Kaufman L, Davis PL, Herfkens R, Lipton MJ, Higgins CB (1984): Cardiac imaging using gated magnetic resonance. *Radiology* 150:121–127.

22. Lanzer P, Barta C, Botvinick EH, Wiesendanger HU, Modin G (1985): ECG-synchronized cardiac MR imaging: method and evaluation. *Radiology* 155:681–686.

23. Lewis CE, Prato FS, Drost DJ, Nicholson RL (1986): Comparison of respiratory triggering and gating techniques for the removal of respiratory artifacts in MR imaging. *Radiology* 160:803–810.

24. Mattrey RF, Higgins CB (1982): Detection of regional myocardial dysfunction during ischemia with computerized tomography documentation and physiologic basis. *Investigative Radiology* 17:329–335.

25. McNamara MT, Higgins CB, Schechtmann N, Botvinick E, Lipton MJ, Chatterjee K, Amparo EG (1985): Detection and characterization of acute myocardial infarction in man with use of gated magnetic resonance. *Circulation* 71:717–724.

26. Mugler JP (1991): Potential degradation in image quality due to selective averaging of phase-encoding lines in Fourier transform MRI. *Magn Reson Med* 19:170–174.

27. Nalcioglu O, Cho ZH (1984): Limits to signal-to-noise improvement by FID averaging in NMR imaging. *Phys Med Biol* 29:969–978.

28. Lenz GW, Haacke EM, White RD (1989): Retrospective cardiac gating: a review of technical aspects and future directions. *Magn Reson Imag* 7:445–455.

29. Parker DL, Caputo GR, Frederick PR (1989): Efficient biphasic spin-echo magnetic resonance imaging. *Magn Reson Med* 11:98–113.

30. Perman WH, Moran PR, Moran RA, Bernstein MA (1986): Artifacts from pulsatile flow in MR imaging. *J Comput Assist Tomogr* 10:473–483.

31. Rubin JB, Enzmann DR, Wright A (1987): CSF-gated MR imaging of the spine: theory and clinical implementation. *Radiology* 163:784–792.

32. Runge VM, Clanton JA, Partain CL, James AE (1984): Respiratory gating in magnetic resonance imaging at 0.5 Tesla. *Radiology* 151:521–523.

33. Schmiedl U, Sievers RE, Brasch RC, Wolfe CL, Chew WM, Ogan MD, Engeseth H, Lipton MJ, Moseley ME (1989): Acute myocardial ischemia and reperfusion: MR imaging with albumin-Gd-DTPA. *Radiology* 170:351–356.

34. Shetty AN (1988): Suppression of radiofrequency interference in cardiac gated MRI: a simple design. *Magn Reson Med* 8:84–88.

35. Spraggins TA (1990): Wireless retrospective gating: application to cine cardiac imaging. *Magn Reson Imag* 8:675–681.

36. Thickman D, Rubinstein R, Askenase A, Cabellero-Saez A (1988): Effect of phase-encoding direction upon magnetic resonance image quality of the heart. *Magn Reson Med* 6:390–396.

37. Thomsen C, Henriksen O, Ring P (1988): In vivo measurements of relaxation process in the human liver by MRI: the role of respiratory gating/triggering. *Magn Reson Imag* 6:431–436.

38. van Genderingen HR, Sprenger M, De Ridder JW, van Rossum AC (1989): Carbon-fiber electrodes and leads for electrocardiography during MR imaging. *Radiology* 171:872.

39. Wendt RE, Rokey R, Vick GW, Johnston DL (1988): Electrocardiographic gating and monitoring in NMR imaging. *Magn Reson Imag* 6:89–95.

40. Winkler ML, Thoeni RF, Luh N, Kaufman L, Margulis AR (1989): Hepatic neoplasia: breath-hold MR imaging. *Radiology* 170:801–806.

41. Wood ML, Henkelman RM (1986): Suppression of respiratory motion artifacts in magnetic resonance imaging. *Med Phys* 13:794–805.

15

Gradient Moment Nulling (GMN)

BASIC PRINCIPLES

Any type of uncoordinated motion gives rise to image artifacts in widely employed two-dimensional Fourier transform spin warp MR imaging for the reasons presented in ROPE. Most commonly, motion is caused by such physiological phenomena as the flowing of blood or moving of an organ. Based on the sources of these various kinds of motion, motion reduction techniques can be divided into two broad categories: one group comprised of techniques such as ROPE and Pause (which are employed to eliminate artifacts caused primarily by the motion of a moving organ); the other group comprised of techniques such as MMORE (which is employed to eliminate artifacts caused primarily by the motion of the flowing blood). Note that techniques such as gating and MAST eliminate both types of motion.

What makes these two groups different with respect to their clinical application is the underlying mechanism of artifact removal. In general, while the first group of techniques tries to match physiological motion with data acquisition by reordering phase encodings or adjusting pulse repetition time, the second group of techniques modifies gradient waveforms of the pulse sequence to refocus flowing spins at the echo time (gradient moment nulling or refocusing).

Before we go further, we will need to review what is meant by intraview and interview motion. The motion that occurs between the application of an excitation pulse and the echo forming pulse (one phase encoding interval) is called the *intraview* motion (eg, blood or CSF flow); the motion that occurs during the cycling of the phase encoding gradient is called the *interview* motion (eg, the motion of the anterior abdominal wall during breathing). Either type of motion can vary the net voxel magnetization because of loss of excited spins. In addition, the presence of a gradient magnetic field causes phase dispersion of the moving spins, and this further attenuates the signal coming from the voxel. While the flow out of the voxel cannot be reversed under normal conditions, the gradient-induced phase dispersion surely can be recovered, at least for the intraview motion of the spins, by modifying the gradients as discussed below.

In the conventional imaging sequences, such as spin echo, gradients are used for three main purposes:

1. for limiting the area of excitation (the slice-select gradient);
2. for attributing different phases to the excited spins (the phase encode gradient); and
3. for attributing different frequencies to the excited spins (the frequency encode or readout gradient).

These three gradients collectively may be called imaging gradients because they are employed primarily for spatially encoding image data. Note that the slice-select gradient may be omitted if exciting the spins nonselectively is desired; and the phase encoding gradient may be omitted if obtaining only a projection of the spins is desired.

It is well known that spins experience variable degrees of dephasing while gradient fields are on (see PBANG). However, if the imaging gradients are designed in such a way that they also rephase the dephased spins, signal loss due to intraview motion can be recovered. In order to do this, the gradient moment (see MMORE for the definition of gradient moment) corresponding to a desired derivative of motion is nullified by modifying the gradient profile, eg, by using a rephasing/dephasing gradient pulse or a bipolar gradient pulse. Any pulse sequence that utilizes gradients to refocus flowing spins significantly, in order to eliminate motion-related artifacts, is called the gradient moment nulling technique. It also has been called gradient moment (motion) rephasing (refocusing) (GMR).

In general, $n + 1$ additional gradient lobes are needed to null n moments (see MMORE). This principle of GMN may be applied to any pulse sequence, and the gradient along any direction may be included, depending upon the clinical application. For example, in a regular spin echo sequence, the readout gradient may be modified by adding two gradient lobes of identical amplitude and polarity on either side of a 180° refocusing pulse (Fig. 15.1) [3,7]. This reduces intravoxel phase dispersion along the read gradient and increases the signal intensity of the voxel. Similarly, GMN also may be incorporated into any gradient echo based technique.

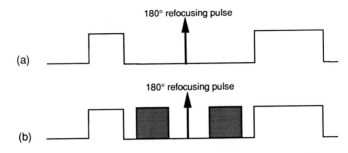

FIG. 15.1 (a) Profile of the read gradient of a conventional spin echo sequence. In the modified read gradient profile **(b)**, the refocusing pulse is sandwiched between two additional gradient lobes of identical amplitude and the polarity, which rephases the spins flowing at a constant velocity in the direction of the gradient.

A simple method for designing the motion compensating gradient waveforms for any order of motion has been proposed by Pipe and Chenevert [11]. Briefly, to compensate for the nth order of motion, an antisymmetric pair of gradients, compensated for the $(n - 1)$th order of motion, is added together (Fig. 15.2).

The addition of extra gradient lobes, however, lengthens the time for which a particular gradient is switched on. This increases motion sensitivity for the higher derivatives of motion (eg, acceleration), which usually are not nullified (VEMORE, see MMORE). Spin dephasing due to these nonnullified moments, therefore, may increase considerably. To avoid the resulting signal loss, an alternative approach has been advo-

FIG. 15.2 (a) Gradient waveform compensated for the static position. In order to compensate for the next order of motion (velocity), its antisymmetric waveform **(b)** is added, to yield the gradient profile, as shown in **(c)**. By time shifting one of the waveforms before performing the addition, different gradient profiles may be obtained.

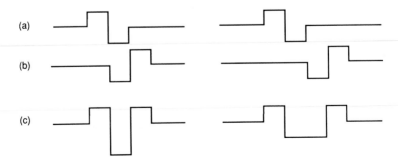

cated, in which instead of nullifying the gradient moment by introducing additional gradient lobes, existing gradient lobes may be "shrunk" to minimize spin dephasing due to any gradient moment [10]. Thus, even though all the moments retain nonzero flow sensitivity, their spin dephasing effects are negligible. This is in clear contrast to the conventional GMN approach.

See also: MAST, MMORE, PBANG.

CLINICAL APPLICATIONS
TISSUE CONTRAST

While the intensity of stationary tissue is unaltered, flowing material, such as the blood, usually appears hyperintense, as the signal loss that would have occurred as a result of motion is now recovered. Depending on the specific clinical situation, this increased signal may either increase or decrease the contrast-to-noise ratio (Fig. 15.3). For example, if blood flowing in the pulmonary vessels is refocused, the contrast-to-noise ratio of the blood/lung is increased because the area surrounding the vessels appears dark, due to the air-filled lungs. However, the situation is quite different only about 5 cm in the left inferior-oblique direction. Normally, the occasional signal void observed on the cardiac SE images gives a good contrast-to-noise ratio with respect to the myocardium (except in end diastole or end systole).[1] As the GMN recovers this signal loss, a point may be reached when the blood and myocardium may appear isointense and at that point, the contrast-to-noise ratio reduces to zero. Beyond this point, the intensity of the blood increases; this increased intensity may result in an increase in the amount of flow-related artifacts. For this reason, spin echo images obtained with GMN often are deteriorated by an increase in flow-related artifacts when compared to non-GMN acquisition.

THE ABDOMEN

If properly employed, abdominal images are free of respiratory artifacts [12]. However, blood flow related artifacts are not effectively suppressed, especially from the aorta and the inferior vena cava. To suppress these vascular artifacts, several presaturating pulses may be applied outside the volume of interest [8].

---

[1] The high signal intensity of blood observed in end diastole or end systole is attributed to slowly flowing blood. In order to suppress the blood signal totally, a nonselective 180° pulse may be applied before the echo readout; when the blood signal reaches its null point following this inversion pulse, the echo is acquired [6].

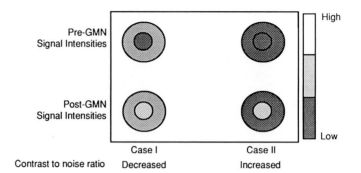

FIG. 15.3 This figure illustrates how the refocusing of the flowing spins may influence the contrast-to-noise ratio for two adjacent tissues. The inner circle represents the vessel lumen surrounded by the tissue (represented by the outer circle). Depending on relative signal intensities, the contrast-to-noise ratio may either increase or decrease. For example, if the blood flow in pulmonary vessels is refocused, the contrast-to-noise ratio will increase, as the lung tissue surrounding the vessel appears as a region of signal void (Case II). However, as shown in Case I, the contrast-to-noise ratio may decrease if the refocused signal becomes isointense with the surrounding tissue.

ANGIOGRAPHY

Moran used the principle of GMN, in its simplest form, to determine flow velocity [9]. Recently, a wide variety of phase-based angiographic techniques that use flow encoding gradients in the form of a bipolar pulse (see PBANG) have been proposed. Laub and Kaiser [5] have presented a three-dimensional form of gradient echo based angiography that uses the GMN principle to minimize artifacts.

ADVANTAGES AND DISADVANTAGES

Motion reduction schemes, such as gating and ROPE, correct only for interview motion; GMN allows us to correct for intraview motion. However, bulk flow-related artifacts are still present even when the higher derivatives of motion are nullified. In such cases, image quality may be improved by employing externally triggered GMN acquisition or, in the case of spin echo technique, by using presaturation pulses (to suppress the signal from incoming spins) [1,2].

One disadvantage of using rephasing gradients is that the rephased spins of a vessel lying obliquely across the phase encoding gradient misregister and appear laterally shifted (Fig. 15.4) [4]. The intensity of this artifact is determined by the time lapse between the application of phase

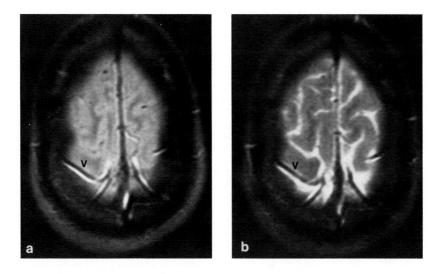

FIG. 15.4 In these flow-compensated images, the signal recovered from the superficial cortical veins (v) appear misregistered and laterally shifted (the bright bands below the veins); see text for details. **(a)** First echo, and **(b)** second echo images. (Courtesy of T.C. Larson; reproduced, with permission, from Larson et al [4].)

encoding and frequency encoding gradients and the degree of dephasing experienced by spins due to uncompensated moments of flow [4]. In addition to GMR, other factors that may determine the intensity of artifacts are:

1. the degree of spin replacement due to the time of flight effect; and
2. the phenomenon of even echo rephasing (see FEER).

As motion along only the rephasing gradient is refocused, three applications of the pulse sequence may be needed if the motion is to be refocused in three directions. This may not apply to global motion such as respiratory motion, which occurs predominantly in the cephalocaudal direction. Moreover, the addition of extra gradient lobes to achieve spin rephasing invariably lengthens the minimum possible TE.

REFERENCES

1. Ehman RL, Felmlee JP (1990): Flow artifact reduction in MRI: a review of the roles of gradient moment nulling and spatial presaturation. *Magn Reson Med* 14:293–307.

2. Felmlee JP, Ehman RL (1987): Spatial presaturation: a method for suppressing flow artifacts and improving depiction of vascular anatomy in MR imaging. *Radiology* 164:559–564.

3. Haacke EM, Lenz GW (1987): Improving MR image quality in the presence of motion by using rephasing gradients. *Am J Roentgen* 148:1251–1258.

4. Larson TC, Kelly WM, Ehman RL, Wehrli FW (1990): Spatial misregistration of vascular flow during MR imaging of the CNS: cause and clinical significance. *Am J Roentgen* 155:1117–1124.

5. Laub GA, Kaiser WA (1988): MR angiography with gradient motion refocusing. *J Comput Assist Tomogr* 12:377–382.

6. Mayo JR, Culham JAG, MacKay AL, Aikins DG (1989): Blood MR signal suppression by preexcitation with inverting pulses. *Radiology* 173:269–271.

7. Metes JJ, Wilner HI, Crowley M, Negendank W, Kelly JK, Lazo A (1989): Gated gradient-motion-refocused (GMR) images with spin-echo sequences. *Am J Neuroradiol* 10:S54–S55.

8. Mitchell DG, Vinitski S, Lawrence DB, Levy D, Rifkin MD (1988): Motion artifact reduction in MR imaging of the abdomen: gradient moment nulling versus respiratory-sorted phase encoding. *Radiology* 169:155–160.

9. Moran PR (1982): A flow velocity zeumatographic interlace for NMR imaging in humans. *Magn Reson Imag* 197–203.

10. Nishimura DG, Macovski A, Jackson JI, Hu RS, Stevick CA, Axel L (1988): Magnetic resonance angiography by selective inversion recovery using a compact gradient echo sequence. *Magn Reson Med* 8:96–103.

11. Pipe JG, Chenevert TL (1991): A progressive gradient moment nulling design technique. *Magn Reson Med* 19:175–179.

12. Runge VM, Wood ML (1988): Fast imaging and other motion artifact schemes: a pictorial overview. *Magn Reson Imag* 6:595–608.

16

Gradient Recalled Acquisition in Steady State (GRASS)[1]

BASIC PRINCIPLES

GRASS is one of the earliest fast imaging techniques based on the generation of fast field echoes (FFE) using the gradient reversal method. It uses small flip angle (less than 90°) RF excitation pulses. As a result, longitudinal magnetization is not flipped all the way to the transverse (xy) plane and, therefore, considerably less time is required for its complete recovery. After several such pulse repetition intervals with a very short pulse repetition time (TR), steady state magnetization is achieved. In this steady state, two signals are generated, one followed by the other (see SSFP). In GRASS, the initial signal is converted into a gradient echo by applying a large dephasing phase encoding gradient that is rephased after the echo is generated (Fig. 16.1). In contrast to FLASH, GRASS employs constant, but nonzero, phase encoding between the echoes.

Variants (A) In what is called spoiled GRASS, transverse magnetization is destroyed just as in FLASH. This occurs when the TR is much less than the tissue T2 value. Ideally, then, the steady state condition does not exist anymore.

(B) A three-dimensional variant of the GRASS pulse sequence has been proposed by Harms et al [11] for obtaining high resolution T1-weighted knee images in a very short time. The characteristics of this pulse sequence (see Fig. 16.2) are:

---

[1] The GRASS pulse sequence basically is similar to the FAST or ROAST pulse sequences. Only those references in which the pulse sequence used is explicitly named GRASS are cited in this section.

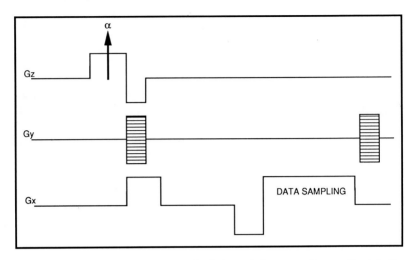

FIG. 16.1 GRASS pulse sequence with a balanced phase encoding gradient. In the "spoiled" GRASS version, the second gradient pulse in the phase encoding direction is omitted. This makes it similar to the FLASH-type pulse sequence.

FIG. 16.2 Three-dimensional FASTER pulse sequence. TR and TE values are much shorter than the GRASS sequence; additional time saving has been achieved by employing asymmetric data sampling in which only partial echo is sampled. (Modified, with permission, from Harms et al [11].)

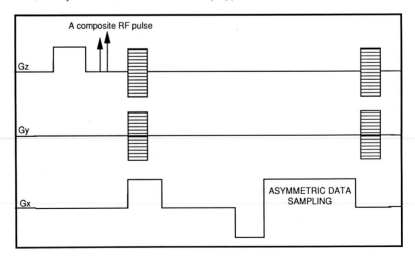

1. a composite RF pulse excitation (20°x–25°y). While the 20° RF pulse is analogous to a low angle RF pulse used in any gradient echo method, the 25° RF pulse destroys residual longitudinal magnetization more completely [10]. In this respect, the latter serves the purpose of spoiler gradient pulses employed in the GRASS sequence.
2. very short TR (16 msec). For a 128 × 128 × 256 data acquisition, this gives a total imaging time of about 4.4 minutes per excitation (128 phase encode in one direction × 128 phase encode in the second direction × 16).
3. very short TE (2.6 msec; only $\frac{3}{4}$ of the full gradient echo is acquired; this is called asymmetric echo sampling).

Very aptly, the above pulse sequence has been called *field echo acquisition with a short repetition time and echo reduction*, or FASTER.
  See also: SSFP.

CLINICAL APPLICATIONS
TISSUE CONTRAST

The image contrast is influenced by the excitation flip angle (EFA) and the pulse repetition time (TR). As the EFA is progressively decreased from 90°, image contrast is increasingly dominated by T1 relaxation, and the very short TR value only increases this T1 dominance. In general, transverse relaxation is determined by the time constant T2*.

THE BRAIN

The cerebrospinal fluid flow void sign [5] (a dark spot on the ungated axial SE images at the site of the aqueduct) signifies that the lumen of the aqueduct is patent. Clinically, this helps in differentially diagnosing CSF flow abnormalities. However, as the flowing CSF appears bright on GRASS images [18], this flow void sign is lost. And as a result, correct identification of various flow abnormalities becomes problematic [1].

THE SPINE

Standard T1-weighted SE often fails to show extradural lesions satisfactorily because both the CSF and adjacent pathology appear isointense (dark). In this situation, short TR, low angle (10°) GRASS has been found as effective as CT and conventional myelography in detecting extradural lesions, such as a herniated disk and bony outgrowths, because the CSF appears brighter than the surrounding tissues [13]. However, the retained iophendylate (an x-ray intraspinal contrast agent) may give false positive results [15].

While three-dimensional Fourier transform GRASS images have a better signal-to-noise ratio (more than a twofold increase) than corresponding two-dimensional Fourier transform images, the contrast between the cord and the CSF or the CSF and the disc has been found inferior to two-dimensional Fourier transform images [9].

THE HEART

GRASS has been used successfully to provide real-time scans (cine-MRI) for the study of cardiac valvular disorders such as mitral and aortic regurgitation or stenosis [24]. The performance of GRASS in this regard has been found comparable to that of the flow Doppler techniques [21]. Cardiac cycle synchronized cine-MRI using GRASS also provides, noninvasively, various physiological parameters, such as left and right ventricular volumes and ejection fraction.

THE LUNGS

As the flowing blood appears as a region of signal void on standard SE images, the clear delineation of vascular malformations becomes difficult as the adjacent air-filled lungs also appear dark. In GRASS (and any other gradient echo technique), the flowing blood has high intensity; this enables easy identification of the pulmonary vessels [7,12]. Unlike SE images, no gating is needed and the images are acquired within a single breath holding interval.

THE ABDOMEN

Total data acquisition times using GRASS are on the order of a few seconds. Therefore, MR examination of the abdominal region can be completed during the span of a single breath holding period [25]. This virtually eliminates respiratory motion artifacts, which usually degrade conventional SE images. The absence of these artifacts and the fact that the flowing blood appears bright enables one to obtain clear visualization of the major abdominal vessels [23].

THE JOINTS

Three-dimensional Fourier transform GRASS images have been found clinically as helpful as standard spin echo images in identifying the meniscal and ligamentous lesions of the knee joint [22]. A similar conclusion has been reached by Schellhas et al and Schellhas and Wilkes [19,20] in the case of the temporomandibular joint, where they found GRASS as sensitive in detecting joint fluid (normal or pathological) accumulations as T2-weighted SE images. The FASTER images also seem to indicate that three-dimensional data acquisition is clinically more rewarding, in terms of the contrast-to-noise ratio, than the two-dimensional implementation of either the GRASS or SE sequences [11].

The faster acquisition times allow one to analyze the dynamics of joint motion. Burnett et al [4] have used "pseudo cine"-GRASS to study normal temporomandibular joints. Briefly, the mouth is opened and closed in fixed increments and decrements, and a series of images thus obtained is displayed in a movie loop mode.

For evaluating the damaged glenoid labrum, multiplanar GRASS has been implemented in such a way that a series of radial slices can be obtained through the glenohumeral joint. This radial series of images provides better visualization of the rotator cuff integrity [17].

THE BLOOD

As GRASS is very sensitive to any inhomogeneity produced in the magnetic field by paramagnetic substances such as hemosiderin, it provides greater sensitivity for the detection of arteriovenous malformations (AVM), such as capillary and cavernous angiomas in the brain.[2] However, certain blood clots may appear hyperintense [8], in which case there is a possibility of confusing the actual flow signal with the clots (see below). Moreover, calcification inside a long-standing AVM may appear as signal loss. This varying pattern of AVM on GRASS makes this pulse sequence less significant for evaluating AVM [2,3].

FLOW

In addition to being rapid, GRASS (or any other GRE) imaging is very sensitive to flow. The signal intensity is increased for laminar flow for three reasons [1]:

1. As the serial sections are acquired in a sequential manner in GRE rather than in an interleaved manner (as in multislice SE), flow-related signal enhancement is observed on each slice

---

[2] The same reason probably is responsible for better images obtained when using Gd-DTPA [6]. Gd-DTPA increases magnetic susceptibility and shortens T2, so that GRASS provides excellent abdominal tissue contrast in addition to what would have been achieved with standard spin echo sequences.

2. The nonselective nature of gradient echo acquisition refocuses even those spins that ordinarily would have left the plane of excitation
3. Quite often, velocity-compensating gradients are introduced in GRE sequences. They also contribute to higher intensity for refocused velocity components

Nonlaminar blood flow, eg, a poststenotic jet, appears as a region of signal void.

Henkelman et al [14] have characterized the appearance of in-plane slowly flowing fluid (0.2 mm/sec) with a relatively long T2 (1600 msec), and they have noticed that band artifacts, which have no diagnostic significance, appear in GRASS images. They reason that these artifacts are caused by modulation of the spatial frequencies in the phase encode direction.

GRASS recently has been used for imaging blood flow in the finger because of its sensitivity to slowly flowing fluid [16]. Interestingly, instead of using conventional linear gradients for flow encoding, RF gradients have been used for detecting spin motion. RF gradients have the following advantages over static gradients:

1. very high amplitude gradients can be generated
2. the gradient rise time is well under a microsecond
3. very slight eddy currents are generated

One other area in which the slow flow sensitivity of GRASS may be clinically important is perfusion imaging. CE-FAST, a variant of FAST (or GRASS), has been employed in this context (see FAST).

ADVANTAGES AND DISADVANTAGES

As small flip angle and short TR values are used, a typical two-dimensional image acquisition takes about 2 to 10 sec. While three-dimensional imaging provides the capability to reconstruct images in any plane, such postprocessing of the data requires additional computer resources.

Like any other gradient echo based imaging technique, GRASS does not use an RF refocusing pulse. So, it is more susceptible to magnetic field inhomogeneities, which occur more often near the base of the skull or the nasal and paranasal sinuses.

GRASS is a standard feature on all GE Signa scanners.

REFERENCES

1. Atlas SW, Mark AS, Frahm EK (1988): Aqueductal stenosis: evaluation with gradient-echo rapid MR imaging. *Radiology* 169:449–453.
2. Atlas SW, Mark AS, Frahm EK, Grossman RI (1988): Vascular intracranial lesions: applications of gradient-echo MR imaging. *Radiology* 169:455–461.

3. Bradley WG (1988): When should GRASS be used? *Radiology* 169:574–575.

4. Burnett KR, Davis CL, Read J (1987): Dynamic display of the temporomandibular joint meniscus by using fast scan MR imaging. *Am J Roentgen* 149: 959–962.

5. Citrin CM, Sherman JL, Gangarosa RE, Scanlon D (1986): Physiology of the CSF flow void sign: modification by cardiac gating. *Am J Neuroradiol* 7: 1021–1024.

6. Choyke PL, Frank JA, Girton ME, Inscoe SW, Carvlin MJ, Black JL, Austin HA, Dwyer AJ (1989): Dynamic Gd-DTPA enhanced MR imaging of the kidney: experimental results. *Radiology* 170:713–720.

7. Dinsmore BJ, Gefter WB, Hatabu H, Kressel HY (1990): Pulmonary arteriovenous malformations: diagnosis by gradient-refocused MR imaging. *J Comput Assist Tomogr* 14:918–923.

8. Dooms GC, Higgins CB (1986): MR imaging of cardiac thrombi. *J Comput Assist Tomogr* 10:415–420.

9. Enzmann D, Rubin JB (1989): Short TR, variable flip angle, gradient echo scans of the cervical spine: comparison of 2DFT and 3DFT techniques. *Neuroradiology* 31:213–216.

10. Freeman R, Kempsall SP, Levitt MH (1980): Radiofrequency pulse sequences which compensate their own imperfections. *J Magn Reson* 38:453–479.

11. Harms SE, Flamig DP, Fisher CF, Fulmer JM (1989): New method for fast MR imaging of the knee. *Radiology* 173:743–750.

12. Hatabu H, Gefter WB, Kressel HY, Axel L, Lenkinski RE (1989): Pulmonary vasculature: high-resolution MR imaging. *Radiology* 171:391–395.

13. Hedberg MC, Drayer BP, Flom RA, Hodak JA, Bird CR (1988): Gradient echo (GRASS) MR imaging in cervical radioculopathy. *Am J Roentgen* 150:683–689.

14. Henkelman RM, McVeigh ER, Crawley AP, Kucharczyk W (1989): Very slow in-plane flow gradient echo imaging. *Magn Reson Imag* 7:383–393.

15. Jack CR, Gehring DG, Ehman RL, Felmlee JP (1988): Cerebrospinal fluid-iophendylate contrast on gradient-echo MR images. *Radiology* 169:561–563.

16. Karczmar GS, Tavares NJ, Moseley ME (1989): Use of radio-frequency field gradients to image blood flow and perfusion in vivo. *Radiology* 172:363–366.

17. Munk PL, Holt RG, Helms CA, Genant HK (1989): Glenoid labrum: preliminary work with use of radial-sequence MR imaging. *Radiology* 173:751–753.

18. Perkins TG, Wehrli FW (1986): CSF signal enhancement in short TR gradient echo images. *Magn Reson Imag* 4:465–467.

19. Schellhas KP, Wilkes CH, Fritts HM, Omile MR, Heithoff KB, Jahn JA (1987): Temporomandibular joint: MR imaging of internal derangements and postoperative changes. *Am J Roentgen* 150:381–389.

20. Schellhas KP, Wilkes CH (1989): Temporomandibular joint inflammation: comparison of MR fast scanning with T1- and T2-weighted imaging techniques. *Am J Roentgen* 153:93–98.

21. Schiebler M, Axel L, Reichek N, Aurigemma G, Yeager B, Douglas P, Bogin K, Kressel H (1987): Correlation of cine MR imaging with two-dimensional pulse Doppler echocardiography in valvular insufficiency. *J Comput Assist Tomogr* 11:627–632.

22. Spritzer CE, Vogler JB, Martinez S, Garrett WE, Johnson GA, McNamara MJ,

Lohnes J, Herfkens RJ (1988): MR imaging of the knee: preliminary results with a 3DFT GRASS pulse sequence. *Am J Roentgen* 150:597–603.

23. Raval B, Kulkarni M, Narayana P, Mehta S (1988): Fast magnetic resonance in vascular diseases of the abdomen. *Magn Reson Imag* 6:473–477.

24. de Roos A, Reichek N, Axel L, Kressel HY (1989): Cine MRI imaging in aortic stenosis. *J Comput Assist Tomogr* 13:421–425.

25. Utz JA, Herfkens RJ, Johnson CD, Shimakawa A, Pelc N, Glover G, Johnson GA, Spritzer CE (1986): Two second MR images: comparison with spin-echo images in 29 patients. *Am J Roentgen* 148:629–633.

17

Gradient Recalled Echo and Spin Echo (GREASE)

BASIC PRINCIPLES

In many cases, T2-weighted (long TR/long TE) and proton density weighted (long TR/short TE) abdominal images provide more clinical information than T1-weighted (short TR/short TE) images. However, acquisition of T2-weighted or proton density weighted images using conventional spin echo sequences usually has been time-consuming. Long TR and long TE also mean that the pulse sequence is highly sensitive to motion-related artifacts. Moreover, the presence of abdominal fat only accentuates the problem by introducing chemical shift effects.

To address this rather complicated situation, a multipronged approach has been suggested in the form of combined gradient echo and spin echo imaging (GREASE). The GREASE approach may be summarized as follows [7].

1. The problem of motion-related artifacts is alleviated by using a gradient echo because it can be obtained in a relatively short period of time (5 to 7 msec) Due to such extremely short echo times, the contribution of T2 or T1 relaxation mechanisms to the gradient echo image is minimal. The rapid reversal of the readout gradient immediately after the RF excitation pulse results in the evolution of a gradient echo.
2. The second echo is obtained following a 180° RF pulse (Fig. 17.1), which, due to its relatively long echo time, furnishes a T2-weighted image. Multiple spin echoes may be obtained by applying a series of 180° RF pulses.
3. To further decrease motion artifacts, multiple averages are utilized. To accomplish this in the shortest possible time, pulse repetition time is shortened.

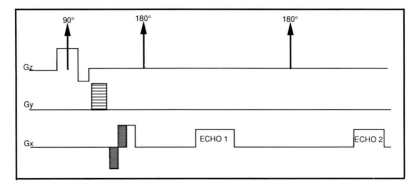

FIG. 17.1 The GREASE pulse sequence is similar to the spin echo sequence with several modifications, as discussed in the text. The excitation pulse angle may be changed from 90° (either increased or decreased) to optimize contrast. The rapid reversal of the frequency encode gradient (the shaded area) gives a gradient echo immediately after the excitation. The remaining echoes are obtained by using 180° refocusing pulses. (Modified, with permission, from Vinitski et al [7].)

4. With short TR, the T1 contribution to the spin echo image may increase. To reduce the latter, the excitation flip angle is optimized.
5. Before executing the sequence, the signal from fat is selectively suppressed by using a fat suppression technique. In one such technique, called CHESS (chemical shift selective), a composite RF pulse brings the longitudinal magnetization of fat protons into the transverse plane, which is then destroyed by a spoiler gradient pulse [3].

Variants   (A) While the above method produces one spin echo and one gradient echo per pulse cycle with a fixed sampling interval, an earlier technique proposed by Vinitski et al [6] produces a spin echo sandwiched by two gradient echoes (Fig. 17.2). In order to understand the essential features of this variant, let us note in passing the following relationships.

$$\text{Sampling rate} \propto \frac{\text{Total number of digitized samples of an echo}}{\text{Total data acquisition time (sampling interval)}} \qquad (1)$$

$$\text{Signal-to-noise ratio} \propto \frac{1}{\text{Sampling rate}} \qquad (2)$$

$$\frac{\text{Chemical shift misregistration artifact}}{} \propto \frac{\text{Chemical shift}}{\text{Bandwidth}} \qquad (3)$$

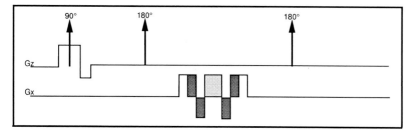

FIG. 17.2 While the shaded gradient profile produces two gradient echoes, a spin echo is formed centered around the dotted gradient lobe. (Modified, with permission, from Vinitski et al [6].)

As the sampling interval is identical to a conventional SE sequence, three times as many samples are collected per unit time. This increases the sampling rate (eq. 1) and, therefore, the signal-to-noise ratio is decreased (eq. 2). However, the increased sampling rate also means that the effective bandwidth is increased. Therefore, from equation 3, the chemical shift misregistration artifacts are reduced. To elevate the signal-to-noise ratio to the normal level, all the echoes are coadded [6]:

$$\text{SNR (Image)} = \sqrt{\text{SNR(echo 1)} + \text{SNR(echo 2)} + \text{SNR(echo 3)}}.$$

(B) An approach related to the GREASE sequence is called spin echo using repeated gradient echoes (SURGE) [1]. Figure 17.3 shows the schematics of the RF pulses and the elicited echoes. Of particular importance are the two gradient echoes and the second spin echo. While the second spin echo yields a conventional T2-weighted image, the images obtained from the gradient echoes are influenced by local field inhomogeneities and are thus T2*-weighted.

FIG. 17.3 This diagram shows the temporal relationship of the echoes produced following each RF excitation in the SURGE technique. In addition to two spin echoes, two gradient echoes (dashed echoes) are produced by gradient reversal.

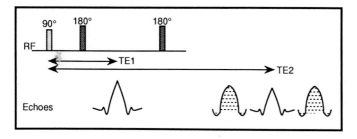

(C) Recently, Oshio and Feinberg [8] have proposed an imaging technique, GRASE (gradient- and spin-echo imaging), which produces multiple gradient echoes for each 180° RF pulse in an otherwise conventional multiple spin-echo sequence (note the similarity of this approach to that proposed by Vinitski et al [6]). Each of these echoes samples a different k-space trajectory, and as the central gradient echo in each RF-refocused echo series occurs precisely at the time of the RF-refocused spin echo, the final image shows RARE-like T2-weighted contrast.

See also: GMN, MAST.

CLINICAL APPLICATIONS
TISSUE CONTRAST

While the gradient echo image is proton density weighted, the spin echo image is primarily T2 weighted. The flip angles of the excitation pulse

FIG. 17.4 (a) A spin echo image (TR = 2.5 sec; TE = 80 msec; 1 average) and **(b)** a GREASE image of the same section obtained with 30° excitation; TR = 650 msec; 4 averages; fat suppression; and bandwidth optimization. Notice an improvement in the image appearance due to elimination of artifacts. Both images were obtained in identical data acquisition times. (Courtesy of S. Vinitski; reproduced, with permission, from Vinitski et al [7].)

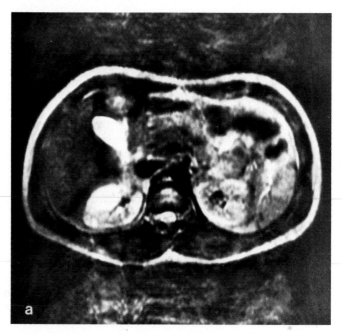

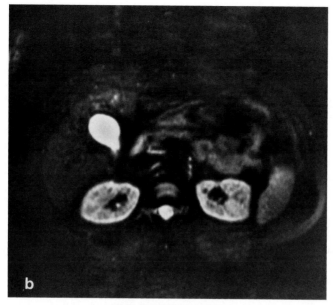

FIG. 17.4 (Continued)

(EFA) and the refocusing pulse (RFA) determine the contrast-to-noise ratio.

For large TR values, EFA of 90° and RFA of 180° produce T2-weighted SE images. As the TR shortens, the contrast is optimized by setting EFA to less than 90° (for an even number of refocusing pulses) or to more than 90° (for an odd number of refocusing pulses). This reduces T1 contribution and increases proton density dependent (and T2-weighted) contrast. It has been observed that an EFA of 135° enhances contrast between the liver and spleen [8]. If EFA is set to 90°, RFA can be decreased to about 135° without affecting image contrast. However, for a non-90° excitation pulse, this reduction in RFA results in a decrease in the contrast-to-noise ratio [8].

THE ABDOMEN

The most useful application of the GREASE technique obviously is in abdominal MR studies. In a limited number of in vivo experiments, it has provided adequate details of intraabdominal organs with the facility for manipulation of image contrast (Fig. 17.4).

ADVANTAGES AND DISADVANTAGES

The gradient echo image of GREASE provides proton density images without a contribution from T2 relaxation. Therefore, unlike a conventional SE image in which muscle appears darker than the surrounding structures, the muscle in this image appears isointense with its surrounding structures. Moreover, the spin echo image is devoid of any motion artifacts, and, even with short TR, exhibits T2-weighted contrast [7].

As shown in equations 1 through 3, the sampling interval, bandwidth, and signal-to-noise ratio have intricate interrelationships. The final balance reached among these variables greatly influences image contrast. Enzmann and Augustyn [2], Simon et al [4], and Vinitski et al [5] have further discussed the influence of the sampling interval and bandwidth on image contrast.

GRASE imaging is fairly rapid (for example, 36 sec for a series of 22 sections with TR = 4 sec) and provides RARE-like image contrast without the need for improved hardware or increasing the amount of RF power deposition [8].

REFERENCES

1. Boyko OB, Pelc NJ, Herfkens RJ, Shimakawa A, Curnes JT, Burger PC (1988): Clinical experience of detecting hemorrhage using an acquisition combining gradient and spin echo imaging generating T2 prime maps [abstr]. Seventh Annual Meeting of the Society of Magnetic Resonance in Medicine, San Francisco, p. 74.

2. Enzmann D, Augustyn GT (1989): Improved MR images of the brain with use of gated, flow-compensated, variable-bandwidth pulse sequences. *Radiology* 172:777–781.

3. Haase A, Frahm J, Hanicke W, Matthaei D (1985): 1H NMR chemical shift selective (CHESS) imaging. *Phys Med Biol* 30:341–344.

4. Simon JH, Foster TH, Ketonen L, Totterman S, Szumowski J, Kido DK, Manzione JV, Joy SE (1989): Reduced-bandwidth MR imaging of the head at 1.5 T. *Radiology* 172:771–775.

5. Vinitski S, Griffey R, Fuka M, Matwiyoff NA, Frost R (1987): Effect of the sampling rate on MR imaging. *Magn Reson Med* 5:278–285.

6. Vinitski S, Mitchell DG, Rifkin MD, Burk DL (1989): Improvement in signal-to-noise ratio and reduction of chemical shift and motion-induced artifacts by summation of gradient and spin echo data acquisition. *J Comput Assist Tomogr* 13:1041–1047.

7. Vinitski S, Mitchell DG, Szumowski J, Burk DL, Rifkin D (1990): Variable flip angle imaging and fat suppression in combined gradient and spin-echo (GREASE) techinques. *Magn Reson Imag* 8:131–139.

8. Oshio K, Feinberg DA (1991): GRASE (gradient- and spin-echo) imaging: a novel fast MRI technique. *Magn Reson Med* 20:344–349.

18

Inversion Recovery (IR)

BASIC PRINCIPLES

The inversion recovery (IR) (also called inversion echo (IE) or inversion spin echo (ISE)) pulse sequence is one of the earliest NMR spectroscopic pulse sequences adopted for NMR imaging experiments. The schematic of the basic pulse sequence has been outlined in Fig. 18.1. The selected image plane is excited by a 180° RF (inverting) pulse. This results in the flipping of the longitudinal magnetization (Mz) onto the −z axis (Fig. 18.2). However, M−z is not stable in this position, and so it tries to regain its original position aligned with the +z axis. In doing so, it releases energy mainly through the T1 mechanism and, therefore, the return of M−z is characterized by the T1 time constant. After about t = 0.7 T1, M−z reaches the horizontal x axis (null point) and in about t = 5 T1, the magnetization is back to its original stable position.

At any time during this recovery period, a 90° RF pulse may be applied to bring the recovering magnetization into the plane of detection and an FID signal is generated. The time interval between the inverting pulse and the first 90° pulse is known as the interpulse inversion time (TI). The generated FID signal can be either collected as such or, better, refocused into a spin echo using a 180° pulse. If the latter is chosen, then the echo delay is kept very short to minimize any influence of T2 relaxation on the image contrast.

Variants (A) Depending on the tissue T1 value, typical TI ranges from 10 to 1000 msec. If the lower range of values (≤200 msec) is employed, the pulse sequence is classified as short tau (*TI*) inversion recovery sequence (see STIR).

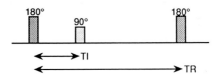

FIG. 18.1 Schematic of the inversion recovery pulse sequence. After the 180° RF pulse inverts the magnetization in the selected region, the 90° RF pulse samples longitudinal magnetization at varying time intervals TI.

(B) In the IR sequence, interpulse time TI determines the recovery of longitudinal magnetization due to T1 relaxation. In the STIR sequence, the TI is made very short in order to suppress the signal from the tissues with very low T1 values, such as fat. Note that the effect of T2 relaxation, in general, is also to decrease the signal. Therefore, the signal (and, therefore, the signal-to-noise ratio) from the tissues with short T1/short T2 is greatly attenuated on the STIR sequences. However, a low T1 value inherently tends to give a larger signal (for example, in SE sequences), due to rapid recovery of longitudinal magnetization. And this usually is negated by the faster T2 relaxation. Therefore, if rapid T2 relaxation is made to yield a larger signal and thus supplement T1 recovery, a higher-than-usual signal may be obtained from the tissues with short T1/short T2 values. The driven inversion spin echo (DISE) is such a pulse sequence (Fig. 18.3), which, unlike the STIR sequence, gives a better signal (and, therefore, a better signal-to-noise ratio) from the short T1/short T2 species [5].

(C) In some instances, it is desirable to use both long as well as short TI values in different excitation cycles. For example, as long TI suppresses the signal from long T1 tissues, such as urine, and short TI suppresses the signal from short T1 tissues, such as fat, a double IR sequence

FIG. 18.2

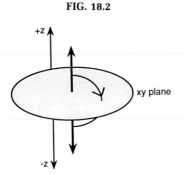

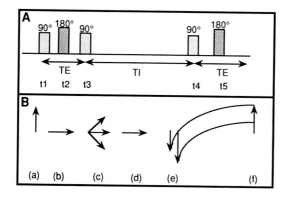

FIG. 18.3 Schematics of the DISE pulse sequence **(A)**. The first RF pulse triplet represents a spin echo configuration in which, at the echo time, transverse magnetization is aligned along the $-z$ axis. After the delay of TI, the recovering longitudinal magnetization is brought into the transverse plane, and a spin echo is formed by a 180° pulse. In order to understand the features of the pulse sequence, it would be helpful to follow the magnetization vector in the rotating frame of reference **(B)**. At time t1, the 90° pulse rotates the longitudinal magnetization **(a)** into the transverse plane **(b)**. During the time interval (t2-t1), the T2 decay dephases the transverse magnetization **(c)**, which is refocused by the first 180° pulse in (t3-t2) time interval **(d)**, and usually a spin echo forms at the time t3. However, instead of reading out the echo at this time, the transverse magnetization is aligned along the $-z$ axis by the second 90° pulse **(e)**. The shorter arrow in (e) shows the transverse magnetization in the case of short T2, and the longer arrow shows the case of long T2. Note that the transition from (a) to (e) can be made by applying a single 180° pulse. However, in that case, T2 decay is not encoded in the inverted magnetization. To encode the T1 relaxation in the present sequence, a variable time interval TI is allowed before applying a third 90° pulse (in a manner similar to the inversion recovery sequence). The tissue with short T1 readily recovers (upper curve) and its magnetization vector is longer than the tissue with longer T1 (lower curve) at the time t4, when the third 90° pulse is applied. Waiting further for time t5, a spin echo is formed by the second 180° pulse, which finally is sampled. Thus, it can be seen that the influences of the short T2 and short T1 are made additive, and a stronger signal is obtained. Recall that the short T2 gives a diminished signal and short T1 gives a higher signal with the standard spin echo sequences. For optimum performance, TE is made equal to the T2 value and TI is made equal to the T1 value.

(DIR), with two different TI, may be clinically useful in regions such as the lower abdomen and the pelvis [3].

(D) To measure the tissue T1 clinically, usually multiple spin echoes are required with varying pulse repetition times (TR), but constant echo time (TE). However, this approach is very time-consuming and, depending on the tissue T1, the total imaging time may take one hour or more. The IR sequence samples several points along the T1 relaxation curve by varying the TI. In a modified fast IR (MFIR), the total TR (from the first inverting pulse to the next inverting pulse) is kept identical, usually at least twice the tissue T1, for all repetitions; but, the waiting period between the 90° pulse and the following 180° pulse is varied between excitations [6,11]. Alternatively, in multiple inversion recovery (MIR), the decaying magnetization is sampled several times along the T1 relaxation curve by applying a series of low angle RF interrogation pulses (see measurement of the relaxation times, MORT) [20].

(E) A type of time-of-flight angiography has been proposed using the IR sequence in a selective mode (see selective inversion recovery, SIR).

(F) Park et al [15] have suggested various versions of the IR sequence for multislice imaging.

See also: IR-FLASH, MORT, SIR, STIR.

CLINICAL APPLICATIONS
TISSUE CONTRAST

In general, image contrast is determined by the values for the TR, TI, and TE.[1] T1 contrast is maximized by a combination of relatively shorter TE and shorter TR values. Depending on the tissue T1 value, TI is either ≤200 msec (STIR) or ≥200 msec (medium and long IR sequences). If TI is chosen such that it selectively suppresses the signal from one tissue compartment, such a sequence is known as t-null inversion recovery sequence. At the tissue null point, the contrast-to-noise ratio is greatest between the tissue and its surroundings. As usual, increasing TE introduces progressive T2 weighting in the image. The effect of decreasing T1 is greater at short TR value than at long TR value. This is demonstrated in Fig. 18.4.

As the conventional modulus reconstruction always assumes that the signal amplitude is positive, it disregards the sign of the IR signal. Hendrick et al [13] have shown that many times the resultant loss of contrast coincides with the area where maximum contrast would have been obtained if the sign of the signal were retained.

---

[1] While evaluating various images with regard to their contrast characteristics, it is useful to remember that the tissue T1 linearly increases with magnetic field strength and, while true T2 is not influenced by the latter, $T2^*$ is determined by the magnetic field (in)homogeneity, which may differ depending on the manufacturer of the scanner (see MORT for additional factors that affect tissue relaxation times).

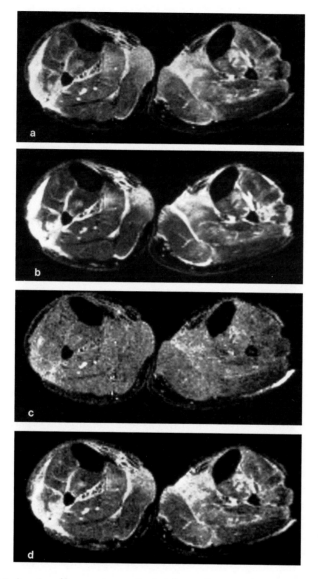

FIG. 18.4 A series of images demonstrating that at short TR, the effect of shortened T1 is more enhanced than at long TR. **(a)** A long TR STIR (TR = 1500 msec; TE = 30 msec; TI = 100 msec) image; **(b)** a postgadolinium image corresponding to (a). Notice little, if any, change in the T1-weighted contrast. **(c)** A short TR STIR (TR = 500 msec; TE = 30 msec; TI = 78 msec) image and the corresponding postgadolinium image **(d)**. Note the remarkable enhancement of the image contrast. (Courtesy of J. Fleckenstein; reproduced, with permission, from Fleckenstein et al [9].)

THE BRAIN

IR images usually show better distinction between the white (short T1) and gray (long T1) matter than the SE images [2,14]. Moreover, edema is better highlighted with IR than with SE sequences. Therefore, in cases where brain neoplasms may have very short T1 and T2 (which is rather unusual), IR images may still show the pathology rather clearly. However, partial volume effects occurring at the boundary between two tissues, eg, white and gray matter, may create unwanted image artifacts, which may appear as a false lesion.

In neonates, phase sensitive IR image display (see below) has been found to be very helpful in studying the maturation process of a developing brain [4]. The properly myelinated areas appear as bright regions on the phase displays.

THE BREAST

Using t-null IR, it is possible to differentiate successfully benign neoplasms, such as fibroadenomas, from carcinomatous growths [18].

THE ABDOMEN

Hepatic pathologies have been most widely studied with IR sequences. In contrast-enhanced studies, gradient echo techniques have proven to be superior to IR in providing maximum lesion contrast [10]. In non-enhanced studies, T1-weighted IR has been found to be superior to the corresponding SE in identifying hepatic lesions [17].

ANGIOGRAPHY

Various MR angiographic techniques have been proposed using the 180° inverting saturation pulses [7] (see SIR).

A report by Young et al [19] compares relative performances of the IR, SE, and partial saturation sequences. They conclude that the IR sequence probably has more diverse clinical applicability than what usually is perceived.

ADVANTAGES AND DISADVANTAGES

Even though the IR sequence has been used in MR imaging since the early days, it has not enjoyed the same level of acceptance as the SE sequence in clinical imaging. Most of the earlier objections were against the medium TI (200 to 500 msec) version of IR, which provided suboptimal image quality in fairly long acquisition times. However, with the introduction and success of STIR, clinical opinion has already begun to change.

IR images provide excellent T1 contrast, but so do T1-weighted SE images, and they are acquired in a shorter period of time. However, even though the TE is decreased in T1-weighted SE images, the contribution to image contrast from T2 relaxation is not completely nullified.

One fundamental pitfall in the IR technique is related to how the raw image data are represented. If the magnetization is sampled at time t (Fig. 18.5), it can be readily seen that the magnetization has a negative amplitude. However, normally employed modulus reconstruction techniques neglect this sign and attribute a positive value to the magnetization. Therefore, the contrast-to-noise ratio for two tissues with different signs (phases) is diminished only on magnitude-based IR image displays. For example, if tissue A has +5 units of magnetization and tissue B has −3 units of magnetization, the range of the true difference (contrast) between them is +5 to −3, or 8 levels. However, in modulus reconstruction, this decreases to +5 to +3, or only 2 levels. Such loss of phase information leads to the generation of line artifacts (usually one pixel wide) at the boundaries of neighboring tissues [8]. Hearshen et al [12] have demonstrated that this artifact appears when two neighboring tissues differ considerably in their T1 values. While such an artifact may help in differentiating between tissues [8], it also may make correct interpretation

FIG. 18.5 Recovery of inverted longitudinal magnetization (Mz) with time (not drawn to scale). The commonly used magnitude reconstruction algorithms fail to differentiate between negative and positive magnetization vectors. As a result, the initial negative curve of the recovery is displayed as a positive curve (broken arrows).

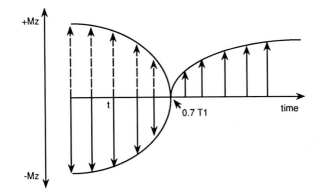

difficult. These artifacts may be removed by adopting various phase-based image display and correction schemes (see UTSS in STIR) [1,16]. The common goal of the various phase correction schemes is to differentiate the negative from the positive signal amplitudes.

REFERENCES

1. Borrello JA, Chenevert TL, Aisen AM (1990): Regional phase correction of inversion-recovery MR images. *Magn Reson Med* 14:56–67.

2. Bydder GM, Steiner RE, Young IR, Hall AS, Thomas DJ, Marshall J, Pallis CA, Legg NJ (1982): Clinical NMR imaging of the brain: 140 cases. *Am J Roentgen* 139:215–236.

3. Bydder GM, Young IR (1985): MR imaging: clinical use of the inversion recovery sequence. *J Comput Assist Tomogr* 9:659–675.

4. Christophe C, Muller MF, Baleriaux D, Kahn A, Pardou A, Perlmutter N, Szliwowski H, Segebarth C (1990): Mapping of normal brain maturation in infants on phase-sensitive inversion-recovery MR images. *Neuroradiology* 32:173–178.

5. Conturo TE, Kessler RM, Beth AH (1990): Cooperative T1 and T2 effects on contrast using a new driven inversion spin-echo (DISE) MRI pulse sequence. *Magn Reson Med* 15:397–419.

6. Crawley AP, Henkelman RM (1988): A comparison of one-shot and recovery methods in T1 imaging. *Magn Reson Med* 7:23–34.

7. Dixon WT, Sardashti M, Castillo M, Stomp GP (1991): Multiple inversion recovery reduces static tissue signal in angiograms. *Magn Reson Med* 18:257–268.

8. Droege RT, Adamczak SM (1986): Boundary artifact in inversion-recovery images. *Magn Reson Med* 3:126–131.

9. Fleckenstein JL, Archer BT, Barker BA, Vaughan JT, Parkey RW, Peshock RM (1991): Fast short-tau inversion-recovery MR imaging. *Radiology* 179:499–504.

10. Fretz CJ, Elizondo G, Weissleder R, Hahn PF, Stark DD (1989): Superparamagnetic iron oxide-enhanced MR imaging: pulse sequence optimization for detection of liver cancer. *Radiology* 172:393–397.

11. Gupta RK, Ferretti JA, Becker ED, Weiss GH (1980): *J Magn Reson* 38:447.

12. Hearshen DO, Ellis JH, Carson PL, Shreve P, Aisen AM (1986): Boundary effects from opposed magnetization artifact in IR images. *Radiology* 160:543–547.

13. Hendrick RE, Nelson TR, Hendee WR (1984): Phase detection and contrast loss in magnetic resonance imaging. *Magn Reson Imag* 2:279–283.

14. MacKay IM, Bydder GM, Young IR (1985): MR imaging of central nervous system tumors that do not display increase in T1 or T2. *J Comput Assist Tomogr* 9:1055–1061.

15. Park HW, Cho MH, Cho ZH (1985): Time-multiplexed multislice inversion-recovery techniques for NMR imaging. *Magn Reson Med* 2:534–539.

16. Park HW, Cho MH, Cho ZH (1986): Real-value representation in inversion-recovery NMR imaging by use of a phase-correction method. *Magn Reson Med* 3:15–23.

17. Steinberg HV, Alarcon JJ, Bernardino ME (1990): Focal hepatic lesions: comparative MR imaging at 0.5 and 1.5 T. *Radiology* 174:153–156.

18. Testa A, Patrizio G, Beomonte ZB, Masciocchi C, Gallucci M, Cardone G, Ciccozzi A, Ventura T, Passariello R (1989): MR characterization of breast pathology using inversion recovery sequence. *Radiologia Medica* 78:329–334.

19. Young IR, Burl M, Bydder GM (1986): Comparative efficiency of different pulse sequences in MR imaging. *J Comput Assist Tomogr* 10:271–286.

20. Young IR, Hall AS, Bydder GM (1987): The design of a multiple inversion recovery sequence for T1 measurement. *Magn Reson Med* 5:99–108.

19

Inversion Recovery—Fast Low Angle Shot Imaging (IR-FLASH)

BASIC PRINCIPLES

Traditionally, T1-weighted images are obtained by preceding a standard SE pulse sequence by an inverting 180° pulse (see IR). The recovery of the inverted magnetization is then sampled at various time points by applying a series of 90° pulses. Even though this method provides excellent T1-weighted contrast, it is prohibitively time-consuming (especially if the tissue T1 is very long), as the pulse repetition time is lengthened by the slow recovery of the magnetization.

Various approaches have been suggested to acquire clinically useful T1 images in practically tolerable time limits. Very fast imaging times in conventional imaging have been achieved by using short TR, short TE, and low angle excitation pulses. The direct implementation of fast sequences such as the snapshot FLASH, however, does not provide the desired tissue contrast because, at very small flip angles (<10°), the image contrast is primarily spin density weighted. Nonetheless, by properly preparing the tissue magnetization (eg, by applying a 180° pulse) and then repeating the fast FLASH imaging experiment n times (Fig. 19.1), a series of n images along the T1 relaxation curve can be obtained within a relatively short period of time (for example, a series of 16 images (64 phase encode ×128), with TR = 3 msec, TE = 1 msec, and flip angle = 5°, takes less than four seconds). This technique of obtaining T1-weighted images is known as inversion recovery FLASH imaging (IR-FLASH) [1,2].

The effective recovery delay (Te) may be defined as the time interval between the excitation and the acquisition of the zero phase encode step. There is a bonafide need for decreasing the Te because a short Te brings

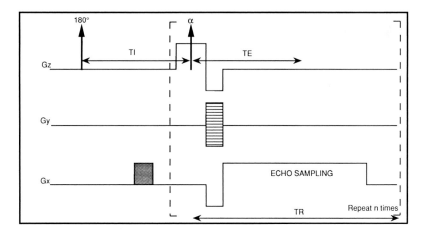

FIG. 19.1 Inversion recovery FLASH sequence. The preceding 180° pulse inverts longitudinal magnetization. The shaded gradient pulse in the frequency encode direction destroys any transverse magnetization that may exist as a result of the incomplete inversion. The snapshot FLASH experiment is then performed n times to sample the T1 relaxation curve and obtain n images with varying T1 contrast.

the zero phase encode line nearer to the excitation pulse and, thus, image contrast is optimized (Fig. 19.2) [2]. In order to decrease the Te, usually the size of the data acquisition matrix is reduced. As a result, unfortunately, the image resolution of IR-FLASH degrades, which undermines the time advantage of the FLASH sequence. However, it is possible to reduce the Te without degrading image resolution, as described below.

Variants   A technique of temporally reordering the phase encoding steps (TOPE) has been proposed by Norris et al [3]. In both IR-FLASH and TOPE, the basic imaging experiment remains the same; but, TOPE manipulates the T1 contrast by reordering the phase encoding steps in such a way that Te is no longer a restriction for image resolution (Fig. 19.3). Note the similarity of this approach to the U-FLARE experiment, in which a similar type of phase shuffling was suggested to improve T2-weighted contrast.

See also: FLASH, IR, MORT.

CLINICAL APPLICATIONS
TISSUE CONTRAST

Excellent T1 contrast is obtained by these rapid T1 imaging techniques. Ideally, T1 contrast should be a factor only of the effective recovery delay

Te. However, the choice of excitation flip angle (EFA) may also affect T1 contrast. Even though larger EFA may provide a better signal-to-noise ratio, it also modulates the T1 contrast. Therefore, the EFA should be small enough to make T1 contrast independent of it.

Klose et al [2] have analyzed the behavior of this technique in brain studies. They have demonstrated that it is possible to vary the contrast of the gray and white matter widely by changing the Te value and, thus, the temporal location of the zero phase encode line.

ADVANTAGES AND DISADVANTAGES

As this technique is a composite of the IR and FLASH sequences, it carries some of their advantages and disadvantages. In general, it provides a series of T1-weighted images in very short time intervals. Such rapid data

FIG. 19.2 A series of coronal images obtained by the alternate phase encoding scheme (5° FLASH excitation; TR = 9.7 msec; TE = 3.8 msec; 4 averages; 2.5 sec for each image) shows the rat kidneys. The time interval between the excitation and the zero phase encode step is **(a)** 250 msec; **(b)** 500 msec; and **(c)** 750 msec. Notice the changes in the relative contrast of the cortex and medulla. (Courtesy of D. G. Norris; reproduced, with permission, from Norris et al [3].)

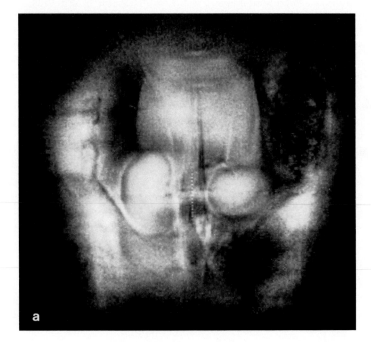

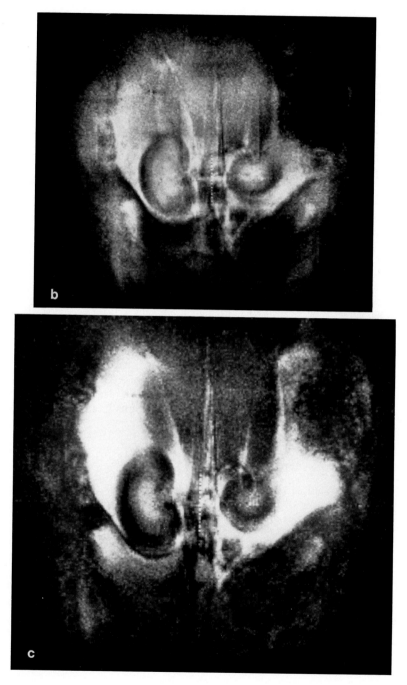

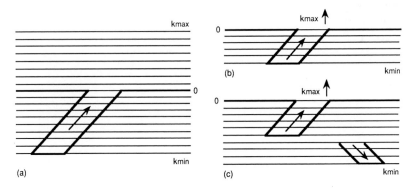

FIG. 19.3 **(a)** The length of the ladder describes the journey from the lowest valued phase step to the zero phase encoding step (dark black lines). The goal of various contrast optimizing schemes for the FLASH sequence is to decrease this transit time. **(b)** In a very simple approach, the total number of phase encoding steps is decreased. As a result, the zero phase encode step is acquired fairly early. However, image resolution also is diminished. In the temporal reordering of the phase encode steps, the total number of phase encode steps is not decreased. However, the length of the ladder is decreased by acquiring the lower valued phase steps later in the data acquisition **(c)**. In either case, Te is minimized, and the T1-weighted image contrast is optimized.

acquisition may help to eliminate the motion-related artifacts that frequently degrade abdominal images. Furthermore, it also may be possible to measure the T1 relaxation curve at several points in a short period of time.

REFERENCES

1. Hasse A, Matthaei D, Bartkowski R, Duhmke E, Leibfritz D (1989): Inversion recovery snapshot FLASH MR imaging. *J Comput Assist Tomogr* 13:1036–1040.

2. Klose U, Nagele T, Grodd W, Petersen D (1990): Variation of contrast between different brain tissues with an MR snapshot technique. *Radiology* 176:578–581.

3. Norris DG, Bottcher U, Leibfritz D (1990): A simple method of generating variable T1 contrast images using temporally reordered phase encoding. *Magn Reson Med* 15:483–490.

20

Line Scan Angiography (LISA)

BASIC PRINCIPLES

In MR imaging, gradient magnetic fields usually are employed in three directions. The purpose of the first imaging gradient is to isolate a section of the object (the slice-select gradient). The purpose of the second (phase encode) and third (frequency encode) gradients is to encode the position of the previously isolated spins in the remaining two directions. Currently, this is the most commonly used imaging strategy.

Alternatively, if the acquired data are not phase encoded, then the signal obtained in the presence of only the frequency encoding gradient yields, after one-dimensional Fourier transform, a line projected onto the axis of the frequency encoding gradient. Therefore, by gradually shifting the position of the line across the isolated section, enough line projections can be obtained to reconstruct the image of the section. This principle for creating an image by using multiple line projections was first proposed by Mansfield and Maudsley [4], and subsequently was extended for simultaneous multiple line acquisition by Maudsley [5]. Note that the projection reconstruction method of Lauterbur [3] had all the lines crossing one another at a common point (Fig. 20.1).

Whereas the earlier line scanning techniques were slow, the availability of fast imaging (such as FLASH) has helped the introduction of rapid angiographic methods using line scanning imaging. Here, we will limit the review to only very fast line scan angiographic techniques.

Frahm et al [2] have used the FLASH sequence to acquire the line projections rapidly. A standard FLASH pulse sequence (minus the phase encoding gradient) is shown in Fig. 20.2. The same slice is excited twice, separated by a time period that is much less than the tissue T1. Therefore,

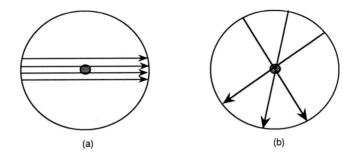

(a)　　　　　　　　　　(b)

FIG. 20.1 Two different types of line projection image reconstruction methods.

the stationary spins remain saturated, while the incoming fresh spins give a very bright signal if the imaging plane is perpendicular to the blood flow. After several such slices are imaged, a projection of the vessel is obtained in the direction of the flow. The data acquisition time is directly proportional to the TR; for the typical TR value of 7 msec, the data for a 128-line angiogram may be obtained in less than one second.

Brown et al [1] have similarly used a gradient echo technique and, incorporating the hardware technology developed for MR fluoroscopy, they have been able to display the angiogram line-by-line as it is being acquired. Typically, in about 220 msec after data acquisition, the reconstructed line is displayed on the monitor.

Both these methods, and line scan angiography in general, rely on the

FIG. 20.2 This pulse sequence produces a projection of the excited spins along the frequency encode direction.

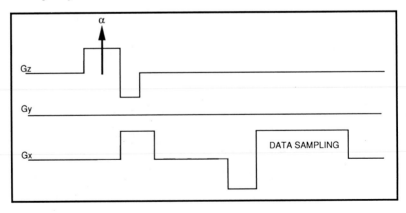

inflow of unsaturated spins for deriving the flow information and, thus, they constitute a subset of the time-of-flight (TOF) angiographic technique.

See also: FANG, PBANG, STREAM in TOF.

CLINICAL APPLICATIONS
TISSUE CONTRAST

As a side benefit for using fast pulse sequences, excellent static tissue suppression is achieved due to very fast repetitions of the pulse sequence with an extremely short TR. At this fast rate, static tissue magnetization

FIG. 20.3 Three stages showing the evolution of the line angiogram. The final angiogram consists of 60 line projections acquired in about 3 min. (Courtesy of D.G. Brown; reproduced with permission, from Brown et al [1].)

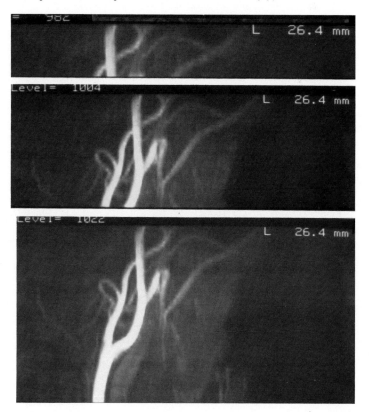

does not have enough time to recover from the preceding RF excitation and remains saturated. While the low excitation pulse angle (10°) provides faster imaging times with adequate flow-related signal, better suppression of static tissue is achieved with a pulse angle closer to 90°. If thin slices are used, the contrast of flowing blood is no longer dependent on the flow velocity; usually, a higher signal is obtained due to inflow of fresh spins after every RF excitation.

A representative LISA angiogram of the carotid arteries is shown in Fig. 20.3.

ADVANTAGES AND DISADVANTAGES

1. LISA can be applied in either spin echo, gradient echo, or stimulated echo mode.
2. As each line is reconstructed immediately after its acquisition, the image can be displayed as it is being acquired.
3. Being a nonsubtraction technique, phase misregistration artifacts, which are common in phase-based angiography, are minimal or absent in line scan angiography.
4. Motion artifacts in the phase encode direction are absent because no gradient is used in that direction. For the same reason, angiograms with arbitrary field of view can be generated using this approach.
5. The LISA technique, in general, is relatively simple to implement on any current MR scanner.

REFERENCES

1. Brown DG, Riederer SJ, Wright RC, Liu Y, Farzaneh F (1990): High-speed line scan MR angiography. *Magn Reson Med* 15:475–482.
2. Frahm J, Merboldt KD, Hanicke W, Gyngell ML, Bruhn H (1988): Rapid line scan NMR angiography. *Magn Reson Med* 7:79–87.
3. Lauterbur PC (1973): Image formation by induced local interactions: examples employing nuclear magnetic resonance. *Nature* 242:190–191.
4. Mansfield P, Maudsley AA (1976): Line scan proton spin imaging in biological structures by NMR. *Phys Med Biol* 21:847–852.
5. Maudsley AA (1980): Multiple-line-scanning spin density imaging. *J Magn Reson* 41:112–126.

21

Motion Artifact Suppression Technique (MAST)[1]

BASIC PRINCIPLES

It is well known that when spins move in the presence of a gradient magnetic field, they acquire phase shifts proportional to the velocity and strength of the gradient. A wide distribution of velocities and phase angles leads to a decrease in the signal, but does not contribute to flow-related artifacts (no signal, no artifact). If, however, a relatively narrow range of velocities exist in a voxel, their vector summation yields a strong signal, but the net phase still remains shifted. Conventional two-dimensional Fourier transform spin warp imaging techniques misregister this phase shifted signal and, as a result, give rise to artifacts in the phase encoding direction.

As a general solution to the above problem, several GMN techniques have been devised (see GMN). MAST also is a gradient moment nulling technique in which the slice-select and frequency encode gradient profiles have been modified to rephase the magnetization of the moving material. Specifically, intraview motion-related artifacts are eliminated.

Fig. 21.1 shows the MAST pulse sequence, which is similar to the standard SE pulse sequence. It consists of a slice-selective 90° RF excitation pulse, followed by a slice-selective 180° RF refocusing pulse. This is similar to the SE sequence. However, as explained below, several additional gradient lobes are introduced in the slice-select and readout gradients. The strategy employed by MAST is explained below.

---

[1] In general, the term motion artifact suppression technique includes such other techniques as signal averaging, cardiac or respiratory gating, and phase reordering. See Gating for more details.

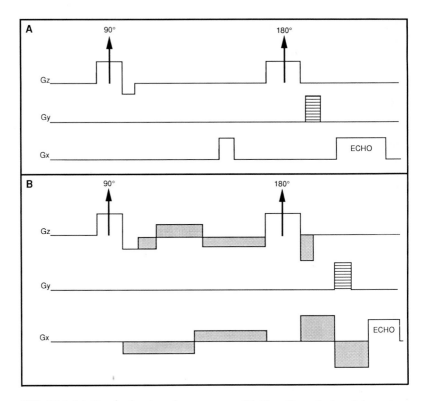

FIG. 21.1 (a) Standard spin echo sequence. **(b)** The slice-select and frequency encode gradients of (a) have been modified to compensate for the moments up to the third order (velocity, acceleration, and pulsatility). Note that four additional gradient lobes (shaded areas) are needed to compensate for three orders of the motion.

   The question is, given the desired degree of motion insensitivity, what is the gradient profile (amplitude and temporal location) of the additional lobes. The general equation to be solved is

   $$[M] \, [A_G] = [MD] - [MI],$$

where [M] is an $n \times n$ matrix of the gradient moments up to and including the desired moment for motion insensitivity; [A_G] is an $n \times 1$ matrix of the gradient amplitudes for the additional lobes; [MD] is an $n \times 1$ matrix comprised of the moment values for the desired order of motion refocusing; and [MI] is an $n \times 1$ matrix comprised of the moment values required for the imaging [4,8].

For simplicity, let us consider only the case of constant velocity. The above matrix equation then becomes

$$
\begin{bmatrix} \int_{a_1}^{b_1} G(t)\, t^0 dt + \int_{a_2}^{b_2} G(t)\, t^0 dt \\ \int_{a_1}^{b_1} G(t)\, t^1 dt + \int_{a_2}^{b_2} G(t)\, t^1 dt \end{bmatrix} \begin{bmatrix} AG_1 \\ AG_2 \end{bmatrix} = \begin{bmatrix} MD_1 \\ MD_2 \end{bmatrix} - \begin{bmatrix} MI_1 \\ MI_2 \end{bmatrix},
$$

where $a_i{}^2$ is the starting time of the gradient lobe and $b_i{}^2$ is the ending time of the gradient lobe. The individual elements of the two 2×1 matrixes on the right-hand side are known. Similarly, the 2×2 matrix on the left-hand side can be solved once the temporal positions of the lobes are finalized. Therefore, the gradient amplitudes can be found out easily by multiplying the right-hand side by the inverse of [M]. Note that the solution will change if the gradient lobes are shifted along the time axis. As is obvious from the above equation, the number of these lobes is determined by the degree of required spin rephasing. In general, $n + 1$ additional lobes in each gradient are needed to correct for n orders of the motion.

The dephasing produced by the phase encoding gradient is ignored by MAST because:

1. as the different phase encoding (monopolar) pulses occupy the identical time interval before the echo readout, the time averaged location of a spin moving with constant velocity is fixed. Conventional two-dimensional Fourier transform image reconstruction, therefore, completely ignores the phase shift [11].
2. the phase encoding gradient is switched on for a very short period of time and the resultant phase shift is negligible.
3. in order to possess imaging capabilities, its zeroth moment cannot be nullified (except when the zero-valued phase step is applied).

The experimental data [3] also support the notion that refocusing along the phase encoding direction is not critical because gradient refocusing along the slice-select and frequency encode directions refocuses motion along any imaging axis.

See also: GMN, MMORE.

CLINICAL APPLICATIONS
TISSUE CONTRAST

The basic contrast characteristics of MAST images are similar to conventional SE images. However, as MAST eliminates motion artifacts, the moving material, such as blood and CSF (which may appear as a region of signal void on T2-weighted SE images), appears uniformly bright on T2-weighted MAST images. As a result, the contrast-to-noise ratio is increased for tissues whose signal is recovered. Most often, MAST is applied in clinical situations where T2-weighted tissue contrast is desired, without the disadvantages (such as lengthy acquisition time and the resulting inferior image quality) of a T2-weighted SE acquisition.

THE BRAIN

Numerous clinical studies implementing MAST in the brain clearly have shown improved image quality when compared to the nontriggered or triggered conventional imaging [4–6,9,10]. This improvement in signal-to-noise ratio mainly results from the elimination of CSF flow-related phase shift artifacts.

THE SPINE

T2-weighted images of the cervical spine and lumbar spine often are corrupted by the presence of motion artifacts (here, the involuntary motion is deglutition and peristalsis, respectively). T2-weighted MAST provides a better contrast-to-noise ratio, and shows greater anatomical detail of the vertebral column, including the spinal canal. This is due to the fact that the CSF has a long T2 value and, on a T2-weighted sequence, it gives an intense signal.

THE ABDOMEN

Usually, the shorter the echo time (TE) and pulse repetition time (TR), the lesser the dephasing influence of the moving material. Therefore, T1-weighted SE images of the abdomen have superior contrast-to-noise ratios than the long TR/long TE (T2-weighted) SE images. Moreover, the upper abdominal T2-weighted images very often are degraded by respiratory or other involuntary motion (eg, peristalsis) artifacts. In such situations, MAST has provided far better delineation of intraabdominal structures, including the pancreas, spleen, liver, and abdominal vessels (see Fig. 21.2) [1,7].

IN-PLANE FLOW QUANTIFICATION

Flow along the direction of the phase encoding and frequency encoding gradients is called *in-plane flow* (Fig. 21.3). Refocusing gradients in the form of MAST have been used to quantitate in-plane flow in the phase

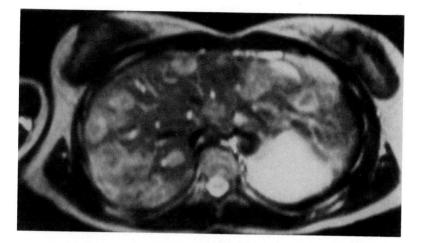

FIG. 21.2 Excellent image contrast is obtained with MAST (TR = 2 sec; TE = 100 msec). Motion artifacts are absent, despite heavy T2-weighting, and the right hepatic metastasis are clearly visualized. (Courtesy of P. Colletti; reproduced, with permission, from Colletti et al [1].)

encoding direction. In comparison to the use of bipolar gradients for quantifying in-plane flow along the frequency encode direction, this modified approach has the following advantages [2].

1. As the higher orders of the motion are effectively suppressed, no signal loss occurs—even due to turbulent flow.
2. As data collection occurs after the spins are phase encoded, the phase evolution during the signal readout is uniform and is independent of the encoding procedure. Note that the simultaneous processes of fre-

FIG. 21.3 In-plane flow occurs in the direction of the phase encode or frequency encode gradients.

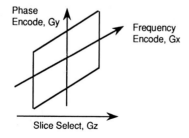

Phase Encode, Gy

Frequency Encode, Gx

Slice Select, Gz

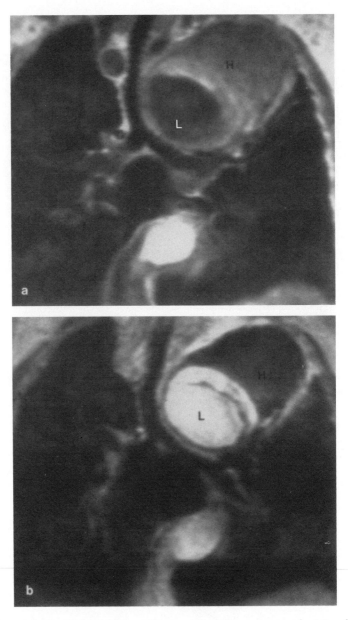

FIG. 21.4 A T1-weighted (TR = 600 msec; TE = 20 msec) spin echo **(a)** and T2-weighted (TR = 2 sec; TE = 100 msec) MAST images showing aortic lumen (L) and dissecting hematoma (H). Note the increased signal intensity of the blood without artifacts. (Courtesy of P. Colletti; reproduced, with permission, from Colletti et al [1].)

quency encoding and data collection may introduce rather large errors in the calculations if flow along the frequency encode direction is encoded [11].

ADVANTAGES AND DISADVANTAGES

MAST suppresses phase shift artifacts ("ghost" artifacts) caused by involuntary motion, including that of blood and CSF. Respiratory gated motion artifact suppression methods result in long scan times, and still do not eliminate phase artifacts introduced by motion that occurs between a 90° RF excitation pulse and data acquisition (commonly called intraview motion). By employing modified gradients, MAST rephases the magnetization of the moving spins in the same time as a conventional T2-weighted SE acquisition. Also, MAST is easy to implement and does not require additional hardware. However, modified gradient waveforms demand more powerful gradients; the placement of additional gradient lobes is subject to the availability of time between the excitation and sampling RF pulses.

As MAST recovers the signal from moving material, blood vessels appear as medium- to high-intensity structures (on T2-weighted sequences) (Fig. 21.4). In some situations, this may result in loss of anatomic detail around the vessel wall (due to similar contrast of perivascular structures).

MAST eliminates only intraview motion artifacts. With the addition of proper physiological gating, interview motion artifacts also may be considerably reduced. This will further enhance the role of MAST, especially in regions such as the thorax.

MAST is available on Picker MR scanners.

REFERENCES

1. Colletti PM, Raval JK, Benson RC, Pattany PM, Zee CS, Boswell WD, Norris SL, Rallis PW, Segall HD (1988): The motion suppression technique (MAST) in magnetic resonance imaging: clinical results. *Magn Reson Imag* 6:293–299.

2. Duerk JL, Pattany PM (1988): In-plane flow velocity quantification along the phase encoding axis in MRI. *Magn Reson Imag* 6:321–333.

3. Duerk JL, Pattany PM (1989): Analysis of imaging axes significance in motion artifact suppression technique (MAST): MRI of turbulent flow and motion. *Magn Reson Imag* 7:251–263.

4. Duerk JL, Simonetti OP, Hurst G (1990): Modified gradients for motion suppression: variable echo time and variable bandwidth. *Magn Reson Imag* 8:141–145.

5. Elster AD (1988): Motion artifact suppression technique (MAST) for cranial MR imaging: superiority over cardiac gating for reducing phase-shift artifacts. *Am J Neuroradiol* 9:671–674.

6. Iwasaki S, Nakagawa H, Uchida H, Fukuzumi A, Otsuji H, Kichikawa K, Watabe Y, Kitamura K, Tsushima J, Hirohashi S (1990): Improvement of T2 weighted images of central nervous system by motion artifact suppression technique (MAST). *Radiation Medicine* 8:13–16.

7. Lipcamon JD, Chiu LC, Phillips JJ, Pattany PM (1988): MRI of the upper abdomen using motion artifact suppression technique (MAST). *Radiologic Technology* 59:415–418.

8. Pattany PM, Phillips JJ, Chiu LC, Lipcamon JD, Duerk JL, McNally JM, Mohapatra SN (1987): Motion artifact suppression technique (MAST) for MR imaging. *J Comput Assist Tomogr* 11:369–377.

9. Quencer RM, Hinks RS, Pattany PH, Horen M, Post MJ (1988): Improved MR imaging of the brain by using compensating gradients to suppress motion-induced artifacts. *Am J Roentgen* 151:163–170.

10. Szeverenyi NM, Kieffer SA, Cacayorin ED (1988): Correction of CSF motion artifact on MR images of the brain and spine by pulse sequence modification: clinical evaluation. *Am J Neuroradiol* 9:1069–1074.

11. Wedeen VJ, Rosen BR, Chesler D, Brady TJ (1985): MR velocity imaging by phase display. *J Comput Assist Tomogr* 9:530–536.

22

Multimoment Refocused Imaging (MMORE)

BASIC PRINCIPLES

In contrast to the standard NMR spectroscopic experiment, magnetic field gradients are used in MR imaging to encode spatially the origin of the NMR signals. In the time interval between RF excitation of the spin system and the beginning of data collection, some loss of signal results due to the interaction between the gradients and excited spins (intraview dephasing).

It is necessary to refocus the dephased spins in order to recover the lost signal at the echo time. Normally, gradient magnetic fields are designed primarily for imaging purposes. However, gradients can be designed in such a way that they spatially encode signals for imaging and also refocus dephased spins at the echo time for the desired order of spin motion. To achieve the latter goal, all moments (up to and including the desired moment) of gradient fields should be equal to zero at the time of data collection. A gradient moment is defined below.

If the moving spins travel for a time interval t, an ith time moment of the gradient G is equal to

$$\int_0^t G(t)\, t_i\, dt,$$

where $i = 0$ means no change in position, $i = 1$ means velocity, $i = 2$ means acceleration, and so forth. Usually, this is achieved by introducing additional gradient lobes, and, in general, it is known as gradient moment nulling (GMN). The MAST was one of the earliest GMN techniques in which additional gradient lobes were introduced for eliminating motion artifacts. The implementation of GMN techniques for single echo sequences, such as MAST, is relatively straightforward. However, as the number of echoes increases (as in multiecho sequences), implementation of gradient moment nulling becomes rather complex. Moreover, the TE is fixed in MAST. If another sequence with different TE is desired, the gradient moments have to be recalculated.

In summary, the MAST-like approach lacks multiecho and variable echo capabilities. Therefore, Duerk et al [1,2] have proposed the following two GMN approaches.

MEMMORE, a multiecho MMORE technique, is based upon the realization that all nullified moments of a gradient remains so even when that gradient waveform is time-shifted by a certain factor (as long as the echo spacing remains constant) (Fig. 22.1) [2]. In other words, nullified gradient moments are independent of their temporal origin. This is very important for designing refocusing gradients for a multiecho pulse sequence because it allows one to calculate the moments for a refocusing gradient, which can then be repeated for the second and subsequent echoes as long as the time between any two adjacent echoes is kept identical throughout the pulse sequence.

VEMMORE, a variable echo MMORE technique, eliminates the constant echo spacing restriction of MEMMORE. If the entire gradient waveform is multiplied by a factor k, then the motion sensitivity of the gradient is increased by a factor $k^{(i+1)}$ [1]. If the original ith moment is zero, then it suggests that the scaled gradient will retain the zero-valued time moment. At the same time, it also suggests that all nonzero moments will increase by a factor equal to $k^{(i+1)}$. For example, a velocity-compensated

FIG. 22.1 Time invariance of the frequency encode gradient profile. The relative positions of the refocusing gradient lobes (shaded areas) are similar in both cases. However, their amplitudes may differ to account for varying echo times. The principle illustrated here also can be extended to the slice-select gradient.

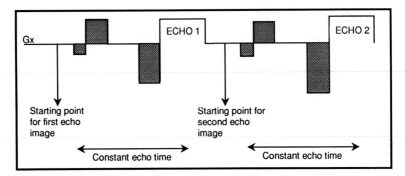

gradient still will be velocity compensated if time scaled, but now it will be more sensitive to acceleration and other noncompensated motion terms. This is not a particularly desirable solution because in order to retain one nullified moment, the dephasing effects of the other moments have been increased. There are only two situations in which the variable echo approach may be useful:

1. if all the desired moments of the original gradient are compensated before time scaling it; or
2. if the gradient scaling factor is less than 1.

If the gradient scaling factor is less than 1, the scaled gradient is shrunk or collapsed, and uncompensated moments in the scaled gradient actually are *decreased* by a factor of $k^{(i+1)}$.

The key point to note is that while the MEMMORE approach is applicable for the time-shifted gradient waveform, the VEMMORE approach is applicable for the time-scaled gradient waveform (Fig. 22.2).

See also: Gating, GMN, MAST.

FIG. 22.2 Three different timing diagrams are illustrated for the same gradient profile. Considering **(a)** as the original gradient waveform, the gradient waveform has been shrunk or collapsed **(b)** and extended in **(c)**. Note that the general outline of the gradient waveform, including the amplitude of the refocusing lobes (shaded areas), remains identical in all three cases.

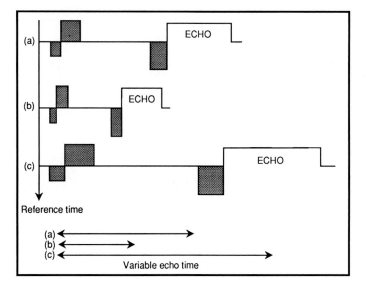

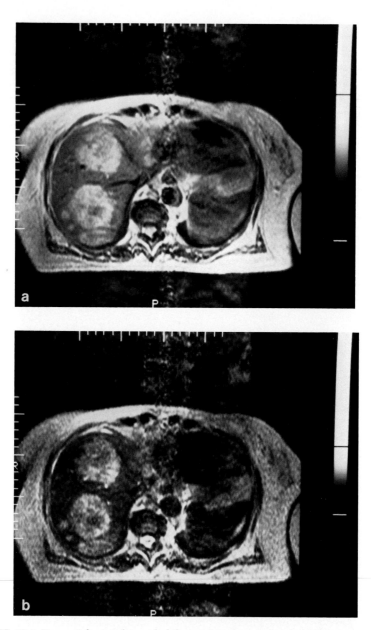

FIG. 22.3 Two axial nonrefocused abdominal images obtained at TE = 80 msec **(a)**, and TE = 160 msec **(b)**. The same images obtained with MEMMORE technique at TE = 80 msec **(c)**, and TE = 160 msec **(d)**. Note the improved image quality and the lesion conspicuity on the refocused images. (Courtesy of J.L. Duerk; reproduced, with permission, from Duerk et al [2].)

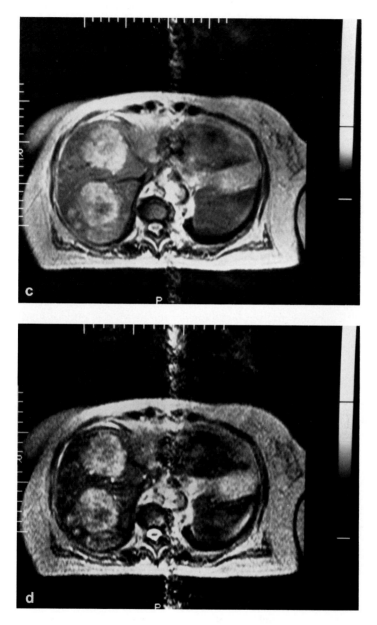

FIG. 22.3 (Continued)

CLINICAL APPLICATIONS
TISSUE CONTRAST

Without any presaturating schemes, flowing blood appears bright and flow-related artifacts are somewhat increased compared to nongradient-refocused (only RF refocused) multiecho images. Such artifacts may be eliminated by applying presaturating RF pulses. The overall signal-to-noise ratio of MEMMORE images is higher than RF refocused multiecho images.

THE ABDOMEN

Multiecho T2-weighted images of the liver have been obtained employing MEMMORE-designed gradient waveforms (Fig. 22.3). When compared to RF refocused multiecho images, these images have fewer physiologic motion induced phase artifacts and, thus, may facilitate identification of the pathology, such as intrahepatic metastasis.

ADVANTAGES AND DISADVANTAGES

Gradient moment nulling techniques, such as MAST, refocus gradient-induced dephasing of moving spins; this decreases motion-induced artifacts. However, GMN techniques are useful only for single-echo sequences. If multiple refocused echoes are required, the sequence has to be reapplied several times; this increases total imaging time.

MMORE is a technique combining multiecho pulse sequences with the benefits of a single-echo gradient moment nulling technique such as MAST. It is relatively straightforward to implement on existing MR scanners.

REFERENCES

1. Duerk JL, Simonetti OP, Hurst GC (1990): Modified gradients for motion suppression: variable echo time and variable bandwidth. *Magn Reson Imag* 8:141–151.
2. Duerk JL, Simonetti OP, Hurst GC, Motta AO (1990): Multiecho multimoment refocusing of motion in magnetic resonance imaging: MEM-MO-RE. *Magn Reson Imag* 8:535–541.

23

Measurement of Relaxation Times (MORT)

BASIC PRINCIPLES

Even before the foundation of MRI was laid down, it was known that tissue relaxation times (T1, T2) change in certain pathologic conditions [8]. In fact, this observation raised the optimism that MRI, once fully operational, would provide tissue-type specific visual information, such as whether a neoplasm is benign or malignant. However, this early optimism did not last long; it quickly became apparent that alterations in tissue relaxation times alone are too nonspecific for deriving definitive clinical conclusions (Table 23.1) [17].

Nonetheless, tissue relaxation times continue to serve as important imaging parameters in MRI. Numerous imaging techniques have been worked out to provide as accurate quantification of these parameters as possible. Based on this quantification, true T1- or T2-weighted images can be calculated retrospectively. While some of these techniques are simple modifications of the spin echo or inversion recovery imaging sequences, others are specialized pulse sequences targeted especially for the task of measuring relaxation times.

T1 MEASUREMENT

T1-weighted imaging is a very loose term used quite often in clinical MRI when short TR/TE images are acquired. It simply signifies that image contrast is predominantly determined by the amount of the recovery of longitudinal magnetization during TR. Commonly, T1 is estimated by acquiring two or more T1-weighted images with different TR values and

TABLE 23.1.

	T1 (msec)[a]	T2 (msec)[a]
Gray matter	640 ± 46	140 ± 16
White matter	414 ± 42	120 ± 12
Pathology		
Pituitary adenoma	728 ± 54	175 ± 21
Perifocal edema	730 ± 91	278 ± 72
Meningioma	765 ± 95	165 ± 35
Meningioma (endotheliomatous)	768 ± 95	167 ± 31
Meningioma (transitional)	723 ± 84	143 ± 37
Meningioma (fibrous)	698 ± 78	135 ± 26
Neuroma	894 ± 74	213 ± 29

[a] At 0.28 T.

Modified, with permission, from Just et al [17].

using the equation

$$SI = k \times e^{-(TE/T2)} \times (1 - e^{-(TR/T1)}),$$

where k is constant. Alternatively, an inversion recovery sequence with different inversion times (TI) or saturation recovery sequence may be employed [39].

The following three factors are of concern: total measurement time, precision of the measurement, and signal-to-noise ratio of the images. While the time efficiency of data collection cannot be easily improved, Sperber et al [42] have proposed a novel algorithm for performing the multiparameter nonlinear least-square fit of the above equation. Although their algorithm is considerably faster, it is less precise. Riederer et al [38] have shown that the precision of the calculation can be increased by 40% by taking into consideration the varying TEs of a multiecho series. Prato et al [34] have concluded that the signal-to-noise ratio can be maximized by optimizing TR. For example, for an estimated T1 value of 500 msec, at least one image should have TR of 400 to 500 msec, as long as the other TR value is between 400 and 1400 msec. Beyond this limit, a better signal-to-noise ratio is obtained by more averaging, rather than length-ening TR. Similarly, in the case of interleaved sign preserved IR/non-IR imaging, Lin et al [21] have demonstrated that for T1 between 150 and 150 msec, TI should be 400 msec, and TR(IR)/TR(non-IR) should be 2.5 to 3.0, as long as the summation of both TRs is 3 to 4 sec. If the latter needs to be increased, then more data averaging should be employed, rather than increasing TR.

In general, approaches based on the above equation are valid only if

longitudinal magnetization fully recovers during TR (TR $\geq$ 5 T1). However, this may not be true for rather long T1 values. Even for shorter T1
values, complete recovery is never reached with clinically employed TR.
In these circumstances, Redpath [36] has proposed the use of a series of
regularly spaced 90° pulses, with every other 90° pulse preceded by an
adiabatic fast passage (AFP, see SIR) pulse (interleaved IR/SR sequence)
(Fig. 23.1). Let us call the signal produced in the absence of the AFP pulse
S1, and the signal obtained in the presence of a 180° pulse S2. Then,

$$S2/S1 = 1 - 2e^{-(TI/T1)}.$$

When TR < 5 T1, the ratio (S1 − S2)/S1 gives better T1 approximation.
Pykett et al [35] have used an interleaved SE/IR sequence and, once again,
the ratio (S1 − S2)/S1 is used for calculations when TR < 5 T1.

All the above approaches are clinically inefficient as they are time
guzzlers. Therefore, a number of schemes have been proposed to decrease
the overall T1 measurement time.

1. Mansfield et al [25] have used an interleaved SR/EPI sequence, not
   only to increase speed, but also to correct for errors in the selection
   of the slice. As shown in Fig. 23.2, when the slice profile is not completely rectangular, spins at the edge of the slice do not experience
   full 90° excitation–rotation. Therefore, a component along the Mz remains, which grows back to M0 during TR. Such edge effects are
   known to introduce errors in T1 calculations [25]. Similarly, if the

FIG. 23.1 In this pulse sequence, every other 90° RF excitation pulse (see inset)
is preceded by inversion of the spins achieved by adiabatic fast passage (AFP).
Thus, it may be considered an interleaved inversion recovery/saturation recovery
pulse sequence.

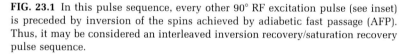

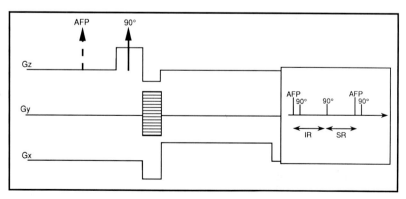

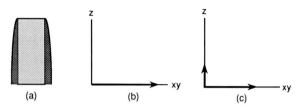

FIG. 23.2 (a) The dotted area shows an ideal slice profile that is perfectly rectangular. In this case, a 90° RF pulse flips all the spins into the transverse xy plane **(b)**. In reality, however, the edges of the slice (shaded areas) do not experience full 90° rotation. And, as a result, some spins relax back in the z direction **(c)**.

inverting pulse is not exactly 180°, the signal is shifted by a factor of $(1 - \cos\phi)$. The measured signal is then given by

$$S(1 - (1 - \cos\phi)e^{-t/T1})),$$

where S is the signal that would have been obtained in the presence of a perfect 180° inverting pulse, and ϕ is the actual nutation experienced by the spins [29].

2. The speed advantage of low flip angle imaging is well established. Fram et al [10] and Wang et al [43] have proposed the use of reduced angle (ϕ) RF pulses for measuring T1. Their technique is fairly simple: for a series of different ϕ, find the quantities

$$x(\phi) = SI/\tan \phi$$

and

$$y(\phi) = SI/\sin \phi,$$

where SI is the signal intensity of a pixel. Then, fit the data in the equation of the form

$$y(\phi) = mx(\phi) + c.$$

The slope, m, of the line equals $e^{-(TR/T1)}$. Therefore, $T1 = -TR/\ln(m)$. Simple as it may look, this approach gives more precise T1 approximation (for T1 > 0.5 TR) than the SR sequence [43]. Wang et al [43] also prove that it is possible to find two optimum ϕ; the estimation thus obtained is comparable to that obtained using multiple ϕ. As the 180° RF pulses are omitted, the imperfect slice profile induced T1 errors also are considerably reduced [16].

3. The approach proposed by Young et al [45] using a multiple inversion recovery (MIR) sequence is shown in Fig. 23.3. T1 can be calculated from the relationship

$$1 = \cos A \times \cos B \times e^{-(T0/T1)} \times (2 - e^{-(Tx/T1)})$$

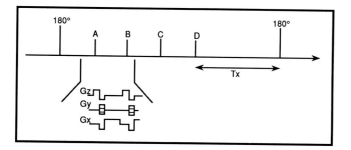

FIG. 23.3 In this multiple inversion recovery sequence, every 180° RF pulse is followed by four interrogation pulses (A, B, C, D). The angles of RF pulses labeled A, B, and C usually are kept less than 90°, and the final pulse D is of 90°.

where T0 is the time when the signal from the region of interest is zero and the others are as explained in the figure. They conclude that the MIR approach is comparable to the IR approach, and also is swift.

4. McVeigh et al [26] have exploited their method for producing stripes (see NIMAT) for measuring the T1. For measuring T1, they produce multiple stripes with different TI values. As the degree of magnetization recovery is different for these stripes, their signal intensities (SI) also are different (Fig. 23.4). These signal intensity values are transformed according to the formula

$$\log (1 - \text{SI/M0}),$$

where M0 is obtained by sampling a noninverted area (area outside the stripes). The transformed SI and corresponding TI are fitted to the line equation

$$y = mx + c,$$

where the slope, m, of the line equals the value $-1/T1$. The T1 values

FIG. 23.4 Each stripe has been produced by using a different inversion time TI. Therefore, their signal intensities are different, depending on how much the longitudinal magnetization has recovered during TI. The tissue T1 is easily derived by using these signal intensity values, as discussed in the text.

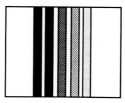

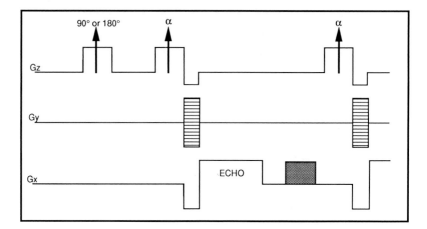

FIG. 23.5 TOMROP pulse sequence. After the initial RF pulse sets the desired magnetization value, a series of interrogation pulses creates gradient echoes. Only two of many interrogation RF pulses of degree α are shown. The spoiler gradient pulse (shaded area) destroys any remaining transverse magnetization after data collection. (Modified, with permission, from Brix et al [5].)

obtained by their approach correlate very well with similar values obtained by the IR approach. In addition, the method proposed by McVeigh et al is very fast (quick $T1$, QT1) and allows for graphical visualization of the T1 recovery curve.

5. TOMROP, *T*-one by multiple readout pulses, is a pulse sequence that allows pixel-by-pixel determination of T1 value by using multiple gradient echo images acquired in a time interval similar to one inversion recovery image [5]. Fig. 23.5 depicts the TOMROP pulse sequence. Initially, a slice-selective RF pulse is used to position longitudinal magnetization to a desired value. A series of low angle RF pulses is then applied, to generate a series of gradient echoes. Any transverse magnetization remaining after each gradient echo acquisition is destroyed by a spoiler gradient pulse. This approach is basically similar to that described by Young et al (see above). An image is created using each gradient echo (Fig. 23.6) and, using a least-square estimation algorithm for nonlinear data fit, curves for the T1 value are obtained from the pixel amplitudes (Fig. 23.7).

T2 MEASUREMENT

For some unknown reason, the spin-spin relaxation time (T2) seems to have been studied less than the T1 relaxation time. In clinical MRI, tissue T2 is obtained by acquiring two or more spin echo images (multiecho

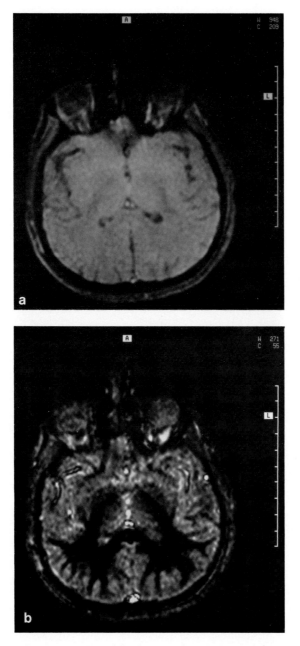

FIG. 23.6 First gradient echo **(a)** and seventh gradient echo **(b)** images obtained by the TOMROP sequence. The white matter is of lower intensity in (b) at the time when its T1 relaxation curve touches the time axis in Fig. 23.7. (Courtesy of G. Brix; reproduced, with permission, from Brix et al [5].)

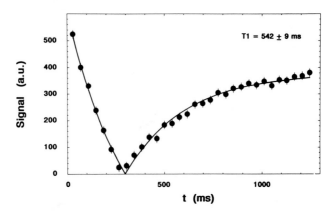

FIG. 23.7 The T1 relaxation curve of the white matter as measured from the intensity values for one pixel across a set of 32 gradient echo images and interpolated by the Lagrange polynomial fit. (Courtesy of G. Brix; reproduced, with permission, from Brix et al [5].)

acquisition) with different TE values. T2 is, then, equal to (TE2 − TE1)/log(E1/E2), where E1 and E2 are the amplitudes of the first and second echoes [19,27,32]. As the TR is kept identical, the T2 measurement time only marginally increases the imaging time of a multiecho series, compared to the single echo series.

Darwin et al [9] have shown that the results obtained by using only a limited number of echoes from a multiecho series give results comparable to those obtained using all the echoes. This suggests that total RF power deposition may be reduced by eliminating some echoes (and the corresponding 180° pulses).

SIMULTANEOUS MEASUREMENT OF T1 AND T2

As we saw previously, separate pulse sequences usually are required for measuring tissue T1 and T2 values. Obviously, the time efficiency of the measurement can be greatly improved by devising pulse sequences that measure both T1 and T2 simultaneously. Many such dual techniques have been proposed [12,28,40]; one of them, simultaneous multiple acquisition of relaxation times (SMART), is described below [12].

In SMART, the standard SE sequence is followed by two additional 90° pulses to generate two spin echoes and a third stimulated echo (Fig. 23.8). While the first echo (S1) is a true spin echo, the second echo (S2) has contributions from both the stimulated third echo (S3) and S1. T1 is,

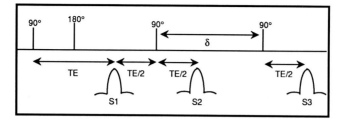

FIG. 23.8 Schematic of SMART pulse sequence. While S1 and S2 are spin echoes, S3 is a stimulated echo. The variable δ should be long enough so that no transverse magnetization persists at the time of third 90° RF pulse, and a pure stimulated echo is obtained.

then, equal to

δ/ln(S2/S3),

and T2 is equal to

TE/ln(S1/2 S2),

where δ = time interval between the last two 90° pulses. (Note that these equations are valid only for a perfect 90° RF pulse profile.)
    See also: IR, IR-FLASH, STEAM.

CLINICAL APPLICATIONS
SYNTHETIC IMAGING

The principle of synthetic imaging is illustrated in Fig. 23.9. As illustrated, it allows one to retrospectively reconstruct a series of images with different contrast characteristics. The concept is very simple: after deriving the T1 and T2 values for all the pixels, feed these values back, along with the newly defined TR and TE parameters, into equation 1. A new pixel value is thus obtained. After repeating the same procedure for all pixels, a new image may be displayed with operator-chosen timing parameters, which also determine the signal-to-noise ratio of the derived images [30].

Bobman et al [3] and Lee et al [20] have formally presented an outline of the system required to successfully implement the procedure for making synthetic images, and have further evaluated the synthetic images in terms of accurate tissue characterization [2]. O'Donnell et al [28] have discussed the influence of various pulse sequences on image contrast and Riederer et al [37] have evaluated the clinical feasibility of such images.

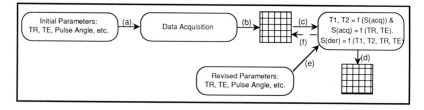

FIG. 23.9 This flow chart explains the principle of synthetic imaging. After choosing the initial timing parameters, data acquisition is performed **(a)**, and an image is reconstructed in the usual manner **(b)**. As the measured T1 and T2 values are some function of the acquired signal (S(acq)), which itself is a function of the pulse parameters (and the tissue relaxation times), a proper mathematical model is chosen for calculating T1 and T2 values **(c)**, and a calculated map is reconstructed pixel-by-pixel **(d)**. Next, the revised pulse parameters are fed into this model for deriving new signal intensity values (S(der)) for all pixels. A "synthetic image" can then be displayed **(f)** without the need for actual data acquisition.

Posin et al [33] have reported that certain pathologies can be made more conspicuous by varying the acquisition parameters. Obviously, the integrity of this approach depends on the accuracy of calculated T1 and T2 values. As discussed below, many factors affect measurement of relaxation times, and thus may unduly alter the characteristics of the synthesized images.

THE BRAIN

It is hoped that T1 and T2 quantification someday will serve as a lesion-specific parameter, and thus provide a "signature" of the involved pathology. Unfortunately, there is considerable overlap in relaxation times of normal and diseased tissues (see Table 23.1). Additionally, T1 relaxation time depends on the location of the white matter sampled [13]. This observation, along with person-to-person variation, accounts for nearly 75% of the total variance [13]. Thus, it seems unlikely that relaxation parameter imaging will become *the* method of choice of the clinical radiologist in the near future. However, a study by Bloch et al [1] indicates that brain tumors always have a higher T2 value than surrounding normal tissue. This is more or less true, except in cases of acute intracerebral hematoma, in which the tumor T2 is decreased [9].

ADVANTAGES AND DISADVANTAGES

Crawley and Henkelman [7] have discussed at length the relative performances of some of the T1 measurement techniques described above in terms of the following figure of merit (FOM):

$$(SI(0) - S(infinity))/(Noise factor \times \sqrt{Acquisition\ time})$$

Using this FOM, they demonstrate that "one shot" methods, such as TOMROP, have efficiency similar to the IR sequence in calculating T1 relaxation time. In addition, TOMROP provides true T1-based image contrast in the brain and excellent differentiation between gray and white matter is achieved.

While many of the newer techniques may decrease T1 measurement time, they have their own limitations, too. As the T1 or T2 values are derived by measuring signal amplitude, any phenomenon that abnormally decreases signal amplitude and/or resolution may adversely affect the derived value. For example, imperfections in the static magnetic field are notorious for lowering the true T2 value [23]. Also, most methods use iterative algorithms for nonlinear data fit, which increase the overall measurement time. In den kleef and Cuppen [15] have proposed a nonlinear noniterative least-square algorithm (RLSQ), which decreases computational time and complexity.

While comparing the T1 and T2 values being reported in the literature, it is important to bear in mind that tissue relaxation times are influenced by the method of measurement (which affects both T1 and T2), field strength (which primarily affects T1) [11,22], diffusion effect (which primarily affects T2) [6], temperature (which affects both T1 and T2) [6], dissolved oxygen concentration (which affects both T1 and T2) [6], and water and collagen content [41]. In a multislice study, the slice interference (when the slice gap is $\leq$ 50% slice thickness) also has been shown to affect the accuracy of measurement of relaxation time [24,44]. In myocardial relaxation time studies, the phase of the cardiac cycle, the heart rate, and the velocity of the cardiac wall have been found to influence the measured T2 [18]. The other concern about relaxation time measurements is how reproducible the results are on a variety of commercial imaging scanners. A study by Breger et al [4] suggests that T1 and T2 values vary by less than 5% over a period of 18 months, despite changeover in imaging software (General Electric Signa, 1.5 T).

The advantage of synthetic imaging is that it allows for retrospective testing of the influence of various imaging parameters on images acquired from a patient. This obviates the need for actually carrying out the imaging experiment repeatedly for different conditions. Moreover, many imaging parameters, such as the use of extremely short TR/TE [30] or variable magnetic field strengths [14,31,33], may not be available at every clinical imaging site.

REFERENCES

1. Bloch P, Lenkinski RE, Buhle EL, Hendrix R, Bryer M, McKenna WG (1991): The use of T2 distribution to study tumor extent and heterogeneity in head and neck cancer. *Magn Reson Imag* 9:205–211.

2. Bobman SA, Riederer SF, Lee JN, Suddarth SA, Wang HZ, MacFall JR (1985): Synthesized MR images: comparison with acquired images. *Radiology* 155:731–738.

3. Bobman SA, Riederer SJ, Lee JN, Tasciyan T, Farzaneh F, Wang HZ (1986): Pulse sequence extrapolation with image synthesis. *Radiology* 159:253–258.

4. Breger RK, Rimm AA, Fischer ME, Papke RA, Haughton VM (1989): T1 and T2 measurements on a 1.5-T commercial MR imager. *Radiology* 171:273–276.

5. Brix G, Schad L, Deimling M, Lorenz W (1990): Fast and precise T1 imaging using a TOMROP sequence. *Magn Reson Imag* 8:351–356.

6. Condon B, Patterson J, Jenkins A, Wyper D, Hadley D, Grant R, Rowan J, Teasdale G (1987): MR relaxation times of cerebrospinal fluid. *J Comput Assist Tomogr* 11:203–207.

7. Crawley AP, Henkelman RM (1988): A comparison of one shot and recovery methods in T1 imaging. *Magn Reson Med* 7:23–34.

8. Damadian R (1971): Tumor detection by nuclear magnetic resonance. *Science* 171:1151–1153.

9. Darwin RH, Drayer BP, Riederer SJ, Wang HZ, MacFall JR (1986): T2 estimates in healthy and diseased brain tissue: a comparison using various MR pulse sequences. *Radiology* 160:375–381.

10. Fram EK, Herfkens RJ, Johnson GA, Glover GH, Karis JP, Shimakawa A, Perkins TG, Pelc NJ (1987): Rapid calculation of T1 using variable flip angle gradient refocused imaging. *Magn Reson Imag* 5:201–208.

11. Gomori JM, Grossman RI, Yu-Ip C, Asakura T (1987): NMR relaxation times of blood: dependence on field strength, oxidation state, and cell integrity. *J Comput Assist Tomogr* 11:684–690.

12. Graumann R, Fischer H, Oppelt A (1986): A new pulse sequence for determining T1 and T2 simultaneously. *Med Phys* 13:644–647.

13. Harvey I, Tofts PS, Morris JK, Wicks DAG, Ron MA (1991): Sources of T1 variance in normal human white matter. *Magn Reson Imag* 9:53–59.

14. Hylton NM, Ortendahl DA (1986): Information processing in magnetic resonance imaging. *Crit Rev Diagn Imag* 26:325–358.

15. In den kleef JJE, Cuppen JJM (1987): RLSQ: T1, T2, and p calculations, combining ratios and least squares. *Magn Reson Med* 5:513–524.

16. Joseph PM, Axel L, O'Donnell M (1984): Potential problems with selective pulses in NMR imaging systems. *Med Phys* 11:772–777.

17. Just M, Higer HP, Schwarz M, Bohl J, Fries G, Pfannenstiel P, Thelen M (1988): Tissue characterization of benign tumors: use of NMR-tissue parameters. *Magn Reson Imag* 6:463–472.

18. Katz J, Boxt LM, Sciacca RR, Cannon PJ (1990): Motion dependence of myocardial transverse relaxation time in magnetic resonance imaging. *Magn Reson Imag* 8:449–458.

19. Kucharczyk W, Brant-Zawadzki M, Lemme-Plaghos L, Uske A, Kjos B, Feinberg DA, Normal D (1985): MR technology: effect of even-echo rephasing on calculated T2 values and T2 images. *Radiology* 157:95–101.

20. Lee JN, Riederer SJ, Bobman SA, Farzaneh F, Wang HZ (1986): Instrumentation for rapid MR image synthesis. *Magn Reson Med* 3:33–43.

21. Lin MS, Fletcher JW, Donati RM (1986): Two-point T1 measurement: wide-

coverage optimizations by stochastic simulations. *Magn Reson Med* 3: 518–533.

22. Lundbom N, Brown RD, Koenig SH, Lansen TA, Valsamis MP, Kasoff SS (1990): Magnetic field dependence of 1/T1 of human brain tumors: correlations with histology. *Invest Radiol* 25:1197–1205.

23. Majumdar S, Orphanoudakis SC, Gmitro A, O'Donnell M, Gore JC (1986): Errors in the measurements of T2 using multiple-echo MRI techniques: II. Effects of static field inhomogeneity. *Magn Reson Med* 3:562–574.

24. Majumdar S, Sostman HD, MacFall JR (1989): Contrast and accuracy of relaxation time measurements in acquired and synthesized multislice magnetic resonance images. *Invest Radiol* 24:119–127.

25. Mansfield P, Guilfoyle DN, Ordidge RJ, Coupland RE (1986): Measurement of T1 by echo-planar imaging and the construction of computer-generated images. *Phys Med Biol* 31:113–124.

26. McVeigh E, Yang A, Zerhouni E (1990): Rapid measurement of T1 with spatially selective pre-inversion pulses. *Med Phys* 17:131–134.

27. Mills CM, Crooks LE, Kaufman L, Brandt-Zamadski M (1984): Cerebral abnormalities: use of calculated T1 and T2 magnetic resonance images for diagnosis. *Radiology* 150:87–94.

28. O'Donnell M, Gore JC, Adams WJ (1986): Toward an automated analysis system for nuclear magnetic resonance imaging: I. Efficient pulse sequences for simultaneous T1-T2 imaging. *Med Phys* 13:182–190.

29. Ordidge RJ, Gibbs P, Chapman B, Stehling MK, Mansfield P (1990): High-speed multislice T1 mapping using inversion-recovery echo-planar imaging. *Magn Reson Med* 16:238–245.

30. Ortendahl DA, Hylton NM, Kaufman L, Crooks LE (1984): Signal-to-noise in derived NMR images. *Magn Reson Med* 1:316–338.

31. Ortendahl DA, Hylton NM, Kaufman L, Watts JC, Crooks LE, Mills CM, Stark DD (1984): Analytical tools for magnetic resonance imaging. *Radiology* 153:479–488.

32. Pope JM, Rapin N (1988): A simple approach to T2 imaging in MRI. *Magn Reson Imag* 6:641–646.

33. Posin JP, Ortendahl DA, Hylton NM, Kaufman L, Watts JC, Crooks LE, Mills CM (1985): Variable magnetic resonance imaging parameters: effect on detection and characterization of lesions. *Radiology* 155:719–725.

34. Prato FS, Drost DJ, Keys T, Laxon P, Commissiong B, Sestini E (1986): Optimization of signal-to-noise ratio in calculated T1 images derived from two spin-echoes images. *Magn Reson Med* 3:63–75.

35. Pykett IL, Rosen BR, Buonanno FS, Brady TJ (1983): Measurement of spin-lattice relaxation times in nuclear magnetic resonance imaging. *Phys Med Biol* 28:723–729.

36. Redpath TW (1982): Calibration of the Aberdeen NMR imager for proton spin-lattice relaxation time measurements in vivo. *Phys Med Biol* 27:1057–1065.

37. Riederer SJ, Suddarth SA, Bobman SA, Lee JN, Wang HZ, MacFall JR (1984): Automated MR image synthesis: feasibility studies. *Radiology* 153:203–206.

38. Riederer SJ, Bobman SA, Lee JN, Farzaneh F, Wang HZ (1986): Improved precision in calculated T1 MR images using multiple spin-echo acquisition. *J Comput Assist Tomogr* 10:103–110.

39. Rosen BR, Pykett IL, Brady TJ (1984): Spin lattice relaxation time measurements in 2D NMR imaging: corrections for plane selection and pulse sequences. *J Comput Assist Tomogr* 8:195–199.

40. Schad LR, Brix G, Zuna I, Harle W, Lorenz WJ, Semmler W (1989): Multiexponential proton spin-spin relaxation in MR imaging of human brain tumors. *J Comput Assist Tomogr* 13:577–587.

41. Scholz TD, Fleagle SR, Burns TL, Shorton DJ (1989): Tissue determinants of nuclear magnetic resonance relaxation times. Effect of water and collagen content in muscle and tendon. *Invest Radiol* 24:893–898.

42. Sperber GO, Ericsson A, Hemmingsson A (1989): A fast method for T1 fitting. *Magn Reson Med* 9:113–117.

43. Wang HZ, Riederer SJ, Lee JN (1987): Optimizing the precision in T1 relaxation estimation using limited flip angles. *Magn Reson Med* 5:399–416.

44. Wong ST, Roos MS (1987): Effects of slice selection and diffusion on T2 measurement. *Magn Reson Med* 5:358–365.

45. Young IR, Hall AS, Bydder GM (1987): The design of a multiple inversion recovery sequence for T1 measurement. *Magn Reson Med* 5:99–108.

24

Magnetization-Prepared Rapid Gradient Echo (MP-RAGE)

BASIC PRINCIPLES

Magnetization-prepared rapid gradient echo (MP-RAGE)-[3] is a volume acquisition technique that uses existing rapid data acquisition pulse sequences. The novelty of this technique lies in the modular nature of the overall imaging experiment.

MP-RAGE can be divided into three distinct modules (Fig. 24.1).

1. During the first module, which is called the magnetization preparation period, the inversion recovery (IR) sequence may be applied to obtain T1 contrast by inverting the longitudinal magnetization of the object [1]. Alternatively, T2 contrast also may be obtained by applying a 90°–180°–90° (DISE) triplet.
2. During the second module, called the acquisition period, any rapid gradient echo sequence, such as FLASH (or its variant, SFI), is applied n times to sample the prepared magnetization. At the end of this period, a selected plane or a part of it (proportional to n) is sampled.
3. In the third module, the magnetization is allowed to recover. The duration of this stage is determined by the tissue T1 value, and the imaging experiment is then repeated, starting with the first module, until data are acquired from the selected three-dimensional spatial volume (k-space).

Overall, the technique is similar to the IR-FLASH approach [1], with the provision that in the MP-RAGE technique, there is a variable waiting period after each cycle of data acquisition.

Total imaging time is determined by the type of pulse sequence employed for data acquisition and the time allowed for recovery of the mag-

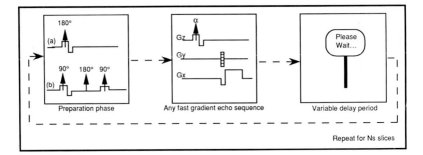

FIG. 24.1 The modular nature of the MP-RAGE approach. During the preparation phase, image contrast may be primed with either T1 **(a)** or T2 **(b)** relaxation. See text for details.

netization. Typically, data acquisition for each image slice takes the time equivalent to the pulse repetition time (TR) multiplied by the number of the phase encoding steps. To this estimate, however, one has to add the time taken for contrast preparation and the recovery period to calculate total imaging time.

See *also*: IR-FLASH.

CLINICAL APPLICATIONS
TISSUE CONTRAST

Tissue contrast depends upon the type of magnetization preparation chosen (see above) and the type of RAGE sequence used to acquire the image data. If the waiting period is relatively long, then each MP-RAGE cycle is effectively decoupled from the previous cycle, and the local perturbations do not become global in nature.

THE BRAIN

Excellent contrast, comparable to T1-weighted SE, between the gray and white matter of the brain has been achieved using this technique (Fig. 24.2). A complete acquisition of head (128 slices, voxel resolution 1.4 mm × 1 mm × 1 mm) in one orientation can be completed in about 6 to 7 minutes using short TR (10 msec) and TE (4.2 msec) with a 10° FLASH sequence. Moreover, magnetic susceptibility artifacts, which frequently arise at or near the interface of the brain mass and the bone, virtually are absent due to extremely short TE.

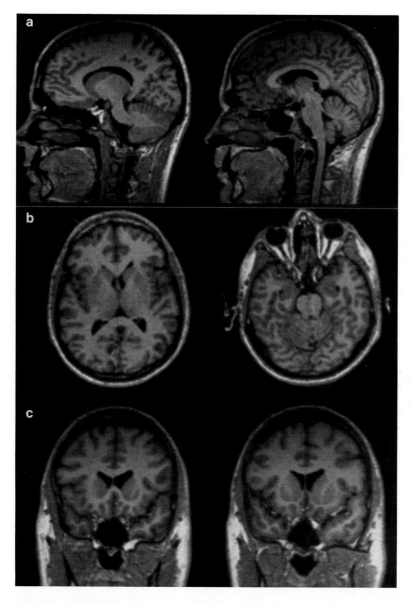

FIG. 24.2 Sagittal acquisition **(a)** reformatted in the transverse **(b)** and coronal **(c)** planes. Magnetization preparation: inversion pulse followed by a 450-msec delay; RAGE acquisition: FLASH (10° excitation; TR = 10 msec; TE = 4 msec). Magnetization recovery: 600 msec. Image matrix; 128 (180 mm) × 128 (250 mm) × 256 (250 mm); effective TR = 2.3 sec; total acquisition time = 5 min. (Courtesy of J. P. Mugler, III; modified, with permission, from Mugler and Brookeman [3].)

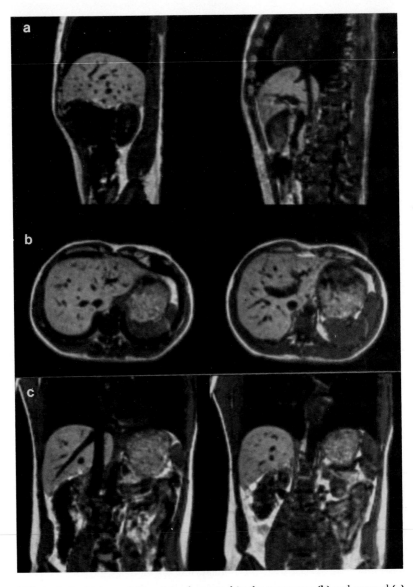

FIG. 24.3 Sagittal acquisition **(a)** reformatted in the transverse **(b)** and coronal **(c)** planes. Magnetization preparation: inversion pulse followed by a 350-msec delay. RAGE acquisition: FLASH (10° excitation; TR = 8 msec; TE = 3.3 msec). Magnetization recovery: 2000 msec. Image matrix: 128 (350 mm) × 128 (350 mm) × 256 (700 mm); effective TR = 3.4 sec; total acquisition time = 3.2 min. (Courtesy of J. P. Mugler, III; modified, with permission, from Mugler and Brookeman [3].)

THE HEART

In principle, it is possible to conduct a cine-MR study of the heart by using cardiac triggered MP-RAGE technique. However, no successful attempt has been reported, so far, to this author's knowledge.

THE ABDOMEN

MP-RAGE has successfully provided complete abdominal three-dimensional MR data sets, devoid of any respiratory artifacts, in about seven minutes (Fig. 24.3). De Lange et al [2] have used the MP-RAGE technique for examining the Morgagni's hernia.

ADVANTAGES AND DISADVANTAGES

Excellent image resolution and contrast are obtained in a fairly short period of time using MP-RAGE. This imaging technique consists of three distinct modules, as outlined above; they are repeated as a group in a periodic manner. Under the control of a proper triggering mechanism, the periodic nature of the sequence can be exploited to obtain three-dimensional image data sets from pulsatile organs, such as the heart, or from stationary organs subject to inadvertent motion, such as the liver, without any significant motion-related artifacts.

REFERENCES

1. Hasse A, Matthaei D, Bartkowski R, Duhmke E, Leibfritz D (1989): Inversion recovery snapshot FLASH MR imaging. *J Comput Assist Tomogr* 13:1036–1040.

2. de Lange EE, Urbanski SR, Mugler JP, Brookeman JR (1990): Magnetization-prepared rapid gradient echo (MP-RAGE) magnetic resonance imaging of Morgagni's hernia. *Eur J Radiol* 11:196–199.

3. Mugler JP, Brookeman JR (1990): Three-dimensional magnetization-prepared rapid gradient-echo imaging (3D MP RAGE). *Magn Reson Med* 15:152–157.

25

Missing Pulse Steady State Free Precession (MP-SSFP)

BASIC PRINCIPLES

Missing pulse steady state free precession (MP-SSFP) is a variant of the more conventional two-dimensional Fourier transform SSFP technique. During the SSFP experiment, if an RF refocused spin echo is desired, this echo would occur at the time when an RF pulse would normally be applied (Fig. 25.1). The advantage of spin echo acquisition is that field inhomogeneities are effectively refocused at the echo time. However, the spin echo cannot be collected at that precise time in its entirety, due to hardware limitations (primarily RF transmitter interference and RF receiver saturation). In Fourier imagining sequences such as FLASH or CE-FAST, therefore, spin echo is transformed into a gradient echo by reversing the readout gradient. However, local magnetic field inhomogeneities—time invariant as well as time varying—are not effectively refocused by the gradient reversal; this results in signal loss. Alternatively, an asymmetric echo acquisition may be performed with some loss in the signal-to-noise ratio.

The general solution to the above problem is to record a spin echo in the absence of the RF pulse, and also to correct simultaneously for field inhomogeneity artifacts. This may be achieved by eliminating RF pulse at some regular interval of time in an SSFP experiment (missing pulse-SSFP, MP-SSFP) and appropriately modifying the imaging gradients [1].

As in an SSFP imaging experiment, a series of equally spaced slice-selective RF pulses is applied to achieve steady state magnetization. However, in MP-SSFP, every third RF pulse is dropped (in general, every nth RF pulse may be dropped; see below). At the time when the dropped pulse normally would have been present, an RF refocused spin echo is

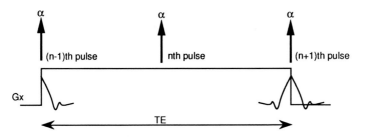

FIG. 25.1 During the SSFP experiment, an RF refocused echo forms at the time when another RF pulse is being applied. Here, the nth RF pulse refocuses the FID following the $(n - 1)$th pulse, just as the $(n + 1)$th pulse is being applied.

formed over a time centered around the missing pulse time, and data acquisition is carried out (Fig. 25.2). Patz et al [1] have theoretically analyzed steady state magnetization and its dependence on interpulse time, interpulse precession angles and the phase, and the angle of RF excitation pulses. As this echo is temporally isolated from RF pulses, it is readily collected by using conventional means.

To understand how field inhomogeneity artifacts are eliminated at the echo time, it is important to realize that such artifacts occur either due to static inhomogeneities (such as local susceptibility changes) or time varying inhomogeneities (such as that due to imaging gradients). In MP-

FIG. 25.2 MP-SSFP pulse sequence, in which every third RF pulse is dropped (indicated by the dashed pulse-gradient complex). (Modified, with permission, from Patz et al [1].)

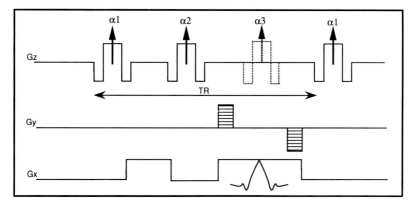

SSFP, the latter are eliminated by keeping the read gradient constant (same direction and amplitude) before and after the spin echo being collected. To eliminate the former, interpulse dephasing of periodic magnetization is made identical for every interpulse interval by appropriately balancing the gradient profiles (see Fig. 25.2).

Variants In syncopated periodic excitation (SPEX), every fourth RF pulse is dropped [3]. Otherwise, the pulse sequence is similar to that in Fig. 25.2.
  See also: SSFP.

CLINICAL APPLICATIONS
TISSUE CONTRAST

Various factors determine the contrast-to-noise ratio of MP-SSFP images. For example, the excitation flip angle (EFA) and the phase of individual RF pulses strongly influence the signal intensity. It has been observed [1] that when the EFA of both RF pulses have identical magnitude and phase (constant phase- or nonphase-cycled case), the pixel intensity is inferior to when the RF pulses have opposite phases (alternate phase or phase-cycled case). However, the phantom studies of Patz et al [1] show that the nonphase-cycled pulse sequence is better for imaging tissues with shorter T1 or T2 values.

As the image contrast depends on the number of RF pulses applied before the dropped pulse, the rank order (n) of the missing pulse also influences image contrast. SPEX images, therefore, would be expected to have different contrast characteristics than MP-SSFP images.

THE KIDNEYS

Perfusion studies of the kidneys provide vital information about the functional status of different regions of the organ. A high-strength main magnetic field is required to obtain high-resolution perfusion images. Unfortunately, local field inhomogeneity artifacts increase with increasing field strengths; commonly employed fast imaging sequences, such as FLASH, are sensitive to these artifacts. MP-SSFP, being insensitive to inhomogeneity artifacts, provides good qualitative assessment (0.3 mm × 0.3 mm) of the cortex and medulla in a fairly short time (about 15 sec for a 128 × 256 image matrix) [4].

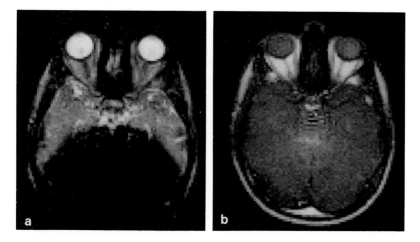

FIG. 25.3 Conventional SSFP (TR = 33.3 msec) **(a)** and MP-SSFP (TR = 33.3 msec; interpulse time = 11.1 msec; every third RF pulse dropped) **(b)** axial images of the head obtained at 0.5 T. A paper clip was placed on the forehead in such a way that the distance between the clip and the imaging plane was 10 cm. The field inhomogeneity insensitivity of the MP-SSFP image is very striking. Also note that the vitreous humor has brighter intensity in **(a)** than in **(b)**; this is due to the reason that MP-SSFP experiences greater loss of signal due to slow flow than the gradient recalled SSFP sequence. (Courtesy of S. Patz; reproduced, with permission, from Patz et al [1].)

ADVANTAGES AND DISADVANTAGES

Unlike the original two-dimensional Fourier transform SSFP, the MP-SSFP technique uses RF refocused spin echo and, therefore, it minimizes the effects of local field inhomogeneities. Because of this, MP-SSFP images obtained in an inhomogeneous magnetic environment (as a result, for example, of metallic prosthesis [2] or widespread areas of hemorrhage) may have fewer artifacts when compared to SSFP images (Fig. 25.3). This advantage becomes more obvious as the main magnetic field strength increases.

The data acquisition rate in MP-SSFP is slower than SSFP technique (by 33% to 75%). Moreover, for the same data sampling rates, MP-SSFP images seem to have less signal intensity than the corresponding SSFP images.

REFERENCES

1. Patz S, Wong STS, Roos MS (1989): Missing pulse steady-state free precession. *Magn Reson Med* 10:194–209.

2. Polak JF, Patz S (1988): Prosthetic cardiac valve imaging: improved performance of missing pulse steady state free precession (MP-SSFP) [abstr]. *Magn Reson Med* 7:S12.

3. Sattin W (1987): Syncopated periodic excitation. *Radiology* 165:S337.

4. Stromski ME, Brady HR, Jakab P, Gullans SR, Patz S. (1989): Imaging of regional renal perfusion using missing pulse steady state free precession (MP-SSFP) [abstr]. *Magn Reson Imag* 7:S26.

26

Multislice Imaging (MUSLIM)

BASIC PRINCIPLES

The feasibility for acquiring multislice MR images was discussed as early as 1977 by Mansfield [17]. His approach was based on the principle of selective excitation and echo planar imaging. In 1984, den Boef et al [6] introduced a three-dimensional Fourier zeumatographic method for obtaining multiple slices. Before discussing multislice imaging in general, let us review how a single slice is obtained and slice characteristics.

A gradient magnetic field establishes a series of planes, each resonating at different Larmor frequencies. The number of such planes is directly proportional to gradient strength (A_G). When an RF field with a frequency range $\pm\omega$ is switched on in the presence of this gradient, only that plane in which the spins resonate at ω is excited. Obviously, the width (thickness, S_{TH}) of the excited slice is determined by the frequency range ($\pm\omega$) of the RF field. In general, the larger the S_{TH}, the greater the signal-to-noise ratio (SNR). A narrowing of $\pm\omega$ decreases S_{TH}. Note that A_G may be increased while keeping the RF frequency the same (Fig. 26.1), achieving the same result. Changes in $\pm\omega$ alter the duration of the RF pulse (a narrower $\pm\omega$ means a larger (longer) pulse). The changing duration of the pulse invariably alters the TE and, therefore, the image contrast [5,11]. In order to prevent the pulse duration from being a variable for image contrast, the gradient amplitude may be modified to achieve thin sections. However, once the maximum gradient amplitude is reached, any further manipulations for obtaining thin sections must consist of narrowing the RF pulse and, thus, the longer RF pulse and the resultant TE penalty. Feinberg et al [11] have discussed the extent to which thin sections may be obtained with adequate signal-to-noise ratio.

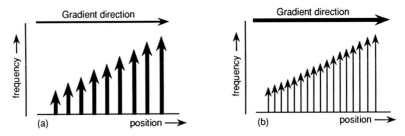

FIG. 26.1 The length of the vertical arrows indicates the Larmor frequency at different spatial locations along the gradient direction; the width of the vertical arrows indicates the thickness of the tissue plane at a given gradient strength (the width of the horizontal arrow). The gradient strength is increased in **(b)** as compared to **(a)**. And, as a result, the resolution along the horizontal position axis has increased. In other words, the width of the tissue slice that can be selectively excited has been effectively decreased.

To change the spatial location of the slice, a fixed offset ($\delta\omega$) is added to (or subtracted from) the RF center frequency ω. In turn, $\delta\omega$ determines the interslice distance (SD), the significance of which will become obvious in the following section. With this scheme, it is simply a matter of sequentially changing the quantity $\delta\omega$ to obtain multiple slices. There are at least two ways in which this may be accomplished (Fig. 26.2): sequential slice propagation (single pass) or alternate slice propagation (two interleaved passes). In the sequential slice propagation approach, the quantity $1 \times \delta\omega$ is added to ω each time ω is incremented (where $1 = 2$ ... number of slices, N). The drawback of this approach is illustrated in Fig. 26.3. To prevent slice interference (see below), either $\delta\omega$ (SD) has to be increased, which decreases N, or $\pm\omega$ has to be decreased, which decreases the signal-to-noise ratio. An alternative approach is to add first the quantity $m \times \delta\omega$, where $m = 3,5,\ldots, N - 1$ and then $n \times \delta\omega$, where $n = 2,4,\ldots N$ (for even N). This is the approach of alternate slice propagation.

In the context of the two-dimensional Fourier transform spin warp imaging sequence, ω is incremented (or decremented) during the pulse repetition time (TR) for the following reason: when the spins in one section

FIG. 26.2 Two approaches for acquiring multiple slices. See text for details.

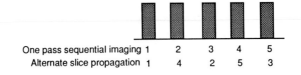

One pass sequential imaging	1	2	3	4	5
Alternate slice propagation	1	4	2	5	3

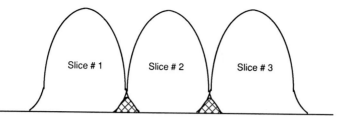

FIG. 26.3 The imperfect slice profile ensures that there is slight overlap (cross-hatched regions) near the edges of the slice if sufficient interslice gap is not allowed.

are relaxing during TR from the previous RF pulse, the spins of the next section can be excited by applying another RF pulse (time multiplexing) [4]. At the end of the TR, the spins are refocused. To keep the TE identical for all the scans, each slice has to be refocused separately. Note that, in this case, the excitatory and refocusing RF pulses must be spatially selective.

Variants   Conventional multislice imaging, as discussed above, is associated with the following inherent limitations.

(A) Clinically, T1-weighted (short TR/TE) and T2-weighted (long TR/TE) multisection studies are performed sequentially. However, any patient movement between studies makes precise anatomic correlation between studies rather difficult. The solution to this problem is to acquire these data sets in an interleaved manner. Farzaneh et al [10] have proposed several pulse sequences with dual pulse repetition times for acquiring both T1- and T2-weighted images in a single run.

(B) The multislice approach discussed above is essentially uniplanar because all the slices are parallel to one another; for example, in a coronal series, all the slices are coronal. However, in certain anatomical areas, such as the cervical or the lumbar spine and the heart, it is often desirable to obtain some slices of a multislice series with a common line of origin (Fig. 26.4). In addition, as the quantity $\delta\omega$ is fixed for one series, S_D also is fixed. Therefore, if more slices are desired in the center of the series than near the ends, it is not possible. While these difficulties may be overcome by extracting slices from a three-dimensional volume data acquisition, the latter requires extended data handling capabilities and may increase total imaging time.

A relatively simple approach, called multiple-angle variable-interval nonorthogonal imaging (MAVIN), has been proposed by Richer et al [26]. As the name suggests, this technique allows multiple slices to be acquired in any plane with varying angles and the interslice distance. In order to achieve this flexibility, it is necessary to rotate conventional imaging

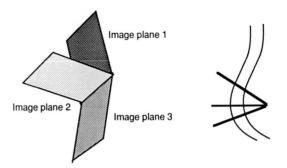

FIG. 26.4 In regions such as the spine, it may be necessary to have multiple imaging planes in nonorthogonal planes. In addition, interslice gap may not be the same throughout the series.

gradients in the logical sense. For a fixed phase encoding gradient in the x direction, the slice-select and frequency encode gradients are rotated by using the following formula [26]:

$$\text{Slice-select gradient} = \cos(\phi)Gy - \sin(\phi)Gz$$

$$\text{Frequency encode gradient} = \cos(\phi)Gz + \sin(\phi)Gy,$$

where Gy and Gz are the conventional directions of the gradients. Note that the interslice gap is indirectly varied by changing the angle ϕ. In order to rotate the gradients sensibly, one should know how three imaging planes normally are defined. Almost universally, the long axis of the gradient (superioinferior) is called z, the anteroposterior direction is called y, and the right-to-left direction is called x. Depending on the individual examination, the functions of slice select, phase encoding, and frequency encoding can be performed along any of these directions. A pictorial article by Slone et al [28] describes this procedure well.

(C) In conventional MR imaging, multiple slices are obtained by time-interleaving RF excitation during the pulse repetition time TR (Fig. 26.5). Therefore, the number of slices in one series is restricted by the effective TR. In general, the minimum number of slices that can be obtained is TR/TE; the maximum number of slices that may be obtained is TR/t, where t = total time for which the RF and the gradients are on. To obtain more slices per TR, two different approaches have been proposed: use of multiple coils and use of multispectral RF pulses.

Multiple coil approach: In order to image two different anatomical regions, such as the shoulders, two surface coils are employed. During the TR of the first coil, the second coil excites the corresponding region.

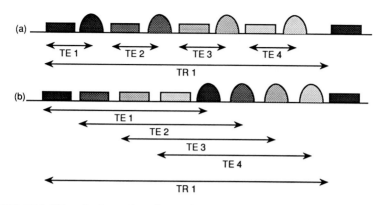

FIG. 26.5 RF excitation and readout pulses (rectangular areas) for multiple slices are intermingled in such a way that during the pulse repetition time TR, many slices can be excited. However, careful attention has to be paid for proper collection of the echoes at their respective echo times. Two permutations are shown **(a)** for short TE; **(b)** for long TE.

These two coils should be mutually uncoupled [13,15], and appropriate changes in the signal receiving software have to be made.

Multispectral RF pulses: The RF excitation pulse is, usually, made up of a single center frequency spectrum and, when applied in the presence of a slice-selective gradient, excites only a specific region of the sample. Most commonly, a sinc shaped RF pulse is used because of near-rectangular slice profile. This sinc function, sin(t)/t, is multiplied by a complex exponential $(i2\pi\gamma GPt)$ [29] to excite a slice located at P offset in the direction of the gradient G (γ = gyromagnetic ratio; t = time). This process may be repeated for any physical offset for any multiple of slices.

It is also possible to compose an RF pulse that can excite two or more slices simultaneously. Such multispectral RF pulses are called *simultaneous multislice frequency excitation* (SIMUFREX) [24], and the corresponding multislice technology is called the *simultaneous multislice acquisition* (SIMA) [29] or *simultaneous multislice imaging* (SIMUSIM) [23–25].

Note that a complex exponential number consists of a real (cosine) term and an imaginary (sine) term. Therefore, a very different situation arises if only one of the terms is multiplied to the sinc function. For example, for (sin (t)/t) $\times$ cos (Pt), two slices located P distance on either side of the gradient isocenter are excited *in phase;* for (sin (t)/t) $\times$ $-$sin (Pt), the same two slices are excited *out of phase* (Fig. 26.6) [29]. By changing P or multiplying the sinc function by additional exponential terms, more slices located at varying offsets can be excited simultaneously. Based on

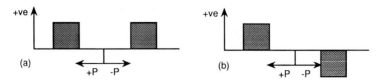

FIG. 26.6 Simultaneous excitation of two slices, located at P distance from the gradient isocenter: **(a)** in-phase; **(b)** out of phase.

this method of SIMUFREX, two different approaches have been extended for SIMUSIM (or SIMA).

In the approach proposed by Muller [23–25] and Souza et al [29], both in-phase and out-of-phase excitations are used sequentially. A subtraction of these data sets yields an image of a slice located at −P offset; an addition of the data sets yields an image of a slice located at +P offset (Fig. 26.7). Note that the intensity of each image is increased by a factor of two (in general, by a factor corresponding to the number of data sets). A similar approach for multiple line scanning has been used by Maudsley [21].

The above approach requires mathematical processing of the data for extracting separate images from the acquired data sets. The complexity of the encoding and decoding of multiple slices increases as the number of slices grows larger. Therefore, two different approaches have been proposed which do not require elaborate data processing.

In the approach by Weaver [30], only an in-phase multiple excitation scheme is used. As each excitation excites all the slices, the echo contains information from all the slices at that phase encoding level. In order to separately identify these different spatial components, the echo is collected in the presence of the slice-select (Gs) and the frequency encode gradients (Gr) (Fig. 26.8). (Just as the combination of the slice-select gradient/SIMUFREX RF pulse selects different planes simultaneously during

FIG. 26.7 On subtraction of (b) from (a) (Fig. 26.6), only the slice magnetization located at −P offset remains. On addition of (a) and (b) (Fig. 26.6), only the slice magnetization located at +P offset remains. Note that the signal amplitude of the remaining slice is increased as a result of this addition–subtraction procedure.

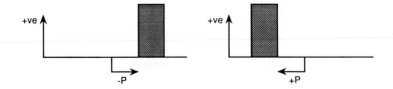

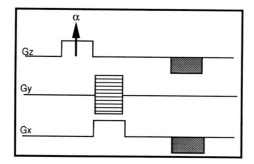

FIG. 26.8 Modified FLASH sequence for simultaneous multislice imaging. Note that both the slice-select and the frequency-encode gradients are on (shaded areas) at the echo time. (Modified, with permission, from S. Muller [24].)

the excitation, the combination of the slice-select gradient and a multi-frequency echo gives a frequency offset to the signal component from each slice.) The image reconstruction algorithm then correctly separates the individual slices and all are displayed in a single image side-by-side, provided that Gs × P ≥ Gr × Field of view (FOV). If this condition is not met, individual slices are overlapped (Fig. 26.9).

In phase offset mutiplanar imaging (POMP), the RF excitation pulse is modulated depending on the phase value (ky) and the desired offset

FIG. 26.9 Recall that in the technique proposed by Weaver, all the slices appear side-by-side in a *single* image. **(a)** Given sufficient field of view, there is no overlap among the slices. However, if the field of view is decreased beyond a certain point, considerable overlap may occur in the final image **(b)**.

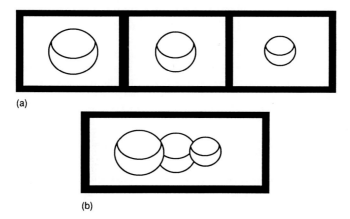

(a)

(b)

(P) of the image, sin (t)/t $\times$ exp(ikyP) [12]. Once again, multiple slices are reconstructed by this approach in a single image within the limits of the image FOV.

(D) As noted while discussing the MAVIN technique above, multiple slices also may be obtained retrospectively from a three-dimensional data acquisition.

(E) Frequency-selective excitation has been the mainstay of conventional MR imaging (including multislice imaging); however, the slice profile obtained seldom is rectangular. It has been shown that the slice profile can be significantly improved by optimizing the selective RF pulses [19]; however, such techniques usually require higher RF power. The method of Conolly et al [2], variable rate selective excitation (VERSE),[1] alleviates this problem by modifying the gradient waveform and RF field in such a way that a better slice profile is achieved, for a given pulse width, without increasing the RF peak amplitude. Mao et al [20] have proposed an alternative technique based upon the conjugate gradient method [18] to produce a better slice profile for a given gradient value, without increasing RF amplitude. On the contrary, their technique makes it possible to decrease the pulse width, which makes its implementation much faster.

CLINICAL APPLICATIONS
TISSUE CONTRAST

In general, the tissue contrast and spatial resolution of multislice images are comparable to those of single slice acquisition. However, if there is considerable overlap of the slices, then the overall intensity of the images is somewhat decreased. In addition, the off resonance effects may further decrease image contrast by the mechanism known as magnetization transfer contrast (MTC) [9,.31]. Dixon et al [7] have studied the effect of MTC on multislice imaging and found an approximate 10% to 20% decrease in the brain gray and white matter intensities as compared fat and water.

As noted above, in the SIMUSIM approach, the intensity of the images is increased due to inherent data averaging. The latter also helps to reduce flow artifacts [24].

---

[1] This is different from VARSE (variable rate spin echo) [33], which is a spin echo imaging technique for obtaining T2-weighted images at a faster rate. The VARSE imaging employs conventional long TR (2000 msec) and long TE (80 msec) values for acquiring the central phase encode values; however, the higher order phase encode steps are acquired with fairly shorter TR and TE values, which decreases the overall imaging time. As the central phase encode steps determine the image contrast, the resultant VARSE image is T2 weighted.

MULTIPLANAR IMAGING

In multiplanar imaging, the restriction of slice parallelism is removed and one way of performing a multiplanar acquisition (MAVIN) was discussed above. Such multiplanar acquisition helps to obtain diagnostic quality images of complex anatomical regions such as the spine (see below). Recently, a new application of multiplanar imaging has been discussed by several investigators [1,32]. In this approach, two or more orthogonal planes are sequentially excited within a period of time much less than the tissue T1. Therefore, the spins lying at the intersection of the planes receive multiple excitations and remain saturated. (Note the similarity to the approach of creating stripes by Zerhouni et al; see NIMAT.) Depending on the number (N) of the planes excited, N-1 stripes appear across the images (Fig. 26.10). The location of these stripes on the images aids in localizing various regions, and thus are very useful as scout images.

THE BRAIN

Muller has obtained highly detailed brain views using SIMUSIM and the snapshot FLASH sequence in a very short period of time (Fig. 26.11) [25].

THE SPINE

The normal anatomical curvature of the spine, particularly in the cervical and lumbar regions, makes it highly desirable to obtain a multislice axial series in which at least one slice is cutting across each vertebra or the disk in its entirety [22]. Using the MAVIN technique, Reicher et al [27]

FIG. 26.10 (a) The volume of interest is preexcited in the transverse and sagittal planes. When a coronal data acquisition is performed on this volume, two stripes, as shown in **(b)**, appear across the image plane.

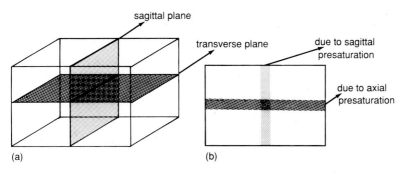

sagittal plane

transverse plane

due to sagittal presaturation

due to axial presaturation

(a)   (b)

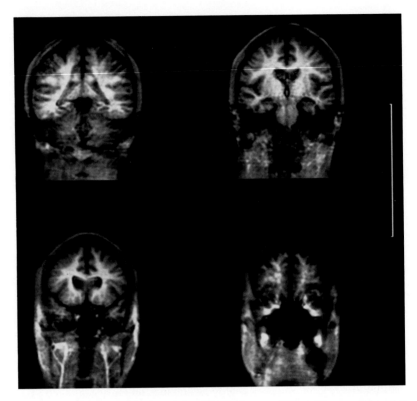

FIG. 26.11 Four coronal IR-snapshot FLASH images (TR = 10 msec; TE = 4.9 msec; TI = 300 msec; 10 mm slice thickness with 10 mm interslice gap; 128 phase encode × 256; total acquisition time 6 sec) obtained using SIMUSLIM technique. (Courtesy of S. Muller; reproduced, with permission, from S. Muller [23–25].)

have demonstrated the usefulness of simultaneous oblique and parallel slices in evaluating spinal pathologies.

THE HEART

Muller also has demonstrated the usefulness of his approach in simultaneously obtaining multiple cardiac slices [24]. When employed in the triggered form, such images offer the advantage of observing several different regions of the heart at the same time.

ADVANTAGES AND DISADVANTAGES

Almost all present clinical studies are performed in a multislice mode. In general, simultaneous multislice acquisition technology offers the following advantages over conventional multislice imaging:

1. The number of slices available for multislice imaging is not limited by the repetition time (TR) of the imaging sequence.
2. If the acquisition is triggered by a physiologic parameter, all slices of interest can be measured at the same point in time.

If enough interslice gap is not allowed, slice interference, as shown in Fig. 26.3, results, which degrades the signal-to-noise ratio, and gives rise to a stimulated echo artifact [3]. Furthermore, the contrast of the T2-weighted image decreases [16]. These altered image characteristics have been found to alter relaxation time measurements [14].

The facility for acquiring some oblique slices in an otherwise conventional series (MAVIN) saves imaging time by eliminating the need for performing two separate acquisitions in different planes. Furthermore, Edelman et al [8] showed that motion artifacts may be effectively pushed out of the region of interest by rotating the direction of the gradient along which such artifacts appear.

Like three-dimensional Fourier transform volume imaging, phase errors in any one slice give rise to artifacts in all the slices, as the data for all slices are acquired during each excitation. However, unlike three-dimensional Fourier transform techniques, the slices do not have to be either contiguous or of similar thickness.

Some consideration has to be given to imaging hardware, such as the transmitter linearity and receiving bandwidth [29]; but otherwise, the implementation of the SIMUSIM technique is relatively straightforward.

REFERENCES

1. Boesch CH, Martin E (1990): Application of interlaced orientation slices in orthogonal planes for system characterization and as a basis of standardized brain sections in multiple-oblique positions. *Magn Reson Med* 15:357–371.

2. Conolly S, Nishimura D, Macovski A (1988): Variable-rate selective excitation. *J Magn Reson* 78:440–458.

3. Crawley AP, Henkelman RM (1987): A stimulated echo artifact from slice interference in MRI. *Med Phys* 14:842–848.

4. Crooks LE, Orthendahl DA, Kaufman L, Hoenninger J, Arakawa M, Watts J, Cannon C, Brant-Zawadzki M, Davis PL, Margulis AR (1983): Clinical efficiency of nuclear magnetic resonance imaging. *Radiology* 146:123–128.

5. Crooks LE, Watts J, Hoenninger J, Arakawa M, Kaufman L, Guenther H, Feinberg D (1985): Thin-section definition in magnetic resonance imaging: technical concepts and their implementation. *Radiology* 154:463–467.

6. den Boef JH, van Uijen CMJ, Holzscherer CE (1984): Multiple-slice NMR imaging by three-dimensional Fourier zeumatography. *Phys Med Biol* 29:857–862.

7. Dixon WT, Engels H, Castillo M, Sardashti M (1990): Incidental magnetization transfer contrast in standard multislice imaging. *Magn Reson Img* 8:417–422.
8. Edelman RR, Stark DD, Saini S, Ferrucci JT, Dinsmore RE, Ladd W, Brady TJ (1986): Oblique planes of section in MR imaging. *Radiology* 159:807–810.
9. Eng J, Ceckler TL, Balaban RS (1991): Quantitative ¹H magnetization transfer imaging in vivo. *Magn Reson Med* 17:304–314.
10. Farzaneh F, Riederer SJ, Djang WT, Cumes JT, Herfkens RJ (1988): Efficient pulse sequences for multisection dual-repetition time MR image acquisition. *Radiology* 167:541–546.
11. Feinberg DA, Crooks LE, Hoenninger JC, Watts JC, Arakawa M, Chang H, Kaufman L (1986): Contiguous thin multisection MR imaging by two-dimensional Fourier transform techniques. *Radiology* 158:811–817.
12. Glover GH, Shimakawa A (1988): POMP (phase offset multi-planar) imaging: a new high efficiency technique [abstr]. Seventh Annual Meeting of the Society of Magnetic Resonance in Medicine, San Francisco, 1988, p. 241.
13. Hyde JS, Jesmanowicz A, Froncisz W, Kneeland JB, Grist TM (1986): Parallel image acquisition from noninteracting local coils. *J Magn Reson* 70:512–517.
14. Kneeland JB, Shimakawa A, Wehrli FW (1986): Effect of intersection spacing on MR image contrast and study time. *Radiology* 158:819–822.
15. Kneeland JB, Jesmanowicz A, Hyde JS (1988): Enhancement of parallel MR image acquisition by rotation of the plane of section. *Radiology* 166:886–887.
16. Kucharczyk W, Crawley AP, Kelly WM, Henkelman RM (1988): Effect of multislice interference on image contrast in T2- and T1-weighted MR images. *Am J Neuroradiol* 9:443–451.
17. Mansfield P (1977): Multi-planar image formation using NMR spin echoes. *J Phys C: Solid State Phys* 10:L55–L58.
18. Mao J, Mareci TH, Scott TN, Andrew ER (1986): Selective inversion radiofrequency pulses by optimal control. *J Magn Reson* 70:310–318.
19. Mao J, Mareci TH, Andrew ER (1988): Experimental study of optimal selective 180° radiofrequency pulses. *J Magn Reson* 79:1–10.
20. Mao J, Yan H, Fitzsimmons JR (1990): Slice profile improvement for a clinical MRI system. *Magn Reson Imag* 8:767–770.
21. Maudsley AA (1980): Multiple-line-scanning spin density imaging. *J Magn Reson* 41:112–126.
22. Modic MT, Masaryk TJ, Ross JS, Mulopulos GP, Bundschuh CV, Bohlman H (1987): Cervical radiculopathy: value of oblique MR imaging. *Radiology* 163:227–231.
23. Muller S (1988): Multifrequency selective RF pulses for multislice MR imaging. *Magn Reson Med* 6:364–371.
24. Muller S (1989): Simultaneous multislice imaging (SIMUSIM) for improved cardiac imaging. *Magn Reson Med* 10:145–155.
25. Muller S (1990): Multislice snapshot FLASH using SIMUSIM. *Magn Reson Med* 15:497–500.
26. Reicher MA, Lufkin RB, Smith S, Flannigan B, Olsen R, Wolf R, Hertz D, Winter J, Hanafee W (1986): Multiple-angle, variable-interval, nonorthogonal MRI. *Am J Roentgen* 147:363–366.

27. Reicher MA, Gold RH, Halbach VV, Rauschning W, Wilson GH, Lufkin RB (1986): MR imaging of the lumbar spine: anatomic correlations and the effects of technical variations. *Am J Roentgen* 147:891–898.

28. Slone RM, Buck LL, Fitzsimmons JR (1986): Varying gradient angles and offsets to optimize imaging planes in MR. *Radiology* 158:531–536.

29. Souza SP, Szumowski J, Dumoulin CL, Plewes DP, Glover G (1988): SIMA: simultaneous multislice acquisition of MR images by Hadamard-encoded excitation. *J Comput Assist Tomogr* 12:1026–1030.

30. Weaver JB (1988): Simultaneous multislice acquisition of MR images. *Magn Reson Med* 8:275–284.

31. Wolff SD, Balaban RS (1989): Magnetization transfer contrast (MTC) and tissue water proton relaxation in vivo. *Magn Reson Med* 10:135–144.

32. Wright SM, Wright RM (1988): A multiphase scout sequence using FLASH imaging. *Magn Reson Imag* 6:105–112.

33. Butts RK, Farzaneh F, Riederer SJ, Rydberg JN, Grimm RC (1991): T2-weighted spin-echo pulse sequence with variable repetition and echo times for reduction of MR image acquisition time. *Radiology* 180:551–556.

27

Navigator Echo Imaging (NAVEC)

BASIC PRINCIPLES

Motion-related artifacts can be classified into two broad categories: artifacts caused by intraview (excitation-readout time lapse) spin displacement and artifacts caused by interview (excitation to excitation time interval) spin displacement. Intraview motion artifacts can be decreased by reducing pulse repetition time (TR) or, more specifically, by reducing echo time (TE). GMN and fast imaging techniques such as echo planar or FLASH mainly decrease intraview motion artifacts. To decrease interview artifacts that occur frequently multislice two-dimensional Fourier transform spin-warp imaging, schemes such as phase reordering of the data (ROPE) or gating (respiratory or cardiac) are employed, which decouple the periodicity of motion from the phase encoding process. In yet another approach, a class of motion rejection techniques (such as SLO-MOTION) exist, in which motion causing data is excluded from the final image reconstruction.

Alternatively, motion-induced image artifacts can be eliminated by implementing appropriate correction methods using motion causing data as a reference model. Some of these methods have been outlined in discussions of retrospective gating (MEGA, see Gating). Here, an adaptive method, the navigator echo imaging (NAVEC), is introduced, which corrects for intraview motion-induced phase shifts as well as interview spin displacement [1]. To accomplish this goal, NAVEC imaging adopts a two-pronged approach: it characterizes the motion by acquiring a special echo and, later on, this echo is used to introduce appropriate correction factors in the image reconstruction algorithm.

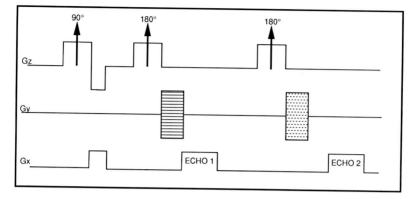

FIG. 27.1 Two-dimensional Fourier transform double spin echo sequence. Here, the first echo is phase encoded for image reconstruction. Alternatively, the second echo may be phase encoded (dashed gradient lobe). In either case, the nonphase encoded echo gives a measure of intraview and interview motion. (Modified, with permission, from R.L. Ehman and J.P. Felmlee [1].)

As shown in Fig. 27.1, a pair of interleaved echoes is obtained by using an otherwise conventional pulse sequence such as the double echo spin echo sequence (any other pulse sequence also may be used).

THE STAGE OF MOTION DETECTION AND MEASUREMENT

As the first echo is obtained without any phase encoding, it gives a projection of the spins along the read gradient. If motion has occurred in this direction during two successive pulse cycles, the spin density projection would vary from one view to another. To calculate this displacement (Δx), a cross-correlation function is obtained for each phase encoding view with one of the navigator echo projections as a reference; the maxima of each function gives the Δx. Similarly, Δy can be obtained by changing the direction of the gradient.

The intraview motion phase shifts the echo and this phase shift can be determined by subtracting the phase angle of the echo obtained in the absence of motion from the phase angle of the echo obtained in the presence of motion. Thus, the first echo serves as a monitor for the motion. By changing the direction of the read gradient, motion along any direction may be monitored.

THE STAGE OF MOTION CORRECTION

The second echo is obtained after switching on the phase encoding gradient so that an image of the object may be derived. The image reconstruction algorithm is properly modified in order to correct for motion. In brief, the algorithm shifts the projected spin density to account for interview motion and it phase rotates the echo to account for intraview motion. In a more general case of the three-dimensional model of the motion, the following formulas give correction phase shifts for interview motion [1,2]:

$$\Delta\phi x = 2\pi\Delta x \, [j - (Nx - 1)/2]Nx^{-1}$$

$$\Delta\phi y = 2\pi\Delta y \, [k - (Ny - 1)/2]Ny^{-1}$$

$$\Delta\phi z = 2\pi\Delta z \, [l - (Nz - 1)/2]Nz^{-1}$$

where Nx is the total number of echo samples; Ny and Nz are the total phase encode steps in two directions; and j, k, and l are the indexes of Nx, Ny, and Nz, respectively. In the case of intraview motion, complex image data are simply phase-rotated by an angle opposite to that obtained during the detection stage. To derive the new pixel value, the old pixel value is multiplied by $\exp(-i\Delta\phi)$, where $D\phi$ is the total phase correction factor for both intraview and interview motion. (Note the similarity to the equation given in the chapter on magnetic resonance fluoroscopy regarding correction for linear motion.)

Thus, the first echo also "navigates" the adaptive algorithm for correct image reconstruction.

See also: MAST, retrospective gating in Gating, ROPE, SLO-MOTION.

CLINICAL APPLICATIONS
TISSUE CONTRAST

The nature of the image echo, and thus the type of pulse sequence, determines image contrast. Note that before the correction for motion, image quality may not be optimum, depending on the degree of motion-induced artifacts.

THE ABDOMEN

The most useful application of the technique may be in the abdominal region, where motion frequently renders images clinically incompetent.

ADVANTAGES AND DISADVANTAGES

Respiratory or cardiac gating is not required for eliminating motion artifacts and, therefore, no additional hardware in the form of sensors or other electronics is needed. Even though the data acquisition time is not increased, this approach requires considerable post-processing of data, which may require additional computer resources and may increase the total time of the study.

REFERENCES

1. Ehman RL, Felmlee JP (1989): Adaptive technique for high-definition MR imaging of moving structures. *Radiology* 173:255–263.
2. Korin HW, Felmlee JP, Ehman RL, Riederer SJ (1990): Adaptive technique for three-dimensional MR imaging of moving structures. *Radiology* 177:217–221.

28

Noninvasive Image Tagging (NIMAT)

BASIC PRINCIPLES

In the past, it was necessary to implant a radiopaque marker directly on the cardiac wall so that individual components of the moving wall could be identified as such accurately on a series of x-ray images [6]. The invasiveness of this procedure made the idea of a noninvasive procedure highly attractive. Moreover, a noninvasive procedure also can be used for other flowing structures such as the cerebrospinal fluid and blood.

The following different approaches have been suggested for producing such noninvasive tissue markers in MRI.

1. *Preinversion pulses*: If the spins of a plane are excited by a 180° RF pulse, their magnetization vector comes to lie parallel with the $-z$ axis. Later on, if a 90° RF pulse is applied in a plane perpendicular to the inverted plane, no transverse magnetization is excited from the spins lying in the inverted plane. Therefore, a line of signal void appears where the imaging plane and the inverted plane coincide (Fig. 28.1). This approach was first proposed by Zerhouni et al [10].

    The inverted planes usually are situated radially around a common line of origin, which is parallel either to the long axis or the short axis of the heart. As the tags persist for only about 400 to 500 msec [4], they have to be reapplied each time the pulse sequence is repeated. Recently, McVeigh and Zerhouni [8] have used multispectral RF pulses (see MUSLIM) to tag several planes simultaneously (Fig. 28.2).

2. *Spatial modulation of magnetization*: A pair of nonselective RF pulses (a composite RF pulse also may be used) separated by a gradient pulse is applied prior to the imaging pulse sequence (Fig. 28.3). While the first RF pulse flips longitudinal magnetization by a degree equal

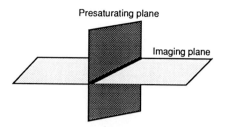

FIG. 28.1 Spins located at the intersection of the presaturating and imaging planes receive multiple RF pulses. As a result, they do not recover rapidly and show up as a line of signal void (black line in the figure).

to the pulse flip angle, the gradient pulse modulates the phase of the resultant transverse magnetization. The following RF pulse (usually of 90° flip angle) returns the magnetization to the z-axis; however, the longitudinal magnetization is now modulated due to previously phase modulated transverse magnetization. When the image is recon- structed, this phase modulation appears as a pattern of parallel bands of alternate intensities. This approach of *spatially modulating* the magnetization (SPAMM) was first proposed by Axel and Dougherty [1,2].

If another such pulse sequence is applied in the direction orthogonal to the first pulse sequence, a grid of bands may be produced. The points of the line intersections appear as if beads were embedded in the myocardium.

3. *Generalized Interferography (GIN)*: It is helpful to review the Fourier shift theorem in order to understand how the technique of interfer- ography produces image stripes. The Fourier shift theorem states that the Fourier transform (FT) of two identical but time shifted signals is a waveform in which one of the signals is superimposed with a mod- ulation, where the time shift determines the frequency of modulation. If the second signal also is phase shifted (ϕ) with respect to the first signal, the modulation is now shifted by the same phase shift ϕ from the previous (time shifted case only) modulation waveform (Fig. 28.4).

To implement this method for two-dimensional Fourier transform MR imaging, two echoes in close temporal proximity, but with dif- ferent phase influences, are elicited by a proper combination of RF and gradient pulses (Fig. 28.5). If a single image is created using these time and phase shifted echoes, the modulation appears across the image plane. This approach for creating stripes on MR images was first proposed by Hennig [5].

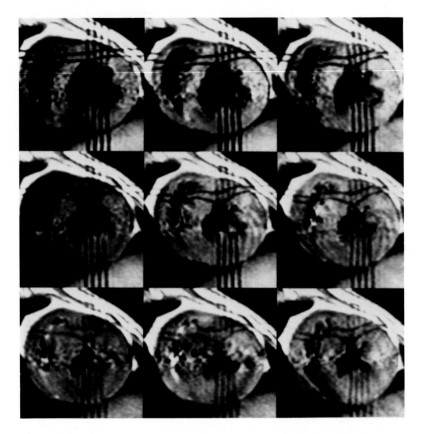

FIG. 28.2 Series of nine systolic cardiac images tagged with multispectral RF pulses beginning at 25 msec after the R wave and every 30 msec thereafter (tag separation 4 mm; 4 averages; total acquisition time 46 min). (Courtesy of E.R. McVeigh and E.A Zerhouni; reproduced, with permission, from E.R. McVeigh and E.A. Zerhouni [8].)

Variants   (A) As illustrated in the Fig. 28.6a, the SPAMM approach yields a pattern of implanted beads in the myocardium. When the technique of preinversion is applied concomitantly with the SPAMM technique (Fig. 28.7), these beads appear only in the inverted plane (Fig. 28.6b). More importantly, now the beads are radially organized. This approach has been called striped *tags* (STAG) [3]. Fig. 28.8 shows a STAG image.

(B) In a simple modification of the original SPAMM sequence, the two RF pulses are substituted by a series of RF pulses whose amplitudes fol-

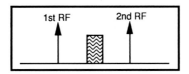

FIG. 28.3 The first RF pulse creates transverse magnetization, as usual. The following gradient pulse modulates the phase of this transverse magnetization, which is returned to the longitudinal axis by the second RF pulse. The magnetization "remembers" the previous phase modulation, and the final image shows the stripes corresponding to the nature of the modulation.

low the binomial distribution (Fig. 28.9) [2]. Between two adjacent RF pulses, a gradient pulse of identical strength is introduced, the purpose of which is to introduce phase modulation. The absolute amplitude of the RF pulses determines the amplitude (intensity) of the stripes, while the stripe width is directly proportional to gradient strength. This modification of SPAMM does not require separate pulse sequences and produces a grid of thinner and crisper stripes, which improves image quality.

(C) Usually, all of the above approaches use cardiac triggering and, after a fixed delay following the R wave, the pulse sequence is applied. However, this prevents data acquisition during the early part of the sys-

FIG. 28.4 **(a)** Two signals with identical phase shifts, S1 and S2, are time shifted. Their Fourier transform is illustrated **(b)**. If these signals are now phase shifted **(c)**, their Fourier transform also is phase shifted **(d)** from that shown in (b).

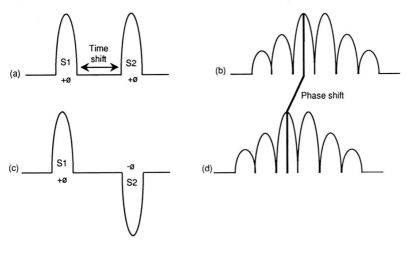

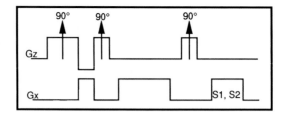

FIG. 28.5 Three 90° pulses produce a spin echo (S1) and a stimulated echo (S2). Obviously, these echoes have differential phase sensitivities to the flow. Therefore, an interferographic image is created by superimposing the data sets corresponding to these echoes. See also Fig. 28.10.

tole. Pearlman and Reese [9] have proposed a tagging pulse sequence in which the tagging occurs before the RF pulse, which allows data acquisition to be performed during the early systole.

(D) In his original article, Hennig suggested a variety of different interferographic pulse sequences for diverse clinical applications ranging from the mapping of field inhomogeneities to flow imaging [5]. Fig. 28.10 shows a cross-section of the heart obtained using one of the variants, the generalized interferography of the spin echo and the stimulated echo (GINSEST).

See also: DOPE.

FIG. 28.6 (a) The SPAMM approach yields a pattern of "beads" across the myocardium (shaded area). These beads actually are the points of intersection of the grid pattern. However, they are located at a variable distance from the endocardial surface. When the SPAMM technique is implemented along with presaturation, these beads are restricted to the planes of the saturation (**(b)**, the arrows). This appearance facilitates the measurement of the transmural thickness in addition to the radial strain.

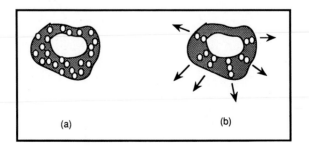

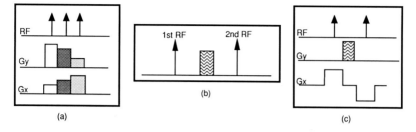

FIG. 28.7 (a) Series of three section-selective RF pulses used to generate three preinversion planes. The locations of these planes are determined by a combination of the y and x gradients. (b) This SPAMM approach generates sinusoidal magnetization over the entire selected plane. The signal from the unwanted transverse magnetization may be canceled by using a spoiler gradient pulse (not shown) after the magnetization is returned to the longitudinal plane by the second RF pulse. (c) In the STAG approach, the sinusoidal pattern is generated only in the preinverted planes. The two 90° RF pulses are applied, first, in-phase, and then out-of-phase. Once again, any unwanted transverse magnetization may be destroyed by a spoiler gradient pulse (not shown). In either approach, the tagging sequence is followed by the imaging sequence. (In this illustration, Gy and Gx do not indicate phase encoding and frequency encoding in the usual sense; they merely indicate two different spatial directions.)

FIG. 28.8 Two STAG images (128 phase encode × 256; 2 averages; total time 25 min per image), obtained 90 msec apart. The heart contracts ongoing from (a) to (b). The tagged lines cross each other at the long axis of the heart on these short axis views. Notice that the beads separate more near the endocardial surface than the epicardial surface, which indicates the transmural dependence of the myocardial thickening during contraction. (Courtesy of E.R. McVeigh and E.A. Zerhouni; reproduced, with permission, from Bolster et al [3].)

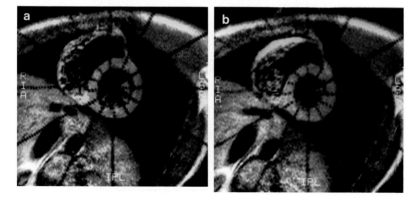

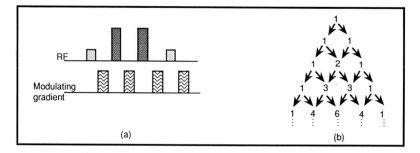

FIG. 28.9 (a) This method for spatially modulating longitudinal magnetization uses a series of RF pulses which follow the binomial distribution (see **(b)** (in this illustration, 1-3-3-1). The modulating gradient, as shown, is applied in two orthogonal directions to create a grid of intersecting lines.

CLINICAL APPLICATIONS
TISSUE CONTRAST

While basic image contrast is not influenced by any of the above techniques, image appearance certainly is altered. For example, SPAMM images show parallel, alternating bands of dark and bright regions. The direction of these bands is determined by the direction of the modulating

FIG. 28.10 MR-interferogram using the GINSEST technique. The image shows a short axis view through the left ventricle of a healthy volunteer during systole (146 msec after R wave). (Courtesy of J. Hennig; reproduced, with permission, from J. Hennig [5].)

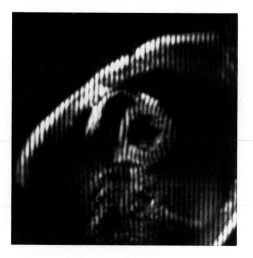

gradient (usually perpendicular to the gradient axis). The width of these bands is directly proportional to the gradient strength and duration.

CEREBROSPINAL FLUID

Any displacement of the bands suggests an abnormality in the motion. Thus, a tumor blocking free CSF flow deforms the bands. However, correct localization of the tumor itself becomes difficult due to the presence of bands and the reduced contrast-to-noise ratio of the images. The DOPE method of MR-myelography is based upon the interferographic principle (see DOPE).

THE HEART

Using various pattern-producing techniques as discussed above, it is possible to successfully track various parts of the myocardium during a cardiac cycle. Such noninvasive tracking may facilitate assessment and differential diagnoses of cardiac motion abnormalities, myocardial wall deformations, and differentiation of static structures from flowing structures. Buchalter et al [4] have measured the torsion and shear strain of left ventricular motion in normal volunteers. Such a database invariably will aid in the understanding of cardiac rhythm abnormalities and the failing heart. In a recent article, McVeigh and Zerhouni [8] have further characterized transmural myocardial strain by using high resolution thin stripes.

THE BLOOD

Flowing blood is demonstrated by the presence of bands curving in the direction of the flow. However, turbulent or nonlaminar flow (for example, near the stenosed valve) may deform the placement of the bands. A thrombus may be identified from flowing blood because the latter usually does not have well-defined stripes [1].

Note that the technique of producing stripes using the preinversion principle has been used for the measurement of T1 relaxation time (see MORT) [7].

ADVANTAGES AND DISADVANTAGES

The original preinversion method of myocardial tagging provides a starlike placement of bands in the imaging plane. Any torsion abnormality (axis disorder) of the ventricular mass alters this starlike pattern and, consequently, may be correctly identified. However, it fails to track alterations in the thickness of the muscular wall itself. Such transmural alterations frequently occur in cases of ventricular hypertrophy or post-ischemic fibrosis.

SPAMM partially corrects this problem by placing a grid of bands across the entire image plane. The relative locations of the intersecting points of the grid help in measuring transmural changes at various time points in the cardiac cycle. However, these points are spread out all over the myocardium without any mutual spatial relationship; this makes image interpretation rather difficult.

STAG images have tagged points, situated at a uniform depth, across the myocardium, in a radial fashion. While the radial orientation of these points helps in identifying torsion abnormalities, any change in the relative locations of these points aids in the assessment of transmural alterations.

These tagging techniques may be followed by any imaging pulse sequence. While the implementation of SPAMM takes only about 10 to 15 msec, the implementation time for the STAG sequence is directly proportional to the number of tags required.

REFERENCES

1. Axel L, Dougherty L (1989): MR imaging of motion with spatial modulation of magnetization. *Radiology* 171:841–845.

2. Axel L, Dougherty L (1989): Heart wall motion: improved method of spatial modulation of magnetization for MR imaging. *Radiology* 172:349–350.

3. Bolster BD, McVeigh ER, Zerhouni EA (1990): Myocardial tagging in polar coordinates with use of striped tags. *Radiology* 177:769–772.

4. Buchalter MB, Weiss JL, Rogers WJ, Zerhouni EA, Weisfeldt ML, Berger R, Shapiro EP (1990): Noninvasive quantification of left ventricular rotational deformation in normal humans using magnetic resonance imaging myocardial tagging. *Circulation* 81:1236–1244.

5. Hennig J (1990): Generalized MR interferography. *Magn Reson Med* 16: 390–402.

6. Ingels NB, Daughters GT, Stinson EB, Alderman EL (1980): Evaluation of methods for quantitating left ventricular segmental wall motion in man using myocardial markers as a standard. *Circulation* 61: 966–972.

7. McVeigh E, Yang A, Zerhouni EA (1990): Rapid measurement of T1 with spatially selective pre-inversion pulses. *Med Phys* 17:131–134.

8. McVeigh ER, Zerhouni EA (1991): Noninvasive measurement of transmural gradients in myocardial strain with magnetic resonance imaging. *Radiology* (in press).

9. Pearlman JD, Reese TG (1990): NMR pulse program for cardiac cine tagging. *Magn Reson Imag* 8:S114.

10. Zerhouni EA, Parish D, Rogers WJ, Yang A, Shapiro EP (1988): Human heart: tagging with MR imaging—a method for noninvasive assessment of myocardial motion. *Radiology* 169:59–63.

29

Pause

BASIC PRINCIPLES

Respiratory motion is a major factor determining the clinical usefulness of an abdominal and thoracic MR image. Many times, such motion renders the acquired images clinically incompetent[1]. While there are many diverse motion reduction schemes [5], none of them is universally applicable with equivocal success.

Pause is a three-dimensional volume imaging technique that uses the conventional Fourier transform (FT) based data acquisition sequence (Fig. 29.1) [4]. It is similar to the breath-hold technique for eliminating motion artifacts. However, the uniqueness of the pause technique lies in the fact that it knowingly allows the subject being imaged to take respiratory

---

[1] Due to a variety of reasons (eg, inadequate sedation in pediatric cases, excessive motion caused by an uncooperative subject, or, simply, overwhelming claustrophobic feelings), an on-going MR examination, sometimes, cannot be completed. Usually, the subject is removed from the scanner in these situations and the scanning procedure is aborted. As the partially collected data are then trashed by the computer, this results in the complete loss of time already spent collecting the trashed data. Lund and Morin [2] suggest that in such circumstances, instead of aborting the scan, data acquisition should continue as usual, even after removing the subject from the scanner. Obviously, the data collected in the absence of the subject mainly is background noise. Therefore, one would expect that the salvaged image would be totally useless because of the excessive noise. However, if data acquisition had proceeded at least beyond the maximum amplitude phase encoding step (zero phase encode step) before the subject was removed, then the image has a tolerable signal-to-noise ratio.

Alternatively, one should be able to locate retrospectively, by the technique of thresholding, the phase encode step after which the motion occurred. The acquired data set then can be stripped off the phase encode steps that occurred in the presence of the motion, and an image can be created from the partial data set, using one of the data undersampling techniques described in the introductory chapter. Elscint's Rollback technique seems to have adopted this approach for displaying data sets affected by inadvertent motion.

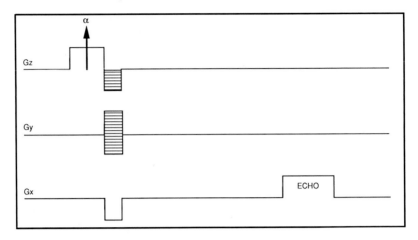

FIG. 29.1 Unlike in two-dimensional Fourier transform imaging, phase encoding is performed in two directions in the three-dimensional Fourier transform pause sequence.

pauses, but otherwise, it lets the subject continue normal breathing. Following is a brief description of the method.

The subject is asked to hold his or her breath for about 20 sec while the data are being acquired. Normal respiration, then, ensues for some time (about 10 sec) before the next period of breath-holding is scheduled. The temporal location of the pauses along the entire imaging experiment is predetermined by the imaging protocol (Fig. 29.2); it is desirable to schedule a pause near the edge of the k-space because the Fourier transform sampling of the data is more sensitive to intensity variations near the center of the k-space, rather than its edge. However, the duration of each pause vary depending on the particular subject's breath-holding capacity. Usually, a single plane through the desired three-dimensional volume is sampled during each respiratory pause.

During the time interval when the subject is respirating, respiration

FIG. 29.2 The temporal location of respiratory pauses is predetermined; however, their duration may vary depending on the subject's breath-holding capacity.

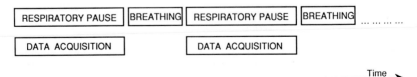

data acquisition is temporarily stopped (paused), and the order of the next phase encoding gradient remains unaltered. A series of RF pulses (as many as 50) are employed to bring longitudinal magnetization back to the steady state level before data acquisition is once again carried out. To keep the image contrast identical for all images, the same number of RF pulses also are employed before initiating the imaging experiment.

In the thoracic region, in addition to respiratory motion, two other sources of motion—namely, cardiac motion and intense blood flow—gives rise to artifacts. Cardiac artifacts are effectively removed by the inherent signal averaging used in the three-dimensional Fourier transform imaging technique. Blood flow related artifacts may be removed by using velocity insensitive gradients (such as those used in MAST).

See also: Gating, GMN, MAST, MP-RAGE, ROPE.

CLINICAL APPLICATIONS
TISSUE CONTRAST

The three-dimensional acquisition gives a better signal-to-noise ratio, and the overall image contrast-to-noise ratio is increased due to elimination of motion artifacts.

THE THORAX

The thoracic region is relatively difficult to image by MRI [3] because it contains numerous sources responsible for physiological motion, such as the heart, lungs, and flowing blood. While gating techniques usually provide clinically useful images, they are prohibitively long and highly susceptible to the irregular rhythm of the heart or respiration.

The technique described herein offers the opportunity for obtaining multiple thoracic images relatively free from cardiac and respiratory artifacts in somewhat lesser time (Fig. 29.3). Total imaging time is determined by a variety of factors, such as the number and duration of pauses, pulse parameters, and the subject's breath-holding capacity.

THE ABDOMEN

It will be most interesting to see the performance of this technique in abdominal images. However, to date, no report has been published indicating its usefulness in abdominal examinations to this author's knowledge.

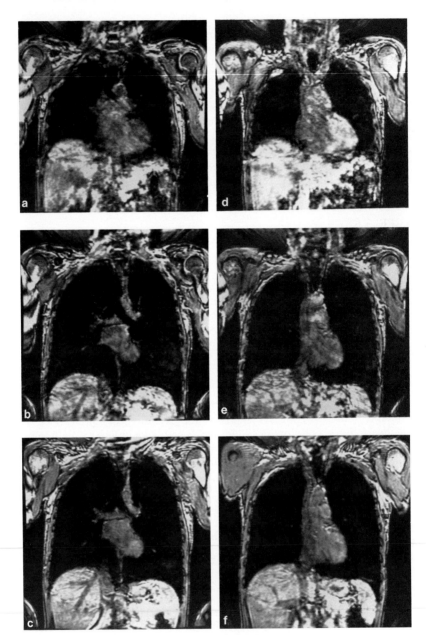

ADVANTAGES AND DISADVANTAGES

Even though the pause imaging technique is supposed to be shorter than gating techniques, the scan times in the range of 40 to 45 minutes still are practically undesirable, especially in the view of other fast imaging techniques, such as snapshot FLASH imaging (turboFLASH) and EPI.

While this technique was designed to eliminate respiratory motion artifacts, it assumes that the abdominal organs return to the same anatomical position after breathing as they were before a breath is taken. However, Kuhns et al [1] have reported that this assumption is far from true. This may limit the degree of artifact elimination achieved by this technique.

REFERENCES

1. Kuhns RK, Thornburg J, Siegel R (1979): *J Comput Assist Tomogr* 3:620.

2. Lund G, Morin R (1986): A technique for image salvage in MR. *Am J Roentgen* 147:1052–1054.

3. Spritzer C, Gamsu G, Sostman HD (1989): Magnetic resonance imaging of the thorax: techniques, current applications, and future directions. *J Thoracic Imaging* 4:1–18.

4. Stern RL, Johnson GA, Ravin CE (1990): Magnetic resonance imaging of the thoracic cavity using a paused three-dimensional Fourier transform acquisition technique. *Magn Reson Imag* 8:747–753.

5. Wood ML, Runge VM, Henkelman RM (1988): Overcoming motion in abdominal imaging. *Am J Roentgen* 150:513–522.

←——————————————————————————————

FIG. 29.3 Series of six coronal images (3 mm slice thickness) of a normal thorax at two different anatomic levels, (a, b, c) and (d, e, f), to illustrate the features of the three-dimensional pause technique. **(a)** and **(d)**: Normal breathing; **(b)** and **(e)**: with pauses and breath-holding intervals; **(c)** and **(f)**: with pauses, breath-holding intervals, and prepulses to restore longitudinal magnetization to the steady state level. Acquisition time was 30 min (with pauses and prepulses) and 20 min (without pauses, but with prepulses), for a total of 64 different anatomic levels. Note the increased clarity of images (c) and (f). (Courtesy of R. Stern; reproduced, with permission, from Stern et al [4].)

30

Phase-Based Angiography (PBANG)

BASIC PRINCIPLES

Like many other signals, the NMR signal is uniquely characterized by its amplitude and phase. The signal amplitude is determined primarily by longitudinal magnetization and reflects the velocity[1] as well as concentration of the spins. There are numerous NMR angiographic techniques that exploit this fact (see TOF). Here, we will study some phase-based angiographic techniques.

The phase of the signal may be defined as the orientation of transverse magnetization in relation to the xy plane (Fig. 30.1). When a gradient magnetic field is applied, the phase of the spins, stationary as well as moving, is altered, and this phase shift ($\Delta\phi$) follows the following simple relationship. For stationary spins:

$$\Delta\phi = \gamma \times A_G \times T,$$

where γ = gyromagnetic ratio; A_G = amplitude of the gradient G; and T = total time for which G is on. For moving spins:

$$\Delta\phi = \gamma \times v \times A_G \times T,$$

where v = flow velocity; and all other parameters are as defined above. In either case, the phase increases nonlinearly with the increasing velocity (for fixed excitation flip angle) or with increasing excitation flip angle (for fixed velocity) [31].

---

[1] The words "flow" and "velocity" have been used interchangeably in this discussion. However, we should not forget that velocity signifies all but only the one term from many describing the flow (the other terms are acceleration, pulsatility, etc.).

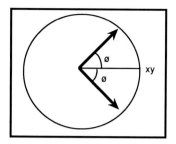

FIG. 30.1 In the transverse plane (xy), two magnetization vectors are shown with their respective phase angles.

While the random and uncontrolled occurrence of such phase shifts is detrimental (due to widespread signal loss) to image contrast, under controlled circumstances, these phase shifts can be creatively exploited for quite useful purposes. For example, the basic technique of NMR imaging itself creates such controlled phase shifts in order to derive the spatial coordinates of the NMR signal. However, it is important to remember that numerous sources, other than velocity and gradient fields, contribute to the observed phase shifts: magnetic field inhomogeneities, eddy currents generated by rapid gradient switching, and local susceptibilities all may introduce undesirable phase effects. If one wants to image selectively only flowing spins, then the above list also should include phase shifts introduced by stationary spins. Therefore, if the phase information is to be used for obtaining flow information, all these nonvelocity-dependent phase shifts should be carefully dissected out from the NMR signal. To this end, various strategies, as described below, have been employed.

1. In its simplest form, a bipolar gradient pulse is incorporated into the pulse sequence (Fig. 30.2) [4,18,19]. While the phase of stationary

FIG. 30.2 A bipolar gradient pulse, as shown, refocuses magnetization of stationary spins, but flowing spins gain a net phase shift proportional to the flow velocity and gradient integral.

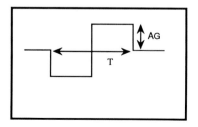

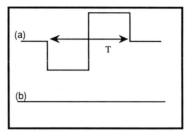

FIG. 30.3 The pulse sequence is repeated twice, once with the flow encoding bipolar pulse on **(a)** and, the second time, without this pulse **(b)**.

spins is restored at the end of the pulse, flowing spins gain a phase shift proportional to the flow velocity. And, instead of a magnitude-based display, a phase map is created to display the phase of each pixel. The disadvantage of this approach is that a greater loss of signal results, due to higher orders of the motion.

Most of the other approaches use subtraction of two data sets with differential flow sensitivity in order to derive the final image. This general approach is known as phase contrast angiography (PCA).

2. O'Donnell [21] and Spritzer et al [24] have used the simplest form of PCA (Fig. 30.3). The flow sensitivity of the sequence can be varied by changing the amplitude of the bipolar pulse. While the technique of O'Donnell is based on spin echoes (velocity imaging with spin echoes, VISE) [21], the flow-compensated image of Spritzer et al [24] is a gradient recalled acquisition and thus exhibits GRASS-like contrast when magnitude reconstructed (velocity imaging with gradient recalled echoes, VIGRE). (Fig. 30.4).

3. Nayler et al [20] have used an asymmetric pair of bipolar pulses (Fig. 30.5). A complex subtraction of the data sets, as explained in the figure, yields a flow image (see FEER).

4. In the velocity compensated/uncompensated (VCUPS) method of Axel and Morton (Fig. 30.6) [2], two magnitude-based projection images are subtracted to reveal the flow-induced phase data.

5. In an approach frequently implemented by Dumoulin and Hart and Dumoulin et al [8–12,29], data acquisition is carried out in the interleaved mode with bipolar pulses of opposite polarity. Therefore, the flowing spins accumulate phase shifts with alternating signs. The net result is that, on the subtraction, the difference signal is bigger than any of the approaches used above (Fig. 30.7).

6. In the approach first used by Wedeen et al [30], the pulsatile nature of the blood is exploited to derive a pair of data sets with different

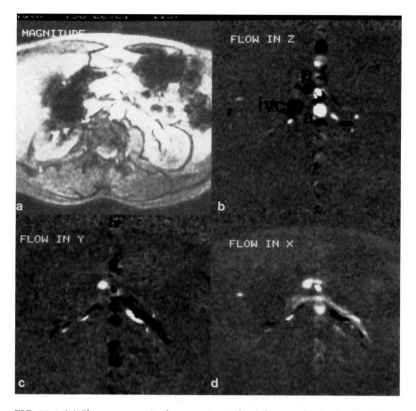

FIG. 30.4 (a) Shows a magnitude reconstructed axial scan, obtained with 30° excitation (TR = 24 msec; TE = 13 msec; 2 averages, 13 sec per acquisition), through the abdomen of a normal volunteer. To derive the following flow images, two acquisitions (flow compensated and flow encoded) were performed, and later subtracted. **(b)** Same section as in (a), but with flow encoding on in the superioinferior (craniocaudal) direction; abdominal aorta (a), inferior vena cava (ivc) and portal vein (p) are visible. **(c)** Same section as in (a), but with flow encoding on in anterioposterior direction. **(d)** Same section as in (a), but with flow encoding on in side-to-side direction. The left renal vein is seen as a bright structure. (Courtesy of C. Spritzer; reproduced, with permission, from Spritzer et al [24].)

flow profiles. In their technique, the ECG-triggered data are acquired in the systole and diastole. Due to different flow rates during these two stages of the cardiac cycle, a magnitude (or cardiac phase) subtraction yields an image of the flow. Fig. 30.8 shows another example of ECG-triggered phase angiography.

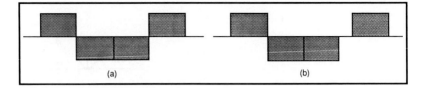

FIG. 30.5 **(a)** A pair of bipolar pulses is joined back-to-back to obtain a gradient profile that is balanced for the velocity. **(b)** When this balanced profile is disturbed, the flowing spins, once again, acquire flow-induced phase shifts.

The common goal of any type of angiographic technique should be to achieve maximum suppression of the stationary spins (background noise) and enhance the signal from the flowing spins in a reasonable amount of time.

Static tissue suppression may be achieved by applying several presaturating pulses ahead of the actual RF excitation pulse. Alternatively, the pulse repetition time (TR) can be made very short. The short TR not only saturates the stationary spins, but also reduces total imaging time. If short TR is combined with low flip angle excitation pulse and gradient echo

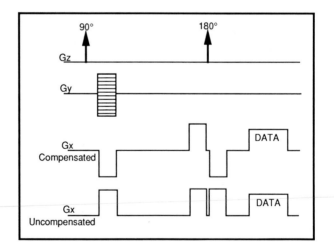

FIG. 30.6 Note that the slice-select gradient is absent. Therefore, a projection of the flowing spins is obtained. The 180° RF pulse effectively makes the first Gx compensated and the second Gx uncompensated. The pulse sequence is run twice: once with the top Gx; once with the bottom Gx. (Modified, with permission, from L. Axel and D. Morton [2].)

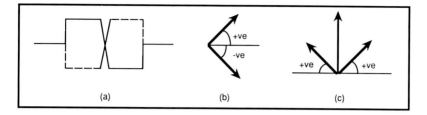

FIG. 30.7 (a) The bipolar gradient pulse, as shown in Fig. 30.2, is applied twice with opposite polarities (solid line and dashed line). (b) The resultant phase angles of the flowing spins for these two gradient pulses are described. (c) When the negative phase angle vector is reversed and added to the positive angle vector, a combined vector is obtained whose amplitude is increased compared to either case taken alone.

acquisition, total data acquisition time can be considerably reduced [9,14,15,24,26]. For example, Tasciyan et al [26] obtained eight images (four in systole and four in diastole) in about 20 to 30 sec by using 30° RF pulses and short TR (22 msec).

To increase the signal-to-noise ratio of the PCA images, a technique of matched filtering has been proposed by Doyle and Mansfield [7] and DeCastro et al [6]. In brief, their approach works in the following way. First, all the images are multiplied by a weighting factor derived from

FIG. 30.8 Two series of ECG-triggered angiographic images of the vessels around the human knee are shown. (a) Rephasing for a constant velocity; and (b) velocity dephasing for spins flowing at more than 50 cm/sec. To obtain these angiographic images, a series of views was acquired by a fast gradient echo sequence at different temporal locations during the cardiac cycle. To achieve better suppression of the stationary spins, the first view was taken right after the R wave was subtracted from each subsequent view. For example, the second angiogram was obtained by subtracting the first view from the third view. (Courtesy of Q. Guo; reproduced, with permission, from Guo et al [14].)

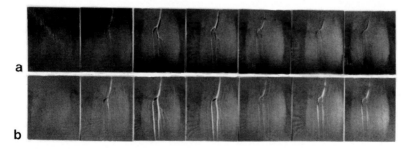

a

b

the spread of the signal intensities over the region of interest, eg, aorta. Second, all the scaled images are coadded. Upon summation, all the static structures are eliminated. The improvement in the signal-to-noise ratio is proportional to the number of images in the series. For example, for a series of 14 images, a 60% increase in the signal-to-noise ratio is achieved [6]. Chenevert et al [5] have suggested a phase correction scheme for further improving subtraction angiogram images. Alternatively, data acquisition can be carried out in three-dimensional space to achieve a higher signal-to-noise ratio, but only at the cost of increased imaging time.

Variants   Almost all the different approaches discussed above use additional bipolar pulses to encode the flow information. However, it is possible to create a phase map simply using the conventional two-dimensional spin warp spin echo sequence where the normal magnitude image is given by the square root of $(R^2 + I^2)$, and the phase map is given by arc tan (I/R) (where I is the imaginary component and R is the real component of the data). Several investigators [23,27] have used such phase maps to differentiate thrombus from flowing blood because while flowing blood shows phase shift on the phase maps, a thrombus does not cause such changes.

See *also*: FANG, FEER, FLAG, LISA, TOF.

CLINICAL APPLICATIONS
TISSUE CONTRAST

In general, vessel appearance depends on the direction as well as the velocity of flow. In the case of laminar flow, usually, high velocities in the direction of the flow encoding gradient show up bright; the opposite is true for lower velocities. The background signal from stationary tissues is annihilated if the contribution of the signal from them is almost totally suppressed, by using either presaturation or subtraction.

THE HEAD AND NECK

This region is relatively easily accessible for MR angiographic examinations because motion artifacts are limited only to the physiological (slow) flow, and the amount of stationary tissue is much less. The carotids, intracerebral (including the circle of Willis), and extracerebral vessels frequently are well-visualized by angiography. Three-dimensional angiography gives a better signal-to-noise ratio and allows smaller vessels to be seen when the maximum intensity projection algorithm is used, and the voxel size is comparable to the vessel dimensions (Fig. 30.9) [22].

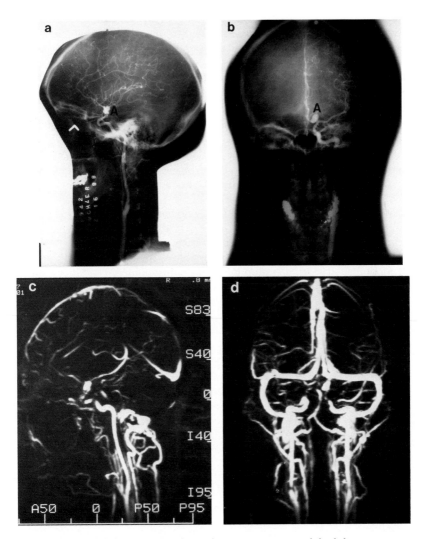

FIG. 30.9 **(a)** and **(b)** Contrast enhanced x-ray angiograms of the left common carotid artery in a patient with the aneurysm (A) at the bifurcation of the internal
carotid artery. **(c)** and **(d)** Corresponding MR angiograms obtained with the three-
dimensional phase contrast technique (15 ° to 30° excitation; TR = 22.3 msec; TE
= 14.7 msec; 2 averages; 12 min acquisition time per flow encoding direction;
total 36 min). The aneurysm is clearly evidence on these MR angiograms. Note
also the richness of the vascular structures that are visualized. (Courtesy of R.
Pernicone; reproduced, with permission, from Pernicone et al [22].)

Alfidi et al [1] discuss the clinical significance of the phase-based angiography in the carotid and peripheral arteries.

THE ABDOMEN

The abdominal region presents the most difficulties, such as the breathing and peristaltic movements, a large amount of stationary tissue, and highly pulsatile blood flow, for any type of angiography. Despite these difficulties, several investigators have been successful in visualizing the normal splenic, renal, mesenteric, and portal vessels [12,25,28].

In general, quantitative measurements of blood flow velocities have been found to agree with the actual flow values. Maier et al [17] have compared abdominal aortic flow velocity with ultrasound Doppler and found a high degree of correlation between them.

In addition to velocity, it is also possible to image higher-order terms of motion such as acceleration and areas of turbulence. The latter is particularly useful in cases of poststenotic valvular disorders, atherosclerotic arteries, and flow near the bifurcation of major arteries.

ADVANTAGES AND DISADVANTAGES

In phase-based angiography, the phase shifts of the flowing spins are directly related to flow velocity alone and, thus, they provide a fairly precise determination of velocity independent of spin density. The dynamic range of flow velocities that can be quantitatively determined varies (from a few mm/sec to 50 cm/sec) according to the individual pulse design. As a general precaution, quantitative information from the vessels, whose anatomical dimensions are in the range of minimum image resolution, should be subject to additional scrutiny.

Many phase-based flow imaging techniques use subtraction at some stage to derive the final image. The advantage of this (and other phase subtraction techniques) is that phase contributions from nonvelocity-dependent phase factors, such as field inhomogeneities, are canceled out upon data subtraction.

In subtraction angiography, only the flow in the direction of the gradient is encoded. Therefore, a total of six pulse applications (three directions multiplied by two applications per flow direction) may be required if total flow encoding is desired. However, recently, it has been reported that PCA angiography may be possible with only four acquisitions, by applying flow-encoding gradients to more than one axis at a time, without degrading the signal-to-noise ratio [16].

As the signal phase is uniquely defined between the values of $-180°$ and $+180°$, any phase rotation in excess of this range is misinterpreted by the image reconstruction algorithm, eg, $\Delta\phi$ 270° is set equal to 270° $- 180° = 90°$ (Fig. 30.10). To avoid the aliasing artifacts (abrupt changes in image intensity) that may occur due to this phase misregistration, the sensitivity of the flow encoding gradient should be adjusted such that the highest predicted velocity gives a phase rotation of no more than $\pm 180°$. However, this may limit the sensitivity of the technique for detecting slow flow velocities. In general, to increase the dynamic range of the velocities that may be imaged, multiecho phase contrast acquisitions have been found useful by enhancing the dynamic range by the square root of the number of echoes (if all the echoes are acquired within a time interval equivalent to the blood T2) [21]. Alternatively, an algorithmic approach, as suggested by Axel and Morton [3], may be employed.

The pixel intensity in a phase map varies according to the velocity; in addition to velocity, spin phase also is affected by other factors, as outlined above. Therefore, unless special care is taken while preparing and/or interpreting a phase map, the information from it may be error-prone. In the subtraction-type of angiographic method, this problem is somewhat corrected. However, these methods still are sensitive to the eddy currents generated by gradient fields; and phase information may be misregistered, even after subtraction. Moreover, in regions such as the abdomen and pelvis, the presence of large amounts of fat, peristaltic motion, and highly pulsatile arterial flow renders subtraction angiography useless. In such cases, projective PCA have been found beneficial. Firmin et al [13] have authoritatively analyzed various phase-based and Fourier-based angiographic techniques.

Almost all major MR scanner manufacturers include some type of phase-based angiographic technique in their standard cardiovascular package.

FIG. 30.10 Magnetization vector M1 is located at 135° from the reference line of detection; magnetization vector M2 is located at 225° from the same line. However, the dashed vector is calculated to be located at $225° - 180° = 45°$ from the reference line.

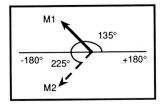

REFERENCES

1. Alfidi RJ, Masaryk TJ, Haacke EM, Lenz GW, Ross JS, Modic MT, Nelson AD, LiPuma JP, Cohen AM (1987): MR angiography of peripheral, carotid and coronary arteries. *Roentgen* 149:1097–1109.

2. Axel L, Morton D (1987): MR flow imaging by velocity-compensated/uncompensated difference images. *J Comput Assist Tomogr* 11:31–34.

3. Axel L, Morton D (1989): Correction of phase wrapping in magnetic resonance imaging. *Med Phys* 16:284–287.

4. Bryant DJ, Payne JA, Firmin DN, Longmore DB (1984): Measurement of flow with NMR imaging using a gradient pulse and phase difference technique. *J Comput Assist Tomogr* 8:588–593.

5. Chenevert TL, Fechner KP, Gelblum DY (1989): Improvements in MR angiography using phase-corrected data sets. *Magn Reson Med* 10:38–49.

6. DeCastro JB, Tasciyan TA, Lee JN, Farzaneh F, Riederer SJ, Herfkens RJ (1988): MR subtraction angiography with a matched filter. *J Comput Assist Tomogr* 12:355–362.

7. Doyle M, Mansfield P (1986): Real-time movie image enhancement in NMR. *J Phys E: Sci Instrum* 19:439–443.

8. Dumoulin CL, Hart HR (1986): Magnetic resonance angiography. *Radiology* 161:717–720.

9. Dumoulin CL, Souza SP, Hart HR (1987): Rapid scan magnetic resonance angiography. *Magn Reson Med* 5:238–245.

10. Dumoulin CL, Souza SP, Walker MF, Yoshitome E (1988): Time-resolved magnetic resonance angiography. *Magn Reson Med* 6:275–286.

11. Dumoulin CL, Souza SP, Walker MF, Wagle W (1989): Three-dimensional phase contrast angiography. *Magn Reson Med* 9:139–149.

12. Dumoulin CL, Yucel EK, Vock P, Souza SP, Terrier F, Steinberg FL, Wegmuller H (1990): Two- and three-dimensional phase contrast MR angiography of the abdomen. *J Comput Assist Tomogr* 14:779–784.

13. Firmin DN, Nayler GL, Kilner PJ, Longmore DB (1990): The application of phase shifts in NMR for flow measurement. *Magn Reson Med* 14:230–241.

14. Guo Q, Fribux L, Nalcioglu O (1990): Investigation of blood flow dynamics by NMR angiography. *Magn Reson Imag* 8:167–172.

15. Lee JN, Riederer SJ, Pelc NJ (1989): Flow-compensated limited flip angle MR angiography. *Magn Reson Med* 12:1–13.

16. Litt AW, Fram EK, Turski PA (1991): MR angiography: second annual workshop, October 19–21, 1990, East Lansing, MI. *Am J Neuroradiol* 12:573–575.

17. Maier SE, Meier D, Boesiger P, Moser UT, Vieli A (1989): Human abdominal aorta: comparative measurements of blood flow with MR imaging and multigated Doppler US. *Radiology* 171:487–492.

18. Moran PR (1982): A flow zeumatographic interlace for NMR imaging in humans. *Magn Reson Imag* 1:197–203.

19. Moran PR, Moran RA, Karstaedt (1985): Verification and evaluation of internal flow and motion. *Radiology* 154:433–441.

20. Nayler GL, Firmin DN, Longmore DB (1986): Blood flow imaging by cine magnetic resonance. *J Comput Assist Tomogr* 10:715–722.

21. O'Donnell M (1985): NMR blood flow imaging using multiecho, phase contrast sequences. *Med Phys* 12:59–64.

22. Pernicone JR, Siebert JE, Potchen EJ, Pera A, Dumoulin CL, Souza SP (1990): Three-dimensional phase-contrast MR angiography in the head and neck: preliminary report. *Am J Neuroradiol* 11:457–466.

23. Rumancik WM, Naidich DP, Chandra R, Kowalski HM, McCauley DI, Megibow AJ, Hernanz-Schulman M, Genieser NB (1988): Cardiovascular disease: evaluation with MR phase imaging. *Radiology* 166:63–68.

24. Spritzer CE, Pelc NJ, Lee JN, Evans AJ, Sostman HD, Riederer SJ (1990): Rapid MR imaging of blood flow with a phase-sensitive, limited flip-angle, gradient recalled pulse sequence: preliminary experience. *Radiology* 176:255–262.

25. Steinberg FL, Yucel EK, Dumoulin CL, Souza SP (1990): Peripheral vascular and abdominal applications of MR flow imaging techniques. *Magn Reson Med* 14:315–320.

26. Tasciyan TA, Lee JN, Riederer SJ, DeCastro JB, Hedlund LW, Herfkens RJ, Spritzer CE (1988): Fast limited flip angle MR subtraction angiography. *Magn Reson Med* 8:261–274.

27. Tavares NJ, Auffermann W, Brown JJ, Gilbert TJ, Sommerhoff C, Higgins CB (1989): Detection of thrombus by using phase-image MR scans: ROC curve analysis. *Am J Roentgen* 153:173–178.

28. Vock P, Terrier F, Wegmuller H, Mahler F, Gertsch Ph, Souza SP, Dumoulin CL (1991): Magnetic resonance angiography of abdominal vessels: early experience using the three-dimensional phase-contrast technique. *Br J Radiol* 64:10–16.

29. Walker MF, Souza SP, Dumoulin CL (1988): Quantitative flow measurement in phase contrast MR angiography. *J Comput Assist Tomogr* 12:304–313.

30. Wedeen VJ, Meuli RA, Edelman RR, Geller SC, Frank LR, Brady TJ, Rosen BR (1985): Projective imaging of pulsatile flow with magnetic resonance. *Science* 230:946–948.

31. Yuan C, Gullberg GT, Parker DL (1989): Flow-induced phase effects and compensation technique for slice selective pulses. *Magn Reson Med* 9:161–176.

31

Rapid Acquisition Relaxation Enhanced (RARE)

BASIC PRINCIPLES

Recently much attention has been given to echo planar imaging (EPI) or one of its several modifications. This is reflected directly in the number of citations that EPI continues to receive. However, a little attention also has been paid to an imaging technique that is basically similar to the original echo planar imaging (see EPI). Rapid acquisition relaxation enhanced (also called rapid relaxation with repeated echoes), or RARE, was first proposed in 1984 by Hall and Sukumar [3], and then by Hennig et al in 1986 [4,5]. Both EPI and RARE (and the recently introduced turboFLASH) reduce planar data acquisition times to less than one second. The major difference between EPI and RARE imaging techniques is the way in which they acquire echoes: while EPI rapidly switches the frequency encoding gradient in the presence of constant amplitude phase gradient to sample the k-space, RARE employs 180° refocusing pulses with variable phase encoding to generate a long series of spin echoes after a single excitation.

Fig. 31.1 shows a representative RARE pulse sequence. After a slice-selective 90° RF pulse excites the spins, a series of 180° RF refocusing pulses is applied, to elicit a long series of spin echoes. Each echo is separately phase encoded and then frequency encoded in the presence of a read gradient. Two things are strikingly different in this pulse sequence from the original EPI pulse sequence:

1. the presence of 180° RF pulses, and
2. the compensating lobes in the phase encoding direction immediately preceding the following refocusing pulse.

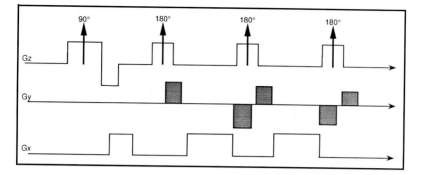

FIG. 31.1 RARE pulse sequence. The initial 90° RF pulse is followed by a series of 180° RF pulses with variable phase encoding between successive pulses. (Modified, with permission, from J. Hennig and H. Friedburg [7].)

The significance of these differences is explained below.

When gradient pulsing is used to refocus the dephasing echo, as in EPI or other gradient-based techniques, it does not correct for local inhomogeneity effects. Moreover, gradient fields have very low homogeneity (by definition, the value of magnetization is different at each point in the course of a gradient magnetic field). Therefore, the signal being observed decays with a rate constant, $T2^*$, which is faster than the true rate constant, $T2$. In a given time, therefore, fewer echoes can be collected per excitation. Classically, 180° RF pulses have been used to refocus all dephasing spins in conventional SE sequences. RARE, therefore, uses 180° pulses to refocus decaying echoes. However, the presence of 180° refocusing pulses limits the minimum spacing (TE) between successive echoes. In turn, this may increase image acquisition time.

A compensating lobe is provided for each phase encoding lobe to bring the spin phase to exactly the same value before each 180° pulse [4]. This simple provision eliminates any stimulated or spurious echoes [7]; however, it also adds to total imaging time.

Variants   Many modifications of the original RARE sequence have been proposed, primarily to achieve contrast flexibility and an improved signal-to-noise ratio.

(A) To achieve variable T1 contrast in RARE images, either TR can be varied or a 180° RF pulse can be applied prior to the 90° RF excitation pulse. The latter approach is known as *inversion recovery* RARE (IR-RARE) (Fig. 31.2) [9]. Note that a similar approach has been employed by others in the cases of FLASH (IR-FLASH) and EPI (IR-EPI) sequences.

(B) To decrease T2 weighting, variants such as *rotated* RARE (RORE),

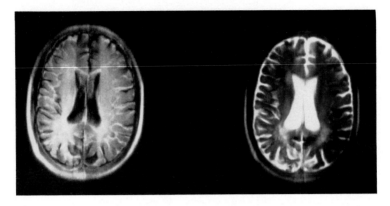

FIG. 31.2 A pair of IRRARE images obtained with T1 = 750 msec **(a)** and T1 = 1 msec **(b)**. Each image was reconstructed from 256 echoes (echo spacing = 12.2 msec), and was obtained in 32 sec (256 sampling points; 2 averages). Note heavy T2 weighting in (b), due to minimal inversion delay. (Courtesy of R. Mulkern; reproduced, with permission, from Mulkern et al [9].)

shuffled RARE (SHARE) or two-shot RARE are suggested. All of these variants differ with respect to the manner in which they sample the k-space (Fig. 31.3) [9]. While RARE samples echoes in a gradually increasing course, starting from the most negative phase value, k_{min}, to the most positive phase value, k_{max} (much like conventional imaging), RORE begins the k-space sampling at a phase value located somewhere between k_{min} and 0. The leftover echoes are measured at the end of the experiment.

FIG. 31.3 The k-space sampling strategy employed in **(a)** RORE and **(b)** SHARE. The direction of the arrowheads, starting from the left-hand side, indicates the order in which phase encode steps are acquired.

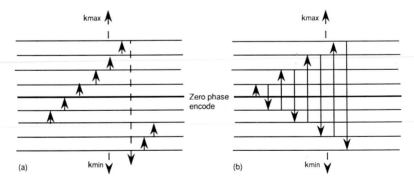

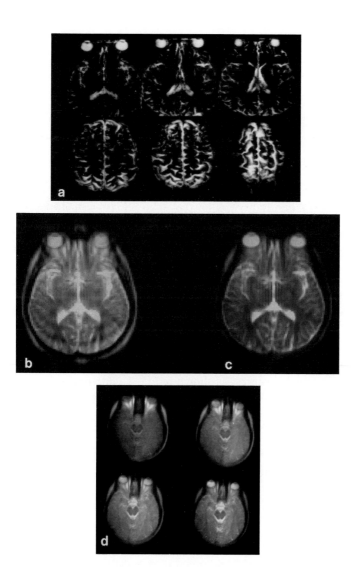

FIG. 31.4 (a) A series of unmodified RARE images of a normal volunteer (TR = 4 sec; 128 echoes; 2 averages; 8.5 sec per section). Note heavy T2 weighting of the images so that only those tissues with long T2, such as the CSF and vitreous, are seen. In order to see the brain tissue, T2 weighting has to be decreased, as discussed in the text. **(b)** RORE and **(c)** SHARE are two variants of the conventional spin warp phase encoding scheme. The zero phase encode step occurs at step number 16 (instead of the usual 64) in both these images. As a result, a considerable amount of brain tissue is visualized. **(d)** The influence of varying TR on the RORE image contrast. TR = 1.5 sec (upper left); TR = 2.5 sec (upper right); TR = 3 sec (lower left); and TR = 4 sec (lower right). (Courtesy of R. Mulkern; reproduced, with permission, from Mulkern et al [9].)

Thus, the echo corresponding to the zero phase value is collected much earlier than in RARE, and it has a relatively smaller T2 influence. As the zero phase valued echo determines image intensity, this time shift in its evolution leads to a reduction in overall T2 influence on image contrast [7]. The effect of the altered k-space sampling strategy on the final contrast and artifact level recently has been analyzed by Mulkern et al [10]. Fig. 31.4 shows the contrast characteristics of these RARE variants.

(C) In *fast low angle RARE* (FLARE), low angle (less then 180°) RF refocusing pulses are used in order to reduce RF power deposition in the subject [7]. When transverse magnetization (Mxy), established by a 90° pulse, is refocused by a pulse of less than 180°, only a part of Mxy is inverted by the first refocusing pulse. The remaining part of Mxy is refocused by later applications of the refocusing pulses. This cumulative effect of the partially refocused Mxy on image contrast is variable, being determined by not only T2, but also the flip angle of the refocusing pulses. The stimulated echoes that would otherwise result from such a pulse sequence are eliminated by including phase encoding compensating pulses [7].

In U-FLARE, an ultrafast variant of the FLARE sequence, rapidly switching (500 μsec) gradients are employed to reduce image acquisition times [11]. In addition, the phase encode steps are temporally rearranged to manipulate T2 contrast as shown in Fig. 31.2 (in a manner analogous to the TOPE approach used with the IR-FLASH experiment to provide variable T1 contrast).

See also: DOPE, EPI, IR-FLASH, SFI.

CLINICAL APPLICATIONS
TISSUE CONTRAST

The tissue contrast obtained using RARE is comparable to that obtained with conventional T2-weighted spin-echo sequences. Typically, RARE provides MR images that are strongly dependent on T2 relaxation time. Thus, tissues with long T2, such as cerebrospinal fluid, joint fluid, and urinary fluid, are better highlighted with RARE, and they appear as regions of high signal intensity on the images. As discussed above in connection with RORE, it is possible to modify this T2 weighting by changing the order of the phase encoding values so that the tissues with short T2 values can be effectively imaged without blurring artifacts (see below).

FLARE image contrast basically is similar to RARE image contrast (heavily T2 weighted), with the provision that the signal-to-noise ratio is less than the corresponding ratio in the RARE images.

T2-weighted images gives better visualization of brain pathologies [12]. However, conventional long TR/TE spin echo acquisition is very time-consuming. Therefore, the chief indication for using RARE is when T2-weighted contrast is desired in a very short period of time. So far, the principal clinical applications of RARE (and its variants) have been in neurological examinations in the form of MR-myelography and in morphological examinations of the urinary tract in the form of MR-urography. The image quality of MR myelograms and MR urograms is highly comparable to that obtained in standard x-ray examinations; but, unlike the latter, there is no need for intravenous administration of contrast agents (Fig. 31.5).

CEREBROSPINAL FLUID

As CSF has a long T2 value, highly T2-weighted myelograms have been obtained with RARE. With three-dimensional implementation, high resolution (256 × 128 × 128) myelograms can be obtained in as little as 11 min [6]. Such myelograms can furnish crucial details regarding mass disorders, such as neoplasms and cysts, and functional disorders, such as CSF flow disorders.

In addition to the detection of intraspinal pathologies, it has been suggested that RARE may be used to obtain quantitative information re-

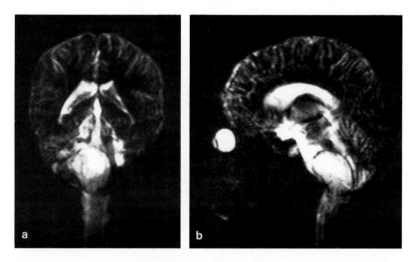

FIG. 31.5 Coronal **(a)** and sagittal **(b)** views of a patient with a spongioblastoma. The pathology has been clearly demonstrated without the need for an invasive contrast agent. Also note a very strong signal from the eye, due to long T2 value of vitreous. (Courtesy of J. Hennig; reproduced, with permission, from J. Hennig and H. Friedburg [7].)

garding CSF flow (see DOPE) [8]. This will help tremendously in the evaluation of disorders like syringomyelia, in which CSF circulation is abnormal, and in the differential diagnosis of disorders such as hydrocephalus and cranial injury.

When compared to standard RARE myelograms, the FLARE image quality is inferior due to diminished signal amplitudes. For example, FLARE myelograms obtained with 60° refocusing pulses have only half the signal intensity of standard RARE myelograms (Fig. 31.6) [7].

THE URINARY SYSTEM

Since the sequence is highly T2-dependent, aqueous material gives off a high intensity signal. Thus, complete urograms obtained with RARE show renal pelvis, ureters, and the urinary bladder as bright structures (Fig. 31.7) [1,2]. Any obstructive or compressive abnormalities can be readily

FIG. 31.6 Comparison of normal 180° RARE **(a)** and 60° FLARE **(b)** images. The images were obtained by the hybrid RARE technique, in which the total number of echoes to be acquired is divided into several series. This approach avoids the blurring artifact caused by the varying T2-weighted signal intensity [7]. For both images, eight excitations were used, each followed by 32 echoes (total 256 echoes) (TR = 3 sec; TE = 30 msec; 25 sec acquisition time). Note that the CSF intensity is relatively the same in both images; however, brain tissue appears less intense on the FLARE image than on the RARE image. (Courtesy of J. Hennig; reproduced, with permission, from J. Hennig and H. Friedburg [7].)

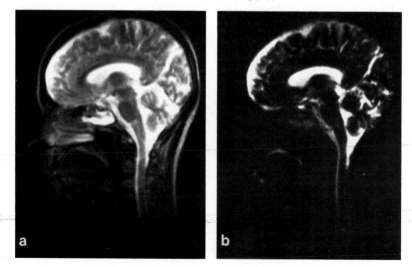

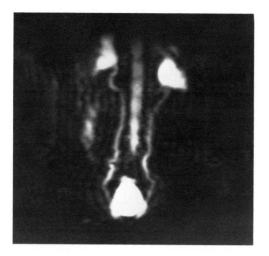

FIG. 31.7 RARE urogram, obtained with 128 echoes, shows the dilated pelvis and ureters. The urinary bladder also is seen. (Courtesy of J. Hennig; reproduced, with permission, from J. Hennig and H. Friedburg [7].)

identified on such MR urograms. As the signal is derived principally from the fluid within the urinary system, the signal-to-noise ratio may degrade if only a small quantity of fluid is present (eg, the distal ureter and bladder may not be properly visualized if the gravid uterus compresses the proximal ureter).

FIG. 31.8 This RARE image shows a developing fetus. The amniotic fluid and the mother's urinary bladder, along with fetal CSF, are visualized. (Courtesy of J. Hennig.)

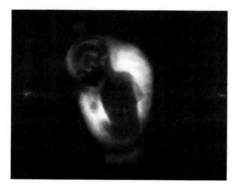

PREGNANCY

Noninvasive MR myelograms or urograms can be particularly useful in pregnancy where ionizing radiation is contraindicated. In addition, amniotic fluid shows up very bright and the profile of the fetus can be identified easily (Fig. 31.8). Therefore, it is possible to detect fetal malformations or certain maternal disorders, such as placenta previa or entangled placental cord.

Various other bodily fluids, such as synovial fluid of the knee joint, have been imaged with RARE or one of its variants [9].

ADVANTAGES AND DISADVANTAGES

The chief advantage of RARE over standard spin echo imaging lies in the fact that RARE considerably reduces image acquisition time (2 to 32 sec) and still provides excellent T2-weighted tissue contrast. Recall that gradient echo techniques also provide fast MR scans, but these techniques suffer from a lack of good image contrast, as no refocusing pulses are used.

With the introduction of U-FLARE, data acquisition times have been reduced considerably and a typical image (64 phase encoding × 128) can be obtained in less than 300 msec [11]. This fact alone puts U-FLARE in direct competition with other fast subsecond imaging techniques such as EPI and turboFLASH (SFI); however, unlike EPI, its implementation is relatively easy and the hardware requirements are not as stringent.

The disadvantage of RARE is that tissues with shorter T2 relaxation times (less than 500 msec) may cause blurring artifacts in the phase encoding gradient. This is because while spin echoes are being collected, the on-going spin-spin relaxation process reduces successive echo amplitudes; echoes corresponding to the higher phase values are most affected (and, thus, the name rapid acquisition relaxation ehanced, RARE).

Additionally, conventional RARE requires that a long series of echoes be obtained using 180° refocusing RF pulses. At high field strengths, this means that above normal RF power may be deposited in the patient. However, when compared to standard RARE, FLARE (with 60° refocusing pulses) deposits only one-ninth as much RF energy in the subject being imaged. Thus, FLARE has been found applicable even at extreme field strengths (as high as 4.7 T).

REFERENCES

1. Friedburg HG, Westenfelder M, Roeren T, Hennig J (1987): MR of the urinary tract in pregnancy. ROFO 147:430–432.

2. Friedburg HG, Wimmer B, Hennig J, Frankenschmidt A, Hauenstein KH (1987): Initial clinical experiences with RARE-MR urography. *Urologe* 26:309–316.

3. Hall LD, Sukumar S (1984): Rapid data-acquisition for NMR imaging by the projection-reconstruction method. *J Magn Reson* 56:179–182.

4. Hennig J, Friedburg H, Stroebel B (1986): Rapid nontomographic approach to MR myelography without contrast agents. *J Comput Assist Tomogr* 10: 375–378.

5. Hennig J, Naureth A, Friedburg H (1986): RARE imaging: a fast imaging method for clinical MR. *Magn Reson Med* 3:823–833.

6. Hennig J, Friedburg H, Ott D (1987): Fast three-dimensional imaging of cerebrospinal fluid. *Magn Reson Med* 5:380–383.

7. Hennig J, Friedburg H (1988): Clinical applications and methodological developments of the RARE technique. *Magn Reson Imag* 6:391–395.

8. Hennig J, Ott D, Adam TH, Friedburg H (1990): Measurement of CSF flow using an interferographic MR technique based on the RARE-FAST imaging sequence. *Magn Reson Imag* 8:543–556.

9. Mulkern RV, Wong STS, Winalski C, Jolesz FA (1990): Contrast manipulation and artifact assessment of 2D and 3D RARE sequences. *Magn Reson Imag* 8:557–566.

10. Mulkern RV, Melki PS, Jakab P, Higuchi N, Jolesz FS (1991): Phase encode order and its effect on contrast and artifact in single-shot RARE sequences. *Med Phys* (in press).

11. Norris DG (1991): Ultrafast low-angle RARE: U-FLARE. *Magn Reson Med* 17:539–542.

12. Smith AS,. Weinstein MA, Modic MT, Pavlieck W, Rogers LR, Budd TG, Bukowski RM, Purvis JD, Weick JK, Duchesneau PM (1985): Magnetic resonance with marked T2-weighted images: improved demonstration of brain lesions, tumor, and edema. *Am J Roentgen* 145:949–955.

32

Rapid Spin Echo (RASE)

BASIC PRINCIPLES

Spin echo sequences, especially those with long pulse repetition times (proton- and T2-weighted), are notorious for excessively lengthy data acquisition times. This disadvantage became more apparent after the introduction of gradient echo based imaging techniques. In order to make SE competitive as far as imaging time is concerned, it may be modified in two simple ways.

1. With every excitation, saturate the magnetization only partially so that less time is required for its recovery. This approach of partial flip imaging already has been discussed in FLASE.
2. Alternatively, shorten the most time-consuming components of the sequence, namely, the pulse repetition time (TR) and the echo time (TE) (Fig. 32.1).

This second alternative is the focus of discussion here. Note that the FLASE approach indirectly decreases TR by employing shallow RF pulses.

RASE may be considered a simple variant of the standard SE pulse sequence. As in the latter, the RASE pulse sequence consists of a 90° excitation pulse followed by a refocusing 180° pulse. However, to achieve faster imaging times, the pulse repetition time (TR) and echo time (TE) are made very short (for example, 110 to 275 msec and 10 to 15 msec, respectively) [4].

To enhance the performance of RASE, several investigators have incorporated half-Fourier imaging in their imaging protocol (see UNSAD). The use of half-Fourier decreases the signal-to-noise ratio. Multiple averages may be obtained to increase the latter; however, this may increase

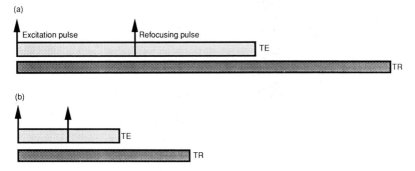

FIG. 32.1 (a) In the conventional spin echo sequence, the excitation pulse is of 90° and the refocusing pulse is of 180°. The echo time is 20 to 80 msec, and the pulse repetition time is 500 to 2000 msec. **(b)** In the rapid spin echo sequence, even though the pulse angles are 90° and 180°, respectively, TE and TR are reduced considerably. However, longitudinal magnetization does not fully recover at short TR values and, therefore, the signal-to-noise ratio is degraded. In contrast, in the FLASE approach, the excitation pulse angle is made very low (10° to 30°) and, therefore, longitudinal magnetization fully recovers even when short TR values are used.

image acquisition time and offset the attractiveness of the RASE approach.

See also: FLASE.

CLINICAL APPLICATIONS
TISSUE CONTRAST

Highly T1-weighted images are obtained with TR values used in this pulse sequence. However, the signal-to-noise ratio is inferior to conventional SE T1 images because of partially saturated longitudinal magnetization (a by-product of the short TR) and the frequent use of the half-Fourier imaging technique.

CONTRAST ENHANCEMENT AND RASE

T2-weighted SE is the most frequently used pulse sequence for abdominal studies. However, long TR/TE makes it very susceptible to motion arti-facts. The primary goal for developing the RASE technique was to com-plete abdominal examinations in a very short time period, possibly a single breath-hold interval, so that motion artifacts do not arise. However, image contrast is undermined at the short TR/TE values employed in

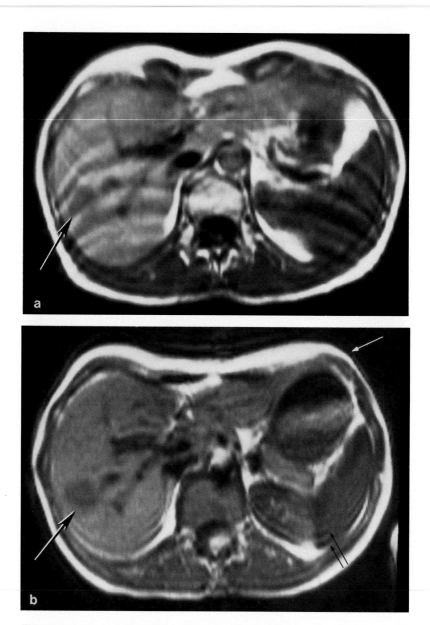

FIG. 32.2 (a) T1-weighted (TR = 300 msec; TE = 10 msec) spin echo (8 averages) and **(b)** T1-weighted (TR = 275 msec; TE = 10 msec) RASE (half-Fourier, 1 average) images of the abdomen. Note the absence of motion artifacts on the RASE image, which clearly shows the hepatic lesion (thick black arrows). Also note that truncation artifacts, which frequently appear on RASE images (thin black and white arrows). (Courtesy of J.K.T. Lee; reproduced, with permission, from Mirowitz et al [4].)

RASE sequences. Therefore, several investigators have attempted to boost image contrast by externally administering contrast agents.

Numerous studies have demonstrated the increased diagnostic capability of contrast-enhanced RASE studies in identifying hepatic pathologies [3,4,8,9,11]. In a study by Greif et al [2], it has been found that RASE (TR = 160 msec; TE = 33 msec) gives the optimum contrast-to-noise ratio for liver when used with a paramagnetic contrast agent, Fe[EHPG]$^-$.

THE HEART

Edelman et al [1] have used the RASE sequence in triggered cardiac imaging where short TE (5 msec) allows the acquisition of up to five slices during the end systole or end diastole. With the conventional SE sequence (TE 30 msec), it is not possible to acquire as many slices. The increased number of slices per unit time increases the temporal resolution of the study and makes functional assessment of cardiac motion more accurate.

THE ABDOMEN

The images of the abdomen obtained using RASE are free of respiratory motion artifacts (Fig. 32.2), which together with the fact that the image contrast is T1-weighted, makes the identification of hepatic metastases easy and reliable. The absence of artifacts also permits clear depiction of the portal and splenic vasculature.

ADVANTAGES AND DISADVANTAGES

With TR of 275 msec, the data acquisition time is about 23 sec for a 128 phase encode × 256 image matrix [4]. If the patient is able to suspend breathing for this relatively longer duration, respiratory motion artifact-free abdominal images are obtained. Stark et al [10] have found short TR/TE RASE to be extremely valuable in attenuating respiratory artifacts and, along with signal averaging, signal-to-noise ratio is considerably improved. By further decreasing the phase encoding steps to 32 and TR to 110 msec, perfusion studies of the liver and kidneys using Gd-DTPA have become possible. Such dynamic studies may provide essential information concerning the functional status of an organ.

One pitfall of the contrast-enhanced RASE is that sometimes vascular artifacts are exaggerated, as longitudinal magnetization recovers sooner from any excitatory or saturating conditions. If half-Fourier data sampling is employed, linear artifacts sometimes appear near the anterior abdominal wall. However, they usually do not extend into the tissue plane [4].

Unlike gradient echo based rapid imaging techniques, RASE images are not susceptible to local inhomogeneity effects, as the 180° pulse refocuses the echo at echo time. Furthermore, no rapid switching of gradients is necessary, and it is very easy to implement on any MR scanner.

Recently, there has been some counter-opinion in the literature, doubting the clinical usefulness of the RASE technique over other means for eliminating motion artifacts and achieving faster imaging times [7]. However, the proponents of the technique [6] still remain confident of the clinical merits of the RASE technique.

REFERENCES

1. Edelman RR, Thompson R, Kantor H, Brady TJ, Leavitt M, Dinsmore R (1987): Cardiac function: evaluation with fast-echo MR imaging. *Radiology* 162: 611–615.

2. Greif WL, Buxton RB, Lauffer RB, Saini S, Stark DD, Wedeen YJ, Rosen BR, Brady TJ (1985): Pulse sequence optimization for MR imaging using a paramagnetic hepatobiliary contrast agent. *Radiology* 157:461–466.

3. Mano I, Yoshida H, Nakabayashi K, Yashiro N, Iio M (1987): Fast spin echo imaging with suspended respiration: gadolinium enhanced MR imaging of liver tumors. *J Comput Assist Tomogr* 11:73–80.

4. Mirowitz SA, Lee JKT, Brown JJ, Eilenberg SS, Heiken JP, Perman WH (1990): Rapid spin echo MR imaging (RASE): a new technique for reduction of artifacts and acquisition time. *Radiology* 175:131–135.

5. Mirowitz SA, Lee JKT, Gutierrez E, Brown JJ, Heiken JP, Eilenberg SS (1991): Dynamic gadolinium-enhanced rapid acquisition spin-echo imaging of the liver. *Radiology* 179:371–376.

6. Mirowitz SA, Lee JKT (1991): Optimizing MR imaging of the abdomen: the case for rapid-acquisition spin-echo MR imaging. *Radiology* 179:612–614.

7. Mitchell DG (1991): Rapid-acquisition spin-echo MR imaging of the liver: a critical view. *Radiology* 179:609–612.

8. Saini S, Stark DD, Brady TJ, Wittenberg J, Ferrucci JT (1986): Dynamic spin-echo MRI of liver cancer using gadolinium-DTPA: animal investigation. *Am J Roentgen* 147:357–362.

9. Schmiedl U, Moseley ME, Ogan MD, Chew WM, Brasch RC (1987): Comparison of initial biodistribution patterns of Gd-DTPA and albumin-(Gd-DTPA) using rapid spin echo MR imaging. *J Comput Assist Tomogr* 11:306–313.

10. Stark DD, Hendrick RE, Hahn PF, Ferrucci JT (1987): Motion artifact reduction with fast spin-echo imaging. *Radiology* 164:183–191.

11. Tanimoto A, Yuasa Y, Endo M, Ohkawa S, Shiraga N, Fujisawa H, Ido K, Ogawa K, Momoshima S, Shiga H (1989): Magnetic resonance imaging of bladder tumors: superiority of serial "fast SE" assisted by Gd-DTPA in tumor staging. *Nippon Acta Radiologica* 49:1552–1566.

33

Resonant Offset Averaging in the Steady State (ROAST)

BASIC PRINCIPLES

ROAST is a variant of the FISP pulse sequence. It is designed to eliminate field inhomogeneity artifacts that occur in the unmodified FISP sequence.

Field inhomogeneity artifacts occur when all the spins in a voxel do not experience the same imposed magnetic field. While a group of spins (an isochromat) occupying a certain voxel precesses faster, another such group may precess slower. The resonant offset of an isochromat (Fig. 33.1) may be defined as the angle through which it precesses before each RF pulse [3] (or, equivalently, during each pulse repetition interval).[1] As the spins can undergo a full rotation around the origin, the resonant offset may range from 0° to 360°. When this angle is constant between any two successive RF pulses, it is said that the phase is coherent. However, due to nonconstant local inhomogeneities, the value of resonant offset (and, therefore, the signal intensity) changes, even for the same spatial position (a voxel). If a particular voxel has a wide range of such resonant offsets, the signal from that voxel fluctuates as the resonant offsets change with fluctuating local inhomogeneities. These widespread fluctuations invariably cause signal loss.

The solution to the above problem is to dephase these resonant offsets in a controlled manner. If this is achieved, then instead of having a range of resonant offset values, each pixel will contain only a single value of the resonant offset. To accomplish this, the frequency encoding and slice-select gradients of the original FISP sequence are made unbalanced (Fig. 33.2), which effectively averages out the wide range of resonant offsets

---

[1] The resonant offset has contributions from the RF phase, imaging gradients phase, phase shift due to spin motion, local inhomogeneities, and pulse repetition time.

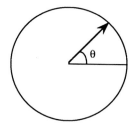

FIG. 33.1 Rotating magnetization vector in the transverse plane. The z direction is perpendicular to this plane. The angle θ describes the resonant offset (or, equivalently, the phase) of the spin magnetization vector.

coexisting in a voxel (resonant offset averaging in steady state, ROAST) [3,5]. Note the similarity of ROAST to the FAST sequence (see FAST). The result of this planned dephasing is that the interfering influences of local inhomogeneities cancel out. The phase encoding gradient is left balanced so that transverse coherence is maintained for stationary spins.

While in FISP both components of the SSFP signal collectively con-

FIG. 33.2 In ROAST, both the slice-select and the frequency encode gradients are made unbalanced (shaded areas). In RARE ROAST, the frequency encode gradient is made balanced by eliminating the shaded gradient pulse and immediately reversing the gradient (dashed area). Interestingly, if the slice-select gradient is made balanced as well (dotted area), the FISP pulse sequence is formed.

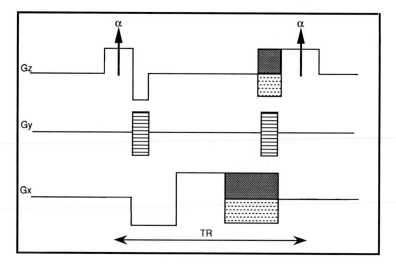

tribute to the acquired echo, the latter has contribution only from the FID part of the SSFP signal in ROAST. The reason is that resonant offset averaging (achieved by extending the readout gradient beyond the echo acquisition) in ROAST effectively prevents the building up of transverse magnetization.

Variants In ROAST, the frequency encoding gradient is made unbalanced, which causes resonant offsets of the moving spins to change for every RF pulse. This ever-changing resonant offset prevents transverse coherence from accumulating; this decreases the signal from flowing spins. To overcome this difficulty, in RARE ROAST (refocused acquisition in the readout direction ROAST), only the slice-select gradient is made unbalanced [3]. This refocuses the pulse sequence, once again, in the read-out direction and is thus useful for imaging in-plane flow. Note that the RARE ROAST sequence still maintains the advantage of diminished sensitivity to local inhomogeneities.

See also: FAST, FISP, SSFP.

CLINICAL APPLICATIONS
TISSUE CONTRAST

As resonant offsets are averaged, the true offset distribution that may exist due to inherent tissue differences is lost. Therefore, the penalty in the form of reduced contrast-to-noise ratio is paid by making the FISP sequence unbalanced (ROAST). This is especially true for the CSF-brain tissue where tissue differentiation is very poor at lower excitation flip angles (EFA) [1]. The RARE ROAST sequence provides better CSF/spinal cord contrast, as the CSF appears very bright (Fig. 33.3).

CEREBROSPINAL FLUID

As no velocity compensation is used by this sequence, free-flowing CSF experiences a velocity-dependent net phase shift in the direction of the gradient. As a result of signal loss due to this phase shift, CSF flowing through regions such as the cervical spine and various foramina of the ventricular system appears dark (note the similarity to FLASH images). This effect is enhanced by using large EFAs [3]. However, stationary CSF, as may be the case with neural cysts and the noncommunicating hydrocephalus, appears bright. This dual appearance of CSF may help in differentiating the various CSF flow abnormalities.

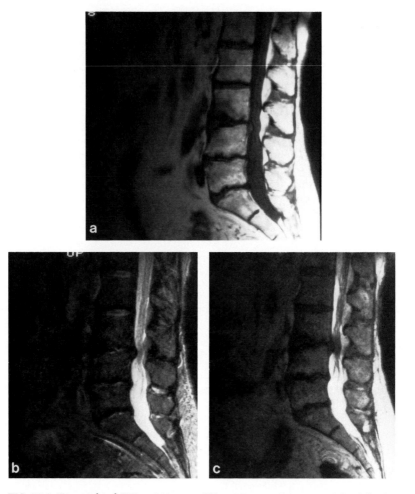

FIG. 33.3 T1-weighted (TR = 500 msec; TE = 20 msec; 4 averages, 8.5 min) spin echo **(a)**, T2-weighted (TR = 4 sec; TE = 90 msec; 1 average, half-Fourier; 9 min) spin echo **(b)**, and three-dimensional RARE ROAST. (35° excitation; 1 average; 1.1 min) **(c)** images of the lumbar spine. Note that all the images clearly show L3-4 disc bulge. Furthermore, the RARE ROAST image shows the nerve roots better than the other two images. (Courtesy of E. M. Haacke; reproduced, with permission, from Haacke et al [3].)

ANGIOGRAPHY

The ROAST sequence may be called the "partially rephased sequence" because the slice-select and frequency encode gradients are deliberately left unbalanced. As a result, flowing spins are not completely rephased at the echo time. While this may result in the loss of signal, the remaining phase shifts, which are proportional to the flow velocity, may be used for displaying the directional flow and its quantification [4]. For example, fast-flowing arterial blood experiences a greater signal loss than slowly flowing venous blood; therefore, the former appears darker and the latter appears brighter on ungated images. If cardiac gating is employed, a sub-traction-type angiography may be carried out, in which arterial structures appear bright. Haacke et al [2] have analyzed the effects of the flip angle, TR, TE, spatial resolution, and image reconstruction method on the quality of the angiograms.

ADVANTAGES AND DISADVANTAGES

Both ROAST and RARE ROAST are insensitive to local field inhomogeneities.

While RARE ROAST is sensitive to motion only along one direction (usually the readout), ROAST is sensitive to motion along two directions. However, no major phase artifacts appear, especially in the case of slow flow. This situation may change at higher velocities when dephasing leads to considerable signal loss.

REFERENCES

1. Darkazanli A, Granstrom P, Unger E, Seeger J, Carmody R, Gmitro A, Toshida T, Suzuki H (1990): Fast scanning of the brain at 0.5 Tesla [abstr]. *Magn Reson Imag* 8:S95.

2. Haacke EM, Masaryk TJ, Wielopolski PA, Zypman FR, Tkach JA, Amartur S, Mitchell J, Clampitt M, Paschal C (1990): Optimizing blood vessel contrast in fast three-dimensional MRI. *Magn Reson Med* 14:202–221.

3. Haacke EM, Wielopolski PA, Tkach JA, Modic MT (1990): Steady-state free precession imaging in the presence of motion: application for improved visualization of the cerebrospinal fluid. *Radiology* 175:545–552.

4. Lenz GW, Haacke EM, Masaryk TJ, Laub G (1988): In-plane vascular imaging: pulse sequence design and strategy. *Radiology* 166:875–882.

5. van der Meulen P, Groen JP, Tinus AMC, Bruntink G (1988): Fast field echo imaging: an overview and contrast calculations. *Magn Reson Imag* 6:355–368.

34

Respiratory Ordered Phase Encoding (ROPE)

BASIC PRINCIPLES

It is well known that the asynchronous respiratory motion of the abdominal wall with respect to the phase encoding gradient (Fig. 34.1) results in ghost artifacts in the phase encoding direction. The ghost artifacts severely degrade the contrast-to-noise ratio of a conventional image. The following paragraph illustrates the reasons for these artifacts.

In commonly used two-dimensional Fourier transform spin warp imaging, the amplitude of the phase encoding step is changed (usually increased) after a full line of data is acquired with the frequency encoding gradient (Fig. 34.2). The time required to collect a line of data is much less than a single respiratory cycle (1/respiratory rate). Therefore, the line acquisition is completed long before the next respiratory cycle begins and, thus, frequency encoding usually is not affected by the motion. However, this is not true in the case of phase encoding, as illustrated with a numerical example. In conventional T2-weighted SE sequences, the pulse repetition time (TR) is about two seconds. As each alteration in the phase encoding value occurs after a time interval equivalent to TR, the fifth such phase change occurs ten seconds after the first one took place. If the respiratory rate is 15/min, then two respiratory cycles have been completed in this ten-second period, and the third cycle is in progress. Clearly, the anatomical structures affected by respiratory motion are not in exact position when the first phase encoding step was applied. If the respiratory rhythm is normal, then every other odd-numbered phase encoding step will be applied when the respiratory cycle is near its peak; every even-numbered phase encoding step will be applied when the respiratory cycle is halfway through the inspiratory or expiratory phase.

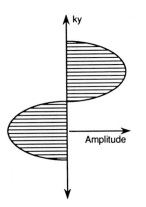

FIG 34.1 The asynchrony between pulse repetition time and respiratory rate gives rise to a sinusoidal variation in signal amplitude along the phase encode axis.

Clearly, the anatomical structures affected by respiratory motion are not at the same position throughout the process of phase encoding. Moreover, the regularity with which successive phase encoding steps see the different phases of motion tends to produce artifacts in the phase encoding direction. These artifacts in the phase encoding direction can be decreased considerably or eliminated by adopting various strategies, as described below. (For other general approaches, see Gating.)

1. Joseph et al [7] have modified the two-dimensional spin warp pulse sequence (Fig. 34.3). As shown in the figure, phase encoding and prephasing is delayed until just before the time for data collection. In this way, the spins remain for a shorter period of time under the dephasing influence of the gradients. While their approach effectively removes

FIG. 34.2 In spin warp imaging, during each readout period the data points comprising one phase encode step (k) (horizontal line) are sampled. The next phase encode step (k + 1) is sampled after the time interval equivalent to the pulse repetition time (TR).

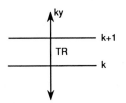

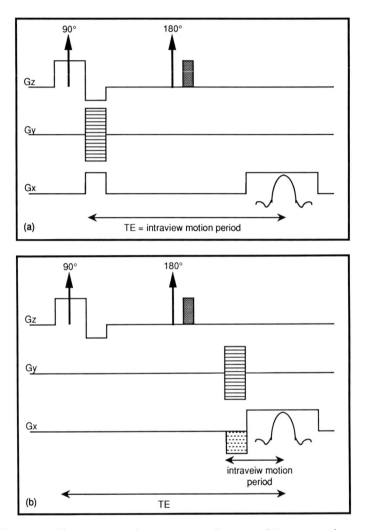

FIG. 34.3 (a) The conventional spin warp two-dimensional Fourier transform spin echo sequence. The shaded gradient pulse is optional; its purpose is to destroy the transverse magnetization that may result due to imperfections in the 180° RF pulse. Note that the period during which intraview motion can occur is same as the echo time. Therefore, sequences with long TE times, such as T2-weighted spin echo sequence, suffer from motion artifacts. **(b)** In this modification of the pulse sequence of (a), the intraview motion period has been considerably reduced compared to echo time by moving the prephasing gradient lobe (dashed area) closer to the readout pulse. Therefore, spins remain for a shorter period of time under the influence of the gradients and, as a result, experience less spin dephasing. (Modified, with permission, from Joseph et al [7].)

intraview motion-related artifacts, the effectiveness for removing the artifacts due to respiration is not known to the author.

2. The principle of artifact separation: If the total number of pixels in the phase encoding direction (the most common direction in which respiratory artifacts appear) is N_{tot}, then the distance (N_d, in pixels) between the image and the artifacts is:

$$N_d = (N_{tot} \times avg \times TR)/(1/f),$$

where TR is the interval between data acquisitions and $1/f$ is the period of the motion. There are three related approaches for separating the artifacts from the image plane ($avg = 1$).

a. In the minimal separation approach, $N_d = N_{tot}$. This is achieved when TR is made equal to the respiratory period. This essentially superimposes all of the artifacts exactly onto the real image (Fig. 34.4b) (pseudo-gating; see Gating).

b. In the maximal separation approach, $N_d = \frac{1}{2} N_{tot}$. This is achieved when TR is made equal to one-half of the respiratory period (Fig. 34.4c). If proper field of view (FOV) is chosen, then this pushes the artifacts out of the image of the subject, and into the black zone [1]. (See also strip scan in UNSAD).

c. In the variable separation approach, the separation between two artifacts is made equal to some multiple of the FOV by properly determining TR in relation to the period of motion. In this case, the artifacts will occur at the same location in the image. By carefully designing the data acquisition, all or most of the artifacts can be superimposed at the same location in the image, away from the region of interest (Fig. 34.4d) [13]. This approach works because of image aliasing. It also suggests that the artifacts will not be removed simply by pushing them out of the image FOV.

3. Fast imaging: If complete data acquisition can be accomplished very rapidly, the adverse influence of motion on image contrast is minimized. To decrease imaging time, short TR and TE values may be adopted (as in RASE or FLASE). However, this restricts the type of

FIG. 34.4 **(a)** Usual image degradation by respiratory artifacts. In **(b)**, all the artifacts are superimposed exactly on the actual image. In **(c)**, the artifacts have been pushed away from the actual image and, in **(d)**, all the artifacts are superimposed onto each other away from the actual image.

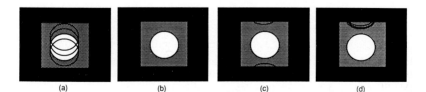

(a)   (b)   (c)   (d)

pulse sequence that may be used and, therefore, the type of tissue contrast that can be obtained. Alternatively, a host of rapid gradient echo techniques are available. However, they are more susceptible to magnetic field inhomogeneities and may require improved hardware.

4. Randomization of the phase steps: If the phase encode steps are totally randomized, then the periodicity of the motion is lost and, as a result, the artifacts break apart. Note that the artifacts are not eliminated from the image; they simply are broken down into smaller pieces and, as such, are not readily appreciable.

5. Changing the direction of the phase encoding gradient sometimes improves image quality by physically separating artifacts from the areas of interest. For example, it has been observed that if the phase encoding gradient is applied in the horizontal direction, respiratory artifacts appear away from the organs, such as kidneys, on the axial scans. This enhances considerably the contrast-to-noise ratio [11]. Similarly, Bock et al [3] have observed that if vertical phase encoding is applied instead of horizontal phase encoding in coronal brain images, then artifacts due to CSF pulsations can be displaced from the temporal lobe, thus providing clear visualization of the latter.

6. The cause of respiratory artifacts is the movement of the anterior abdominal wall. Therefore, Edelman et al [4] have proposed a technique, called FRODO (flow and respiratory artifact obliteration with directed orthogonal pulses), in which the anterior abdominal wall is presaturated prior to the imaging experiment (Fig. 34.5). While this effectively removes artifacts, a loss corresponding to the slab thickness in the image field of view occurs. As the name suggests, in addition to eliminating respiratory artifacts, flow-related artifacts also can be removed by properly placing the presaturating slab.

A different approach has been adopted in the technique presented here, respiratory ordered phase encoding (ROPE), in which the phase encoding steps are not acquired in a fixed order from k_{min} to k_{max}; however, the number of the phase encoding step to be acquired next is determined by measuring respiratory motion. This technique works in the following way [2].

As we saw above, motion artifacts occur due to the fact that many respiratory cycles occur before all the phase encoding steps are completed. The purpose of ROPE is to make it appear that only one such cycle occurred during the examination. In order to do this, ROPE matches the amplitude of abdominal motion with a phase encoding value in such a way that the lowest amplitude of motion corresponds to the most negative phase encoding value. The remaining phase encoding values are paired with the motion amplitudes in an increasing order. This means that higher-valued phase encoding occurs during the end inspiration and

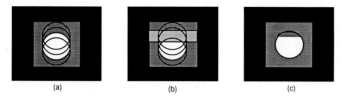

(a) (b) (c)

FIG. 34.5 **(a)** The image is degraded by motion of the anterior abdominal wall. In **(b)**, a presaturating pulse is applied to this region (dotted area), therefore, the artifacts are removed **(c)**. However, note that structures in the vicinity of the presaturated region also are not visualized.

lower-valued phase encoding occurs during the end expiration. If the amplitude of motion steadily increases in a time-dependent manner during inspiration, this reordering of the phase values makes the period of motion very slow through the data acquisition and simulates the situation as if only a single respiratory cycle occurred over the course of the entire data acquisition. ROPE thus decreases the effective frequency of the respiratory cycle.

To obtain respiratory amplitudes, a suitable sensor is placed near the level of the diaphragm. It is assumed that the motion of the anterior abdominal wall represents the summation of all the moving structures in the abdomen (mathematicians call it a point spread function). Two different algorithmic approaches may be implemented to determine the order of the phase encoding steps in the final image:

1. The respiratory signal (r) is sampled n times at regular intervals for a period of a few minutes. Each sample will then have an amplitude value (rA). If m ($m \le n$) samples have identical rA values, then the probability of a sample with rA will be equal to m/n. Now this is determined before beginning the actual MR examination. Based on this probability distribution information, the correct order of the phase encoding value is chosen during data acquisition.
2. The data are acquired without any prior knowledge of the respiratory signal, which is obtained after the data are acquired. By postprocessing, the phase encoding steps are then properly arranged.

While the first approach yields a data set with properly arranged phase encoding steps, the phase encoding steps have to be arranged after the data are acquired in the second approach.

Variants (A) While ROPE reorders data from the lowest phase encoding value to the highest value, centrally ordered phase encoding (COPE) reorders the data from the central region of the phase axis (ky) outward [6].

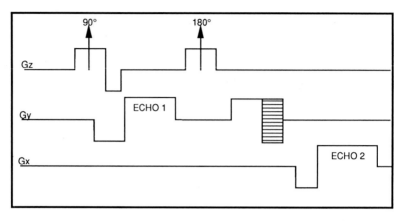

FIG. 34.6 A conventional spin echo pulse sequence has been modified to acquire a projection of the respiratory motion (ECHO 1). ECHO 2 is the usual phase encoded image echo. (Modified, with permission, from Kim et al [8].)

FIG. 34.7 **(a)** Prior to the actual imaging, a prescanning of abdominal motion is performed to determine certain landmarks of the motion curve (for example, points 1 through 5). Once the actual imaging is begun, the amplitude value of the line projection is compared to these landmarks and the status (or phase) of the motion is determined. For example, if the value of the projection amplitude falls between points 1 and 2, it indicates that the motion amplitude is on the rising edge. The value of the next phase encode step is immediately derived from the already prepared look-up table, and the image data are acquired for that projection. After all the phase encode steps are acquired, they are rearranged before performing the Fourier transform. This treatment of the data makes it appear that motion amplitude changes monophasically in only one direction **(b)**.

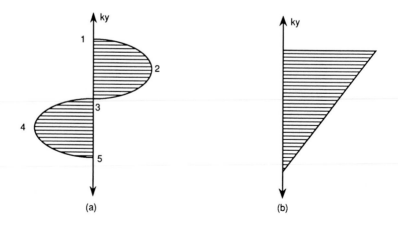

(B) To eliminate the need for explicit measurement of respiratory motion amplitudes in ROPE, a modified ROPE technique acquires a line projection of the abdominal movement immediately before the standard echo is acquired during each repetition of the pulse sequence (Fig. 34.6). Depending on the magnitude of this projection, the rank of the next phase encoding step along the respiratory cycle can be determined (Fig. 34.7). This method of phase ordering with projection data is called projection ordered phase encoding (POPE) [8].

See also: COPE, Gating, MAST.

CLINICAL APPLICATIONS
TISSUE CONTRAST

The tissue contrast characteristics are determined by the pulse sequence and imaging technique employed. However, the contrast-to-noise ratio is significantly improved due to elimination of ghost artifacts in the phase encoding direction. COPE images usually have better spatial resolution and less noise than the corresponding ROPE images [6].

While MMORE and GMN are chiefly employed for eliminating blood flow related artifacts, ROPE is applied primarily in clinical situations where respiratory motion is undesirable but unavoidable.

THE ABDOMEN

The visualization of intraabdominal lesions, such as liver metastasis, is far improved [5]; the boundaries between neighboring organs become more conspicuous due to elimination of respiratory motion-related artifacts [9]. Fig. 34.8 shows the improvement in the abdominal image obtained using the POPE technique.

ADVANTAGES AND DISADVANTAGES

The ROPE technique eliminates motion artifacts caused by periodic motion such as respiration. However, it does not improve spatial blurring— and may even increase it [12,13]. In addition, it does not correct for peristaltic or blood flow effects. A study by Mitchell et al [10] suggests that proper use of this technique, along with the GMN technique, would considerably eliminate vascular artifacts that predominantly degrade upper abdominal long SE images.

ROPE requires pre- or postprocessing of the data; this may increase total imaging time even though the data acquisition time may not be prolonged. Additional hardware in the form of a suitable sensor is re-

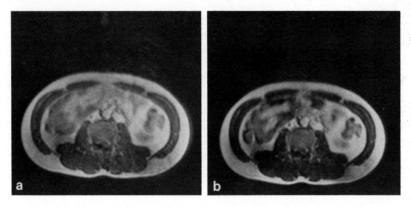

FIG. 34.8 Conventional spin echo **(a)** and POPE **(b)** images (TR = 600 msec; TE = 30 msec; 128 phase encode × 256.4 averages) of the abdomen. (Courtesy of W.S. Kim; reproduced, with permission, from Kim et al [8].)

quired to obtain respiratory motion amplitude values independently from the NMR signals. However, a recent modification of the pulse sequence (POPE) [8] may permit the required phase reordering without the need for such a sensor (see above).

Wood et al [14] have diligently reviewed major motion reduction schemes, including the ROPE technique.

A software package (EXORCIST) that uses the ROPE technique is available from GE Medical Systems.

REFERENCES

1. Axel L, Summers RM, Kressel HY, Charles C (1986): Respiratory effects in two-dimensional Fourier transform MR imaging. *Radiology* 160:795–801.

2. Bailes DR, Gilderdale DJ, Bydder GM, Collins AG, Firmin DN (1985): Respiratory ordered phase encoding (ROPE): a method for reducing respiratory motion artifacts in MR imaging. *J Comput Assist Tomogr* 9:835–838.

3. Bock JC, Neumann K, Sander B, Schmidt D, Schorner W (1991): Prepontine artifacts due to cerebrospinal fluid pulsation in the T2-weighted coronal MRT picture: clinical significance, frequency, technique for artifact suppression. *ROFO* 154:202–205.

4. Edelman RR, Atkinson DJ, Silver MS, Loaiza FL, Warren WS (1988): FRODO pulse sequences: a new means of eliminating motion, flow, and wraparound artifacts. *Radiology* 166:231–236.

5. Foley WD, Kneeland JB, Cates JD, Kellman GM, Lawson TL, Middleton WD, Hendrick RE (1987): Contrast optimization for the detection of focal hepatic lesions by MR imaging at 1.5 T. *Am J Roentgen* 149:1155–1160.

6. Haacke EM, Patrick JL (1986): Reducing motion artifacts in two-dimensional Fourier transform imaging. *Magn Reson Imag* 4:359–376.

7. Joseph PM, Shetty A, Bonaroti EA (1987): A method for reducing motion induced errors in T2-weighted magnetic resonance imaging. *Med Phys* 14: 608–615.

8. Kim WS, Mun CW, Kim DJ, Cho ZH (1990): Extraction of cardiac and respiratory motion cycles by use of projection data and its applications to NMR imaging. *Magn Reson Med* 13:25–37.

9. Mitchell DG, Vinitski S, Lawrence B, Levy D, Rifkin MD (1988): Multiple spin-echo MR imaging of the body: image contrast and motion-induced artifact. *Magn Reson Imag* 6:535–546.

10. Mitchell DG, Vinitski S, Lawrence DB, Levy D, Rifkin MD (1988): Motion artifact reduction in MR imaging of the abdomen: gradient moment nulling versus respiratory-sorted phase encoding. *Radiology* 169:155–160.

11. Reicher MA, Gold RH, Halbach VV, Rauschning W, Wilson GH, Lufkin RB (1986): MR imaging of the lumbar spine: anatomic correlations and the effects of technical variations. *Am J Roentgen* 147:891–898.

12. Runge VM, Wood ML (1988): Fast imaging and other motion artifact reduction schemes: a pictorial overview. *Magn Reson Imag* 6:595–608.

13. Wood ML, Henkelman RM (1986): Suppression of respiratory motion artifacts in magnetic resonance imaging. *Med Phys* 13:794–805.

14. Wood ML, Runge VM, Henkelman RM (1988): Overcoming motion in abdominal MR imaging. *Am J Roentgen* 150:513–522.

35

Snapshot FLASH Imaging (SFI)

BASIC PRINCIPLES

Snapshot FLASH imaging (also known as turboFLASH) was first proposed by Haase [6], and is a variant of the more conventional FLASH imaging.

In both FLASH and SFI, the basic pulse sequence remains the same. However, by implementing modified gradient hardware, a more than fourfold reduction in total image acquisition time as achieved. The pulse repetition time (less than 3 msec), echo time (less than 2 msec), and excitation flip angle (less than 5°) are extremely low when compared to the FLASH sequence; a typical image (64 phase encoding × 128) takes less than 200 msec.

Variants In the segmented turboFLASH approach [3], the total number of phase encoding steps (t) is divided into several segments (n) of identical size (t/n). The first segment, then, contains the encoded steps numbered $1, n + 1, 2n + 1, \ldots, t - n + 1$; the second segment contains the encoded steps numbered $2, n + 2, 2n + 2, \ldots, t - n + 2$; and the nth segment contains the encoded steps numbered $n, 2n, 3n, \ldots, t$ (Fig. 35.1).

See also: EPI, FLASH.

CLINICAL APPLICATIONS

TISSUE CONTRAST

At very low excitation angles (less than 5°), TR (less than 4 msec), and TE (1.5 msec), the signal is influenced predominantly by the proton density. So, snapshot FLASH images do not possess any specific contrast

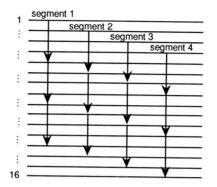

FIG. 35.1 In this illustration, the total number of phase encoding steps is 16, which is divided into four segments (represented by a vertical column of arrows), each containing four phase encoding steps. See text for the advantage of this approach.

characteristics. However, the desired contrast weighting may be incorporated by preceding the SFI experiment by either a 180° RF pulse (for T1 weighting) [5,11] or a 90° − 180° − 90° (DISE) triplet (for T2 weighting).

The magnetization in this snapshot imaging technique has not reached equilibrium or the steady state at the time of first data collection because of very short pulse timing parameters. The steady state is reached only during the ongoing imaging experiment. Therefore, the time course of the magnetization trying to attain equilibrium determines image contrast (7,10). As the zero phase encode step determines image contrast, Jones and Rinck [10] have analyzed various schemes of reordering this step in order to achieve optimum contrast. They conclude that if the zero phase encode step coincides with the null point following the inversion pulse, then optimum image contrast is obtained. Holsinger and Riederer [9] also discuss the importance of early acquisition of the low frequency phase steps when the TR value approaches that used in SFI so that image contrast matches that of the preparatory phase. Figure 35.2 demonstrates the effect of varying the delay time between excitation and the zero phase encoding step on image contrast.

THE BRAIN

It is of the utmost importance for neurosurgeons to determine, with great precision, the relative locations of blood vessels with respect to brain tissue so that blood loss from major vessels can be avoided during surgery. With MRI, it is possible to image the soft tissue and vessels with high specificity. Ehricke and Laub [4] have demonstrated that using snapshot

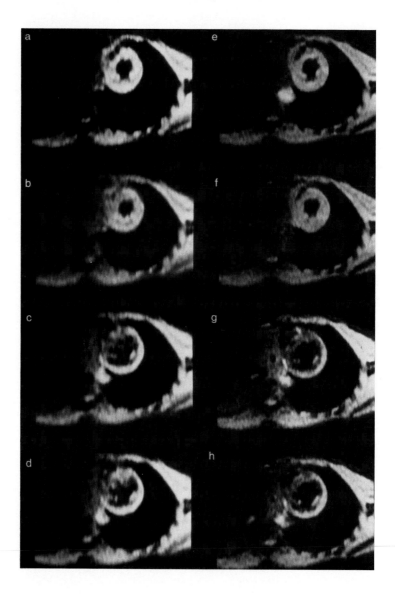

FLASH imaging, the entire human brain (128 slices) can be imaged in about six minutes with a 10° FLASH and 10 msec TR. The three-dimensional reconstruction of this data set, then, shows the complete brain profile in three dimensions. Moreover, in order to image the blood ves-

FIG. 35.2 Series of eight snapshots illustrating the influence of the time delay between excitation and the zero phase encode step. For all images, TR = 4.4 msec; TE = 2.8 msec; 8 mm slice thickness; and the standard phase encoding scheme (k_{min} to k_{max}). The images (a), (b), (c), and (d) were acquired in 139 msec (32 phase encode × 128) and the images (e), (f), (g), and (h) were acquired in 209 msec (48 phase encode × 128). The delay time between the R wave and the application of the zero phase encode step were: 350 msec (a) and (e); 400 msec (b) and (f); 625 msec (c) and (g); 650 msec (d) and (h). The time delay for images (a), (b), (e), and (f) represents the systolic phase; the time delay for images (c), (d), (g), and (h) represents the diastolic phase. (Courtesy of J. Frahm; reproduced, with permission, from Chien et al [2]).

←——————————————————————————————

sels, they used flow-compensated two-dimensional FLASH sequences and the maximum intensity projection algorithm to obtain complete arteriograms and venograms of the brain. The superimposition of these angiograms on the three-dimensional brain profile allows one to interactively examine the intricate structure of the brain before undertaking a major invasive procedure.

THE HEART

Numerous studies have demonstrated the clinical utility of snapshot imaging [1,2,8,12]. The ability to acquire detailed cardiac snapshots with high temporal resolution will benefit the examination of dynamic cardiac disorders.

THE ABDOMEN

Subsecond imaging times would naturally result in the elimination of breathing artifacts. However, to this author's knowledge, no successful abdominal series has been reported using SFI.

ADVANTAGES AND DISADVANTAGES

While the standard cine-FLASH requires 10 to 30 minutes to complete one cine study, the snapshot FLASH imaging approach results in greatly reduced data acquisition times and performs the complete cardiac cine study in about 30 seconds (Fig. 35.3).

The advantage of the segmented SFI is that it can completely nullify the signal from fat and the liver. For example, snapshot imaging takes about 900 msec with TR of 7 msec and 128 phase encoding step. As this value is longer than the T1 values for many organs (including fat and the

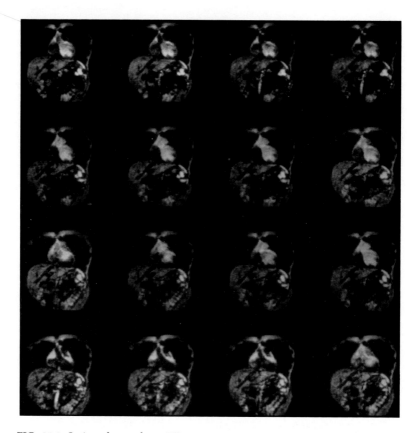

FIG. 35.3 Series of snapshots (TR = 3 msec; TE = 1.5 msec; 128 × 128 × 32) of the human heart obtained using three-dimensional snapshot FLASH imaging in 32 R-R intervals (only 16 frames are shown). Each snapshot takes less than 400 msec (128 phase encode × 3 sec). Note the high intensity of blood in comparison to the myocardium. (Courtesy of D. Henrich.)

liver), true T1 contrast is not achievable except at considerably longer TI time (500 to 700 msec). In the segmented approach, each segment is obtained in about 220 msec (32 phase encode × 7 msec), which is very close to the T1 of fat (≈200 msec) and liver (≈300 msec). Therefore, the signal from fat and the liver is nullified at comparably lower TI values. This results in a higher contrast-to-noise ratio for the liver at greatly reduced data acquisition times [3].

No time gaps in the sequence are available for time interleaved acquisition of multiple slices. Therefore, snapshot FLASH basically is restricted to single slice imaging. However, this hardly poses a grave difficulty, as additional images can be obtained very rapidly. Recently, Muller [13] obtained simultaneous multiple snapshot FLASH slices using the SIMUSIM technique (see MUSLIM).

Similar to the EPI technique, snapshot FLASH imaging also requires improved gradients but it is slower than EPI by a factor of 2.

REFERENCES

1. Atkinson DJ, Edelman RR (1991): Cineangiography of the heart in a single breath hold with a segmented turboFLASH sequence. *Radiology* 178:357–360.

2. Chien D, Merboldt KD, Hanicke W, Bruhn H, Gyngell ML, Frahm J (1990): Advances in cardiac applications of subsecond FLASH MRI. *Magn Reson Imag* 8:829–836.

3. Edelman RR, Wallner B, Singer A, Atkinson DJ, Saini S (1990): Segmented turboFLASH: method for breath-hold MR imaging of the liver with flexible contrast. *Radiology* 177:515–521.

4. Ehricke HH, Laub G (1990): Integrated 3D display of brain anatomy and intracranial vasculature in MR imaging. *J Comput Assist Tomogr* 14:846–852.

5. Haase A, Matthaei D, Bartkowski R, Duhmke E, Leibfritz D (1989): Inversion recovery snapshot FLASH MR imaging. *J Comput Assist Tomogr* 13: 1036–1040.

6. Haase A (1990): Snapshot FLASH MRI: applications to T1, T2, and chemical shift imaging. *Magn Reson Med* 13:77–89.

7. Hanicke W, Merboldt KD, Chien D, Gyngell ML, Bruhn H, Frahm J (1990): Signal strength in subsecond FLASH magnetic resonance imaging: the dynamic approach to steady state. *Med Phys* 17:1004–1010.

8. Henrich D, Haase A, Matthaei D (1990): 3D-snapshot FLASH NMR imaging of the human heart. *Magn Reson Imag* 8:377–379.

9. Holsinger AE, Riederer SJ (1990): The importance of phase-encoding order in ultrashort TR snapshot MR imaging. *Magn Reson Med* 16:481–488.

10. Jones RA, Rinck PA (1990): Approach to equilibrium in snapshot imaging. *Magn Reson Imag* 8:797–803.

11. Klose U, Nagele T, Grodd W, Peterson D (1990): Variation of contrast between different brain tissues with an MR snapshot technique. *Radiology* 176: 578–581.

12. Matthaei D, Haase A, Henrich D, Duhmke E (1990): Cardiac and vascular imaging with an MR snapshot technique. *Radiology* 177:527–532.

13. Muller S (1990): Multislice snapshot FLASH using SIMUSIM. *Magn Reson Med* 15:497–500.

36

Selective Inversion Recovery (SIR)

BASIC PRINCIPLES

When excited spins flow during an imaging experiment, they appear either bright or dark. In addition to the phase changes experienced by them, certain time-of-flight effects determine their final appearance (see TOF). Under normal imaging conditions, these TOF effects are not controlled and, hence, the depiction of blood vessels is inconsistent (for example, on conventional spin-echo images). However, by systemically exploiting the TOF effects, a variety of MR flow imaging techniques have been made possible; one of the simplest approaches is to presaturate the stationary spins and/or selectively tag the flowing spins [8]. The selective inversion recovery (SIR), a type of subtraction angiography, uses this approach [3,4].

Figure 36.1 illustrates the principle of this technique. The basic inversion recovery (IR) sequence is applied twice. In the first application of the IR sequence, the 180° inverting pulse is made nonselective. Therefore, it inverts both the flowing and stationary spins in a selected slice. The inverted blood entering the selected region of a slice (slab) has a small signal amplitude because the inverted spin magnetization has decreased due to T1 relaxation during the inversion period TI (Fig. 36.2). Remember that only the inverted spins experience T1 relaxation because, in the inverted position, longitudinal magnetization is not stable, and it decays while trying to regain its original position. Unperturbed longitudinal magnetization of the uninverted spins is stable and, when brought into the plane of detection by a 90° RF pulse, it gives off a strong signal. Next, the IR sequence is applied in the slab selective mode. During TI, inverted blood in the slab is replaced by uninverted blood entering from

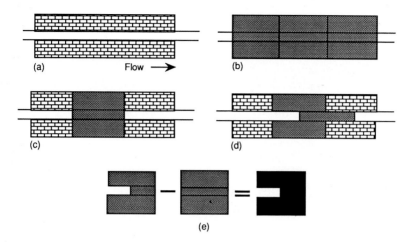

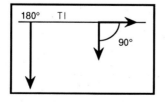

FIG. 36.1 (a) A vessel surrounded by stationary tissue. **(b)** When a 180° pulse is applied in a nonselective mode, it inverts the magnetization for the entire region (shaded area). Therefore, the blood entering the slab of interest (area bordered by two inner vertical lines) is already saturated and yields a low signal. **(c)** Next, the 180° pulse is applied in the selective mode, whereby it inverts the spins only in the region of the slab of interest. Therefore, when the signal from the slab is read out after a lapse of a certain time interval, a greater signal is obtained because the unsaturated blood enters the slab during this time interval and replaces the previously saturated flowing spins **(d)**. The degree of this spin replacement is directly proportional to the time and flow velocities. Then, a subtraction of (b) from (d) cancels out the signal contributions from stationary spins, and leaves an image of only flowing spins **(e)**. The illustration presents, of course, an ideal situation in which complete subtraction of stationary spins has been achieved. In reality, factors such as slice thickness and magnetic field inhomogeneities prevent total elimination of stationary spins.

FIG. 36.2 During inversion time TI, the inverted magnetization experiences T1 relaxation and, therefore, when a 90° RF pulse is applied, the signal amplitude is diminished.

either side of the slab; the degree of this replacement is purely a function of the flow velocity and TI. As uninverted blood has a large magnetization value, the signal from the slab is very strong. During both applications of the IR sequence, the stationary spins yield identical signal amplitudes. Therefore, a complex subtraction of these two projective data acquisitions leaves a difference signal only from the flowing spins. The interpulse time TI regulates the degree of the washing-in effect and, thus, the signal amplitude.

However, Nishimura et al (4) have shown that the difference signal (the signal obtained after the subtraction of two data sets) is inversely proportional to TI. Therefore, an intermediate value of TI has to be adopted for optimum signal strength. In a related approach by Dixon et al [2], inversion of the flowing spins is accomplished by adopting the principle of adiabetic fast passage (AFP). Figure 36.3 illustrates the main differences between conventional RF pulse and AFP inverting pulse.

Variants   Several modifications of the original SIR approach recently have been introduced for enhancing the performance of the technique.

(A) All the gradients in the SIR sequence are made flow-insensitive to minimize the signal loss due to gradient-induced spin dephasing. However, the higher-order terms of motion exist near such anatomical areas as the bifurcation and stenosis. To further enhance its performance in these situations, in a modified sequence, all the imaging gradients are collapsed in the time domain; in other words, the duration of each gra-

FIG. 36.3 **(a)** Shows an ideal RF pulse consisting of a single frequency. In **(b)**, a range of frequencies is applied during the time interval t. The pulse in (a) has the following features: it can be made section-selective in combination with a gradient; due to nonideal circumstances, the inversion achieved may not be exactly 180°, and, lastly, it requires higher RF power deposition than (b). The adiabetic fast passage pulse of (b) has the following features: it cannot be made section-selective due to the fact that it contains a range of frequencies; the maximum inversion that can be achieved is not more than 180°; and, lastly, it requires less RF power deposition than (a).

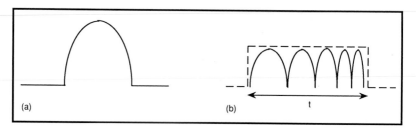

dient lobe is made as short as possible [5]. With this modification, while no moment is completely nullified, the dephasing effects of all of the moments, including those of acceleration and turbulence, are minimized (Fig. 36.4).

(B) SIR may be employed in either single readout or multiple readout mode. In the multiple readout mode [6], a series of 90° interrogating pulses follows one inverting pulse (Fig. 36.5). Multiple signals thus obtained may be used to project the same vessel from different angles or to image the same vessel at different points in time. When the earlier approach is employed, less than 90° interrogating pulses have been used in order to avoid spin saturation and obtain uniform vessel intensity in all of the projections. In either mode, some kind of cardiac triggering is used to trigger the sequence.

FIG. 36.4 Digital subtraction angiogram **(a)** of the stenosed internal carotid artery and the corresponding MR angiogram (TI = 500 msec; 128 phase encode × 256; 4 min), obtained with the SIR technique **(b)**. (Courtesy of D. Nishimura; reproduced, with permission, from Nishimura et al [5].)

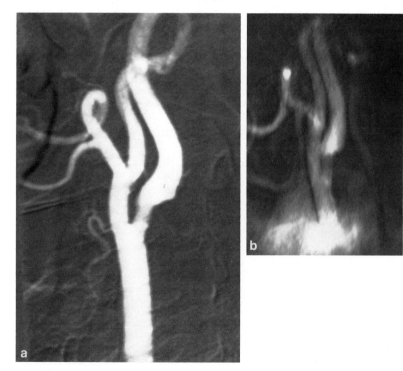

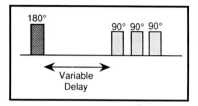

FIG. 36.5 In the multiple readout mode, a series of readout pulses is applied at a variable delay time following the inversion pulse.

(C) A typical SIR angiogram takes on the order of 3 to 4 minutes. This is enough time for motion artifacts, such as those due to cardiac blood flow induced carotid displacement, to creep into the carotid angiograms. A faster version of the SIR sequence, which uses extremely short (13 msec) and TE (4 msec), in addition to the low flip angle interrogating pulses [7] recently has been proposed. By concomittantly decreasing the number of phase encoding steps to 96, the total scan time for a single image has been brought down to approximately 20 seconds (Fig. 36.6).

See also: IR, TOF.

FIG. 36.6 (a) Oblique view of the heart along the long axis of the left ventricle, showing the left anterior descending and the diagonal branches of the left coronary artery (2 averages, each taking 24 R-R intervals). Pulmonary artery (P) and ascending aorta (A) also are seen. **(b)** Shows the unsubtracted image for reference. (Courtesy of S. J. Wang; reproduced, with permission, from Wang et al [6].)

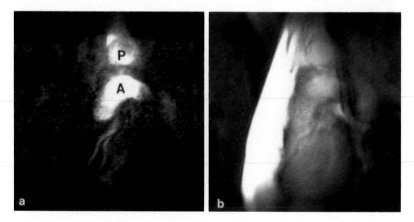

CLINICAL APPLICATIONS
TISSUE CONTRAST

On subtraction–projection images, flowing blood appears bright. Primarily, the contrast-to-noise ratio of the angiogram depends on the degree of suppression of the static background and the amount of motion-related artifacts. In cardiac gated acquisitions, CSF shows signal intensity that varies in relation to the phase of the cardiac cycle [1].

CEREBROSPINAL FLUID

MR-myelograms have not been successfully obtained using spin tagging techniques, such as the one described herein (or any other TOF technique). One reason is that the flow velocity of CSF is very slow (only a few mm/sec), which minimizes the washing-in effect. However, the pulsatile nature of CSF flow has been successfully documented using the gated SIR sequence; it has been shown that the CSF signal intensity varies systematically at different stages of the cardiac cycle [1].

THE ANGIOGRAPHY

MR angiograms of various vessels, such as the left coronary artery, carotids, aortic arch, and leg arteries, have been obtained using the SIR technique (Fig. 36.6). In the cardiac-triggered mode, a typical single readout SIR angiographic image (128 phase encode $\times$ 256) takes about 40 minutes. However, in the same time, four or more images can be obtained if multiple read gradients are applied. This raises the possibility of visualizing the same vessel from different angles or at different points in time in the cardiac cycle. The latter may be useful in studying flow dynamics.

ADVANTAGES AND DISADVANTAGES

As SIR is a TOF-based MR angiographic technique, it has, in general, the same advantages and disadvantages as other TOF techniques (see TOF).

By appropriately varying the inversion of the spins, it is possible to attribute directional sensitivity to the flow. This directional sensitivity aids in isolating the arteries from the veins, which is clinically quite useful. Moreover, if sufficient time is allowed for the washing-in effect to take place, not only the vessels perpendicular to the imaging plane, but also the vessels lying in any other plane (eg, curving vessels such as the arch of aorta) can be visualized. Note that the latter is not possible in phase based gradient-sensitive MR angiography unless the pulse sequence is repeated with different velocity-sensitive directions.

REFERENCES

1. Bergstrand G, Bergstrom M, Nordell B, Stahlberg F, Ericsson A, Hemmingsson A, Sperber G, Thuomas KA, Jung B (1985): Cardiac gated MR imaging of cerebrospinal fluid flow. *J Comput Assist Tomogr* 9:1003–1006.

2. Dixon WT, Du LN, Faul DD, Gado M, Rossnick S (1986): Projection angiograms of blood labeled by adiabetic fast passage. *Magn Reson Med* 3:454–462.

3. Nishimura DG, Macovski A, Pauly JM, Conolly SM (1987): MR angiography by selective inversion recovery. *Magn Reson Med* 4:193–202.

4. Nishimura DG, Macovski A, Pauly JM (1988): Considerations of magnetic resonance angiography by selective inversion recovery. *Magn Reson Med* 7: 472–484.

5. Nishimura DG, Macovski A, Jackson JI, Hu RS, Stevick CA, Axel L (1988): Magnetic resonance angiography by selective inversion recovery using a compact gradient echo sequence. *Magn Reson Med* 8:96–103.

6. Wang SJ, Nishimura DG, Macovski A (1991): Multiple-readout selective inversion recovery angiography. *Magn Reson Med* 17:244–251.

7. Wang SJ, Hu BS, Macovski A, Nishimura DG (1991): Coronary angiography using fast selective inversion recovery. *Magn Reson Med* 18:417–423.

8. Wehrli FW, Shimakawa A, MacFall JR, Axel L, Perman W (1985): MR imaging of venous and arterial flow by a selective saturation-recovery spin echo (SSRSE) method. *J Comput Assist Tomogr* 9:537–545.

37

Spatial Localization for Motion-Rejected Imaging (SLO-MOTION)

BASIC PRINCIPLES

Many different strategies, as discussed previously, have been employed to defeat motion in MRI. One of the strategies (NAVEC) derives information regarding motion from the image data and then applies a correction factor before performing the final Fourier transform. In order to do so, the pulse sequence acquires a nonimaging (nonphase encoded) echo during each pulse repetition cycle. As discussed in NAVEC, the total phase correction factor can be calculated from this echo, and an artifact-free corrected image obtained.

Yet another class of imaging techniques for avoiding motion artifacts is not to acquire the image data while motion takes place (motion-rejection techniques). For example, the pause technique is a motion-rejection technique in which data are acquired only during periods of breath-holding. SLO-MOTION is a motion-rejection technique that combines the features of the NAVEC and pause techniques. Like NAVEC, it also acquires an additional echo before the phase encoded echo is acquired; like pause, it proceeds with the RF application only if motion has not occurred. However, it also has some important differences from these techniques, as described below.

In SLO-MOTION [1], the motion-monitoring echo is acquired from an external marker attached to the region being imaged. Initially, this marker is placed a few centimeters away from the region of interest (ROI) (Fig. 37.1).

Before each data acquisition from the ROI, a spatial localization technique is used to acquire the signal from the external marker (Fig. 37.2). As long as the object does not move and cause the signal from the marker

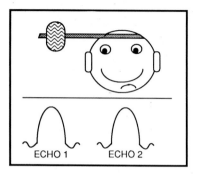

FIG. 37.1 An external marker is attached via a head strap to the subject's forehead. During each pulse cycle, the echo from this marker is measured (ECHO 1). If the echo amplitude is below the preset threshold value (which may occur if the subject's head moves), the acquisition of the image echo (ECHO 2) is halted. The data acquisition is resumed only when the amplitude of the marker echo rises above the threshold value.

to fall below a present level, data acquisition is continued. However, if the ROI moves, then the marker also moves out of the localized slice and its signal amplitude will diminish. Only if the signal attenuation is below the preset threshold value, data acquisition from the ROI is halted until the signal from the localized slice returns to the preset level.

FIG. 37.2 The SLO-MOTION pulse sequence acquires two echoes: ECHO 1 is a gradient recalled FID whose amplitude determines whether the external marker has shifted from its position; ECHO 2 is the standard phase encoded spin echo. (Modified, with permission, from S.J. Blackband [1].)

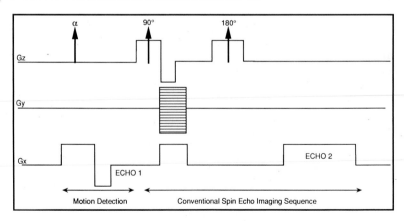

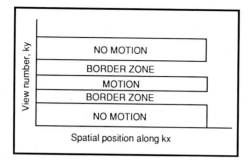

FIG. 37.3 Schematics of data after one-dimensional Fourier transfer. By visually inspecting the plot, the regions of excessive motion and the unaffected regions often can be differentiated. However, in order to correctly demarcate the upper and lower limits of the phase views corresponding to motion, edge detection and thresholding techniques are used.

Variants   (A) A recently proposed technique also uses an external marker to monitor the subject motion [2]. However, unlike the SLO-MOTION approach, it does not halt data acquisition if motion occurs; but, the data that occurred in the presence of motion are retrospectively identified during the postprocessing of the image, and eventually corrected, as explained below.

A one-dimensional Fourier transform of the acquired data along the frequency encode axis gives a plot as shown in Fig. 37.3. Through edge detection and thresholding maneuvers, the most likely spatial frequency region corresponding to the object is identified. With the phase encode step of the highest signal-to-noise ratio (usually the zero phase encode step) as a reference, the displacements are calculated. Once these displacements are calculated, a phase correction factor is determined by an approach described in NAVEC or MR fluoroscopy.

Even though the performance of this approach is not as good as the navigator echo approach, most of the image detail can be recovered, especially with use of a marker [2].

See also: Gating, NAVEC, ROPE.

CLINICAL APPLICATIONS

The SLO-MOTION technique has not yet been tried in the clinical setting. It should be most useful in eliminating random motion artifacts associated with regions such as the head and extremities.

Fig. 37.4 shows a phantom experiment in which image improvement is evident by using the SLO-MOTION technique.

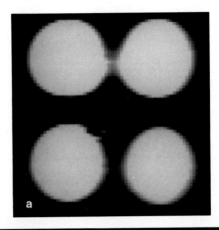

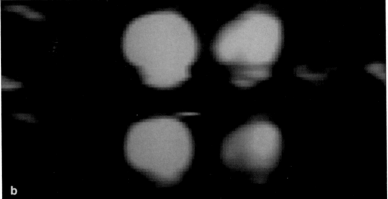

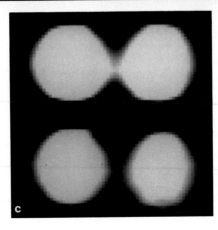

ADVANTAGES AND DISADVANTAGES

The implementation of SLO-MOTION requires logical decision making during the execution of the pulse sequence. In other words, the computer has to decide on-line whether motion has occurred and, accordingly, either apply the next pulse or halt the execution. Conceptually, this does not seem very difficult to accomplish; however, the present generation of scanners does not allow such flexibility during the execution of the pulse program. Note that interruptions in the pause approach are under operator control, and they are predetermined.

If sporadic motion occurs too often, it may halt data acquisition for extended periods of time, and this may increase total imaging time considerably if the SLO-MOTION technique is employed.

REFERENCES

1. Blackband SJ (1990): Spatial localization for motion-rejected NMR imaging: SLO-MOTION. *Magn Reson Med* 13:263–270.

2. Felmlee JP, Ehman RL, Riederer SJ, Korin HW (1991): Adaptive motion compensation in MR imaging without use of navigator echoes. *Radiology* 179: 139–142.

FIG. 37.4 (a) Image (TR = 750 msec; TE = 35 msec) of a stationary phantom consisting of four water-filled bottles. **(b)** The phantom was manually moved 10 mm during data acquisition. **(c)** This image is reconstructed only from those phase encoding steps that occurred when the signal from the motion detect slices was the largest (and thus indicated that the external marker had moved from its original position during data acquisition). Note the absence of motion artifacts. (Courtesy of S.J. Blackband; reproduced, with permission, from S.J. Blackband [1].)

38

Steady State Free Precession (SSFP)

BASIC PRINCIPLES

By steady state, we mean that the magnetization achieved at the end of an RF pulse does not experience alterations in its amplitude in an amount of time less than the tissue relaxation times. By free precession, we mean that the precession is immune from the influence of the external oscillating RF magnetic field and is determined only by the static main magnetic field strength. Much of the initial NMR imaging [2,8] was done using sequences based on this principle of steady state free precession first reported by Carr in 1958 [3]. Hinshaw's sensitive-point method of NMR imaging used the SSFP condition [10]. However, due to the poor contrast of earlier images and the T2 coherence effects (carrying over of the transverse magnetization from one repetition cycle to the next cycle), they were replaced by the spin echo techniques. In recent times, various technological improvements, such as the use of low excitation flip angle (EFA) pulses and gradient focused echo acquisition, have brought SSFP-based imaging techniques back into the clinical domain.

In the traditional spin echo based imaging techniques, a steady state magnetization is established only in the longitudinal direction (if TR $\geq$ 5 T1). If, however, a volley of phase coherent RF pulses is applied with very short pulse repetition times (TR $\ll$ T1, T2), a periodically varying steady state magnetization is established in both the longitudinal and transverse directions (Fig. 38.1).

In this particular sequence, the SSFP signal is essentially a projection of the plane along the constant gradient, and a projection image is created by combining multiple such projections obtained by rotating the constant gradient. This type of projection SSFP imaging requires individually

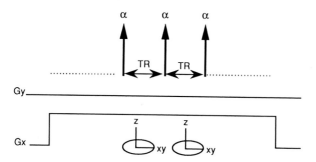

FIG. 38.1 Conventional SSFP imaging experiment in which the very short pulse repetition time (TR ≪ T1, T2) establishes steady state magnetization in both the longitudinal and transverse planes. As TR is very short compared to the T2 value, transverse magnetization is not completely lost during the interpulse period, and some amount of magnetization persists along the xy plane. After several pulse repetitions, the amount of unrecovered transverse magnetization becomes stable, and a steady state is achieved.

phase-corrected projections and the collection of the signal very close to the time of RF application. The latter poses grave technological adjustments for RF circuitry.

To overcome the difficulties of the original SSFP imaging, several Fourier-based fast imaging techniques (two-dimensional Fourier transform-SSFP) recently have been proposed in which the frequency encode gradient is nonconstant and, additionally, a phase encode gradient has been included. With these modifications, the SSFP signal may be split into its two inherently different components (Fig. 38.2). The first component is an FID arising from the nth RF pulse (due to recovery of longitudinal magnetization). The second component is a refocused echo (due to persistence of the transverse magnetization) produced by the nth pulse, which refocuses the FID produced by the $(n - 1)$th pulse (not shown). Note that either or both components of the SSFP signal may be conveniently acquired as gradient echoes by appropriately altering the imaging gradients. Based on this, two-dimensional Fourier transform-SSFP techniques can be divided into the following broad categories (Fig. 38.3).

1. Group 1: It constitutes techniques in which the FID part of the SSFP signal is acquired as an echo during the first half of the pulse repetition period (Fig. 38.3a), eg, FLASH. The phase encoding gradient is not reversed following data acquisition. As the gradient profile is not symmetric in the time domain, it prevents the development of steady state transverse magnetization [17]. In order to suppress the remaining transverse magnetization, it is destroyed by a dephasing gradient pulse

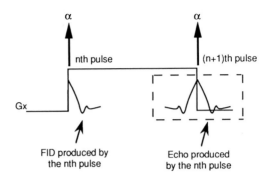

FIG. 38.2 In the presence of the unbalanced frequency encode gradient, the SSFP signal can be separated into two components. The dashed boxed area shows the echo produced as a result of refocusing of the FID following the $(n - 1)$th pulse (not shown) by the nth pulse.

after each echo acquisition (see below). In contrast to this spoiled FLASH version, the refocused FLASH reverses the phase encoding gradient before the pulse sequence repeats and, thus, restores transverse magnetization. Obviously, spoiler gradient pulses are excluded from the refocused FLASH sequence.

2. *Group 2:* While in FISP all the gradients are balanced, in GRASS, FAST, and ROAST, only the phase encoding gradient is balanced (Fig. 38.3b). As in group 1, only the FID part of the SSFP signal is collected. If the frequency encode gradient also is balanced, the sequence has been called RARE ROAST (see ROAST) [7]

3. *Group 3:* The second component of the SSFP signal is acquired during the latter part of TR (Fig. 38.3c), eg, CE-FAST [5] and SSFP, as described by Hawkes and Patz [9].

4. *Group 4.:* Transverse magnetization is preserved by employing a bipolar balanced phase encoding and slice-select gradients (Fig. 38.3d), eg, FISP. In addition, both the SSFP signal components are superimposed onto one another because of the balanced frequency encode gradient.

5. *Group 5:* The SSFP signal produced in each pulse repetition is decomposed into its two inherent components and two separate images are derived using each individual component (Fig. 38.2), eg, FADE.

6. *Group 6:* Recently, it has been reported that steady state transverse magnetization may be Fourier expanded into several higher-order echoes [13]. By reconstructing images from individual echoes, a series of images with variable image contrast can be obtained. Zur et al [18] have used these echoes to design motion-insensitive SSFP pulse sequences.

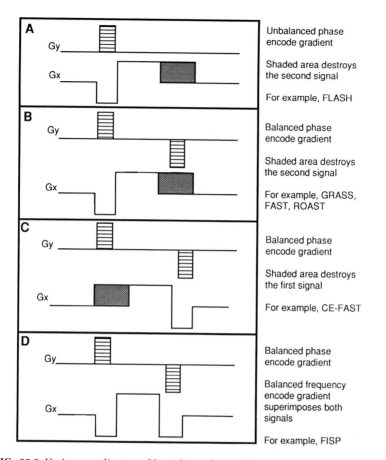

FIG. 38.3 Various gradient profiles (slice-select gradient is not shown) for acquiring SSFP signals. For details, refer to the individual sequence.

Collectively, all of the above grouped sequences may be called fast field echo (FFE) sequences. Zur et al [17] have analyzed the steady state conditions for the refocused variety of SSFP techniques and have demonstrated that, in order to obtain artifact-free images, it is critical to achieve either precise overlap of the two components (FISP-like approach) or enough temporal separation between them so that only one component falls in the sampling window at a given point in time.

Normally, the refocused echo formation and the application of the next RF pulse are two very closely occurring events. Therefore, the pulse that produces FID also may transfer some transverse coherence from the previous repetition to the newly excited FID signal (especially when TR $\ll$ T2) [4]. Obviously, this corruption of the FID is not desirable for fast imaging sequences such as FLASH and FAST, which use FID for image reconstruction. Additional spoiler gradient pulses, therefore, may have to be employed in order to disrupt this transfer of the information.

To keep the phase coherence identical for all pulse intervals and, thus to ensure motion insensitivity, the net effect of any applied gradient should be nullified for any pulse interval. However, this may also result in the appearance of strip artifacts across the image. These artifacts can be removed by either leaving one of the gradients, usually readout gradient, unbalanced (in which case, the motion along that gradient decreases the SSFP signal intensity) or by adopting a scheme proposed by Wood et al [16], which preserves the signal intensity of the flowing spins. In either case, flow sensitivity of the SSFP sequences is determined by the wavelength of the periodically varying steady state magnetization. SSFP imaging is particularly sensitive to slow flow; this fact has been used for imaging diffusion/perfusion in the brain (see FAST). Patz [15] has quantified the SSFP flow sensitivity and has derived the following relationship:

$$\phi = \gamma v G \tau,$$

where ϕ represents spin dephasing proportional to the gyromagnetic ratio (γ), the flow velocity (v) and the gradient integral (Gτ). Note also that the quantity $1/\gamma G \tau$ represents the wavelength of the periodic steady state transverse magnetization. Therefore, for a given flow velocity, the slow flow sensitivity of the SSFP experiment may be altered by changing the wavelength which means, primarily, the gradient integral [15].

Variants   In two-dimensional Fourier transform SSFP, usually a gradient echo formation occurs during the pulse repetition time. However, field inhomogeneities are not effectively refocused at this time. To overcome this difficulty, two basically identical approaches recently have been proposed in which every nth RF pulse is dropped, and an RF refocused echo formation occurs at the time when the dropped RF pulse normally would have been been present (syncopated periodic excitation, SPEX; and missing pulse SSFP, MP-SSFP; see MP-SSFP).

See also: FADE, FAST, FISP, FLASH, GRASS, MP-SSFP, ROAST.

CLINICAL APPLICATIONS
TISSUE CONTRAST

In two-dimensional Fourier transform SSFP imaging, usually both the longitudinal and transverse magnetizations are preserved. The signal amplitude depends on the excitation flip angle (EFA), TR, T1, and T2 values.

The relative contributions of the T1 and T2 values to the observed contrast are determined by the flip angle of the RF pulses and the signal component used for creating the image. Low angle RF pulses provide the maximum contrast-to-noise ratio and T1-dependent images, while EFA closer to 90° provide diminished differentiation between adjacent tissues (Fig. 38.4). The interpulse time (TR) also modulates image contrast. A report by Haacke and Tkach [6] excellently reviews the basic features of various SSFP techniques and their signal and contrast behaviors.

THE BRAIN

The non-two-dimensional Fourier transform implementation of SSFP resulted in images that failed to differentiate white matter from gray matter. However, with the implementation of low flip angle fast gradient echo techniques, the clinical utility of SSFP in brain studies has been enhanced. Short EFA RF pulses provide the best contrast-to-noise ratio in the brain; the distinction between normal gray and white matters is optimum. However, certain pathologies, such as lipoma, are better visualized with 90° RF pulses.

FIG. 38.4 A 30° **(a)** and 90° **(b)** SSFP images in which only the second signal is acquired. Note the higher contrast-to-noise ratio in (a) than in (b). Acquisition times were 100 msec for (a) and 50 msec for (b). More data averaging was employed in (a) to account for the decreased signal as a result of the lower flip angle. (Courtesy of S. Patz; reproduced, with permission, from R.C. Hawkes and S. Patz [9].)

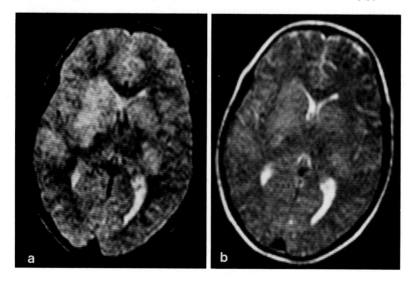

CEREBROSPINAL FLUID

The slowly flowing CSF and CSF trapped in cysts exhibit flow patterns that are difficult to visualize because of very slow velocity. Using SSFP-based techniques, it is possible to image CSF flowing at a velocity of less than 1 mm/sec [11,14]. Depending on the configuration of the imaging gradients and the flow velocity, the areas of flow are represented either by lower or higher signal intensity. Two-dimensional Fourier transform SSFP images show CSF very bright, which is clinically useful in regions such as the cervical spine in order to achieve the maximum contrast-to-noise ratio [4]. However, if a pathologic cyst exhibits the slow flow pattern similar to CSF, the anatomical differentiation between them may become problematic [1].

THE ABDOMEN

Due to rapid data acquisition rates, it is possible to complete abdominal MR studies within a time span of approximately 25 sec (128 phase encode × 256 image matrix). Thus, without resorting to respiratory gating or other motion-compensation schemes, motion artifact-free images are obtained in a relatively short period of time.

THE BLOOD

The contrast of the flowing blood is influenced by, among many other variables, the EFA [12]. For EFA values less than 40°, the flowing blood appears bright (due to steady state longitudinal magnetization) and contrast with the surrounding fat may be lost. As the EFA approaches 90°, the flow-related signal loss becomes apparent, and the distinction between the vessel and the fat is made more obvious.

ADVANTAGES AND DISADVANTAGES

In general, various SSFP-based imaging techniques provide variable contrast characteristics and fairly rapid examination times, from a few seconds to about a minute. Refer to the individual sections for further details.

SSFP images are degraded by inhomogeneity artifacts, which are accentuated at higher main magnetic field strengths. To improve the signal-to-noise ratio, more averages of the data may be needed, which may increase total acquisition time. However, MP-SSFP, a variant of two-dimensional Fourier transform SSFP, minimizes the effects of field inhomogeneities and makes the implementation of SSFP techniques possible even at high magnetic field strengths (see MP-SSFP).

REFERENCES

1. Brooks ML, Jolesz FA, Patz S (1988): MRI of pulsatile CSF motion within arachnoid cysts. *Magn Reson Imag* 6:575–584.
2. Buonanno FS, Pykett IL, Kistler JP, Vielma J, Brady TJ, Hinshaw WS, Goldman MR, Newhouse JH, Pohost GM (1982): Cranial anatomy and detection of ischemic stroke in the cat by nuclear magnetic resonance imaging. *Radiology* 143:187–193.
3. Carr HY (1958): Steady-state free precession in nuclear magnetic resonance. *Phys Rev* 112:1693–1701.
4. Edelstein WA, Bottomley PA, Hart HR, Smith LS (1983): Signal, noise and contrast in nuclear magnetic resonance (NMR) imaging. *J Comput Assist Tomogr* 7:391–401.
5. Gyngell ML (1988): The application of steady-state free precession in rapid 2DFT NMR imaging: FAST and CE-FAST sequences. *Magn Reson Imag* 6:415–419.
6. Haacke EM, Tkach JA (1990): Fast MR imaging: techniques and clinical applications. *Am J Roentgen* 155:951–964.
7. Haacke EM, Wielopolski PA, Tkach JA, Modic MT (1990): Steady-state free precession imaging in the presence of motion: application for improved visualization of the cerebrospinal fluid. *Radiology* 175:545–552.
8. Hawkes RC, Holland GN, Moore WS, Worthington BS (1980): Nuclear magnetic resonance (NMR) tomography of the brain: a preliminary clinical assessment with demonstration of pathology. *J Comput Assist Tomogr* 4:577–586.
9. Hawkes RC, Patz S (1987): Rapid Fourier imaging using steady-state free precession. *Magn Reson Med* 4:9–23.
10. Hinshaw WS (1976): Image formation by nuclear magnetic resonance: the sensitive-point method. *J Appl Phys* 47:3709–3721.
11. Jolesz FA, Patz S, Hawkes RC, Lopez I (1987): Fast imaging of CSF flow/motion patterns using steady-state free precession (SSFP). *Invest Radiol* 22:761–771.
12. Jolesz FA, Patz S (1988): Clinical experience with rapid 2DFT SSFP imaging at low field strength. *Magn Reson Imag* 6:397–403.
13. Kim DJ, Cho ZH (1991): Analysis of the higher-order echoes in SSFP. *Magn Reson Med* 19:20–30.
14. Patz S, Hawkes RC (1986): The application of steady-state free precession to the study of very slow fluid flow. *Magn Reson Med* 3:140–145.
15. Patz S (1988): Some factors that influence the steady state in steady-state free precession. *Magn Reson Imag* 6:405–413.
16. Wood ML, Zur Y, Neuringer LJ (1990): SSFP technique with zeroth moment nulled for insensitivity to motion. *Magn Reson Imag* 8:S25.
17. Zur Y, Stokar S, Bendel P (1988): An analysis of fast imaging sequences with steady-state transverse magnetization refocusing. *Magn Reson Med* 6:175–193.
18. Zur Y, Wood ML, Neuringer L (1989): Motion-insensitive, steady-state free precession imaging. *Magn Reson Med* 16:444–459.

39

Stimulated Echo Acquisition Mode (STEAM)

BASIC PRINCIPLES

Originally a pulse sequence for the NMR spectroscopy, stimulated echo acquisition mode (STEAM) recently has been adopted for magnetic resonance imaging [5,7,10].

The basic STEAM pulse sequence consists of at least three RF pulses of 90° or less. In the following discussion the interpulse timing intervals are as noted in Fig. 39.1, and it is assumed that all RF pulses are of 90°. The first RF pulse flips longitudinal magnetization into the transverse xy plane. During the time interval p1, magnetization decays by T2 relaxation. The second RF pulse then aligns the transverse magnetization excited by the first RF pulse along the −z axis. The inverted magnetization is thus stored along the −z axis, where it decays by the T1 relaxation during the time interval p2. The third RF pulse flips back the decaying magnetization into the transverse plane and when p3 = p1, a stimulated echo is evolved. Note that when p2 = p1, a spin echo also is produced, which usually is destroyed by using additional gradient crusher pulses during the p2 interval. The intensity of the stimulated echo is ½ of the spin echo or gradient echo [7] because of magnetization lost during the preparation period (Fig. 39.2).

A close inspection of the STEAM pulse sequence of Fig. 39.1 reveals that it is not much different from the 180°−90° (IR) pulse sequence. However, the presence of three separate RF pulses and three interpulse intervals gives wider access to the contrast and more functional flexibility for designing diverse clinical applications. The following points should be noted from the above discussion.

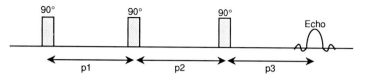

FIG. 39.1 Schematic of a simple STEAM sequence showing three 90° RF pulses. A stimulated echo forms when p3 = p1. The p2 time interval is variable depending on the specific application, but generally is longer than the p1 time interval.

1. p1 and p2 can be varied independently of each other to manipulate either the T2 contrast or T1 contrast, respectively.
2. As the velocity-dependent phase shift of the moving spins is proportional to the gradient integral and the excitation readout interval, usually the latter is lengthened in spin echo based slow flow (diffusion) imaging in order to increase flow sensitivity. However, this also means that a greater part of the signal is lost due to T2 decay. This concern is not valid for the STEAM pulse sequence because the p2 time interval can be arbitrarily increased without an additional loss of signal.
3. Furthermore, by employing bipolar gradients during the time interval p2, the velocity can be encoded in the form of the amplitude of stored magnetization.
4. If all the RF pulses are made slice selective in mutually orthogonal

FIG. 39.2 Magnetization vector at different time points during the STEAM pulse sequence. **(a)** The first 90° pulse flips the entire longitudinal magnetization into the plane of detection. E1 shows the echo if it had been obtained at this time. However, during the p1 time interval, transverse magnetization undergoes T2 decay **(b)**. Therefore, when the second 90° pulse is applied, it flips only a part of the original transverse magnetization along the -z axis **(c)**. Waiting further for time interval p2, the negative longitudinal magnetization undergoes T1 decay. Therefore, when the third 90° pulse is applied, the transverse magnetization vector is comparably small **(d)** and the elicited stimulated echo amplitude has diminished considerably (E2).

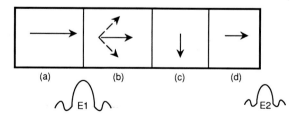

directions, then it is obvious that only that fraction of the volume lying at the intersection of the three slices is uniquely selected.

Each of the above features has been utilized for distinct clinical applications, as will be discussed below. For the clinical goal, the pulse sequence of Fig. 39.1 may have to be modified in the following manner.

For T1 Measurement   Similar to the inversion recovery method for T1 measurement, multiple points along the T1 relaxation curve may be obtained by repeatedly flipping the inverted magnetization into the transverse plane using the third RF pulse [3,15] (see also SMART in MORT).

For Flow Measurement   For measuring the slow flow (~0.1 mm/sec), a relatively longer p2 is employed. A representative pulse sequence is shown in Fig. 39.3. For measuring the blood flow, note that it is not necessary to have a p2 interval as long as that shown in Fig. 39.3. Two different approaches have been proposed for STEAM angiography:
1. In the approach based on the time of flight effect, the first and third RF pulses excite different slices located some distance apart [12]. Only those spins excited in the first slice are detected by the third RF pulse. The projective method of STEAM angiography proposed by Foo et al [4] is different; the distinction is made graphically clear in Fig. 39.4.
2. In the approach proposed by Lehrech et al [8,9], a 180° RF pulse is

FIG. 39.3 In this STEAM pulse sequence, the velocity component along the z direction is measured by the dashed gradient lobes along the slice-select direction. Usually, long p2 values are used for slow flow sensitivity. The spoiler gradient pulse (shaded area) is used for eliminating any nonstimulated echoes. (Modified, with permission, from Caprihan et al [1].

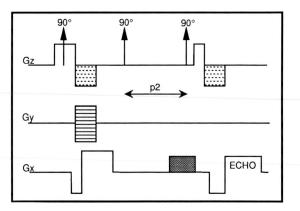

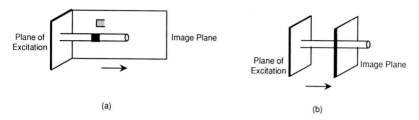

(a)   (b)

FIG. 39.4 (a) The projective STEAM angiography in which the excitation and imaging planes are perpendicular to each other and the direct visualization of flow is obtained [4]. **(b)** In this approach, the excited bolus is detected in a slice located downstream [12].

placed between the second and third RF pulses (Fig. 39.5). If the 180° pulse is applied along the x-axis of the rotating frame, then the amplitude of the stimulated echo is attenuated (amplitude = 0 when T1 = T2; otherwise, variable intensity depending on the ratio T1/T2). However, this is true only for stationary spins. Flowing spins acquire a phase shift proportional to the velocity, and their signal intensity varies with this velocity-dependent phase shift. Note that a flow image

FIG. 39.5 The STEAM pulse sequence for projective angiography uses nonselective RF pulses as shown. The flow encoding bipolar gradient pulses are applied in the same direction as the frequency encode gradient. The spoiler gradient pulse (shaded area) destroys incidental magnetization in the flow insensitive direction (Modified, with permission, from Lahrech et al [9].)

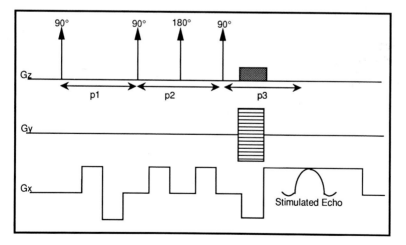

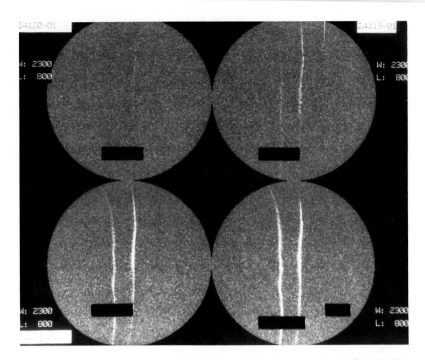

FIG. 39.6 Series of flow images of two water-filled pipes embedded in CuSO₄ solution. The images were obtained by using the technique of projective STEAM angiography. The flow encoding amplitudes (mT/m) were 0.5 **(a)**, 1 **(b)**, 1.5 **(c)**, and 2 **(d)**. (Courtesy of H. Lahrech; reproduced, with permission, from Lahrech et al [9].)

FIG. 39.7 As the slice-select direction for each RF pulse is different (dotted areas), the stimulated echo arises from the volume element at the intersection of these three planes. The spoiler pulses are shown by the shaded areas. (Modified, with permission, from Mills et al [13].)

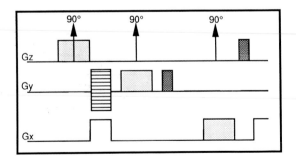

is thus obtained without the need for the subtraction of different images (Fig. 39.6).

For volume localization   The sequence consists of three 90° RF pulses applied in the presence of three mutually orthogonal slice-selective gradient magnetic fields (one RF pulse per gradient magnetic field, Fig. 39.7). This results in the evolution of a stimulated echo arising from a voxel at the intersection of the mutually orthogonal planes. To acquire the data, the phase encoding gradient is turned on immediately after the first RF pulse and the data are sampled in the presence of the frequency encoding gradient. An excellent degree of localization is thus achieved using the STEAM technique [13].

See also: MORT.

CLINICAL APPLICATIONS
TISSUE CONTRAST

Just as p1 determines T2 contrast, p3 also determines T2 contrast. Variations in the timing between the second and third pulses (p2) provide T1-dependent contrast because transverse magnetization from the first RF pulse is transformed into longitudinal magnetization by the second RF pulse (Fig. 39.8). In general, the signal-to-noise ratio of STEAM images is somewhat inferior to inversion recovery T1 images [3], as half the magnetization is lost in the form of a spin echo.

DIFFUSION

Using velocity encoding gradients in conjunction with the stimulated echoes, flow velocities as low as 0.1 mm/s have been accurately imaged [1].

LOCALIZATION

The STEAM sequence is extremely reliable for localizing ^{1}H NMR signals when the three gradients are mutually orthogonal. In what is called inner volume imaging, an imaging experiment is performed on the volume of interest previously localized using a localizing pulse sequence such as STEAM. Then the field of view (FOV) is decreased to match the dimensions of the volume of interest. In other words, the total number of phase encodings and frequency encodings remains the same even though the imaging volume has been decreased. If an imaging experiment is carried out on this localized volume, it results in a zoomed image of the selected region. Unlike the zoomed images obtained using linear interpolation, these images have far better spatial resolution, and the main magnetic field is very homogeneous in this small volume. For example, when the

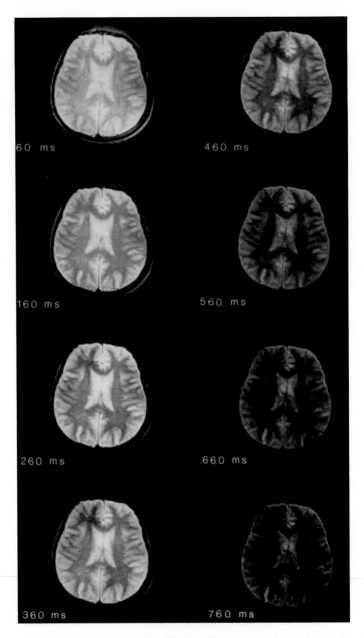

FIG. 39.8 Series of STEAM images obtained following a 25° readout pulse (the third RF pulse) at varying time intervals, as indicated. Note the changes in the T1-weighted image contrast with increasing time delay. (Courtesy of A. Haase, reproduced, with permission, from Haase et al [7].)

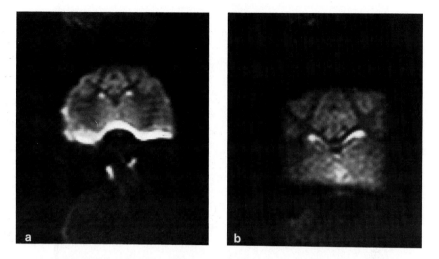

FIG. 39.9 (a) Section of a cat brain obtained with TR = 5 sec; TE = 62 msec; 4 averages; FOV = 80 × 80 mm. **(b)** Selected region of interest from (a) has been imaged with FOV = 40 × 40 mm and 16 averages. The image matrix is 64 × 64 in both images. The echo planar imaging technique was MBEST. (Courtesy of R. Turner; reproduced, with permission, from Turner et al [16].)

EPI is performed on the localized volume [16], excellent resolution is obtained without blurring artifacts (Fig. 39.9).

Just as a passing note, recently, the STEAM sequence has been used for in vivo human proton spectroscopy of the brain [6].

ADVANTAGES AND DISADVANTAGES

Spin echo based diffusion imaging requires very long TE, which ultimately results in a poor signal-to-noise ratio due to T2 decay. In this situation, the stimulated echoes method may be used, as T1 relaxation is more prominent than T2 decay in this method. However, Prasad and Nalcioglu [14] recently proposed a modified spin echo based imaging technique with shortened data acquisition times. As a result, their pulse sequence is less sensitive to motion artifacts due to macroscopic (non-diffusion) motion [14].

When using the STEAM sequence in the chemically selective form, Matthaei et al [11] have found that the separation of the fat and water signals is far better than conventional CHESS imaging.

The uncontrolled occurrence of stimulated echoes may give rise to image artifacts. For example, it has been reported that when the slice gap in a one-pass multislice series is less than 50% of the slice thickness (see MUSLIM), image artifacts occur from the evolution of stimulated echoes [2].

REFERENCES

1. Caprihan A, Griffey RH, Fukushima E (1990): Velocity imaging of slow coherent flows using stimulated echoes. *Magn Reson Med* 15:327–333.
2. Crawley AP, Henkelman RM (1987): A stimulated echo artifact from slice interference in magnetic resonance imaging. *Med Phys* 14:842–848.
3. Crawley AP, Henkelman RM (1988): A comparison of one-shot and recovery methods in T1 imaging. *Magn Reson Med* 7:23–34.
4. Foo TKF, Perman WH, Poon CSO, Cusma JT, Sandstrom JC (1989): Projection flow imaging by bolus tracking using stimulated echoes. *Magn Reson Med* 9:203–218.
5. Frahm J, Merboldt KD, Hanicke W, Haase A (1985): Stimulated echo imaging. *J Magn Reson* 64:81–83.
6. Frahm J, Bruhn H, Gyngell ML, Merboldt KD, Hanicke W, Sauter R (1989): Localized high-resolution proton NMR spectroscopy using stimulated echoes: initial applications to human brain in vivo. *Magn Reson Med* 9:79–93.
7. Haase A, Frahm J, Matthaei D, Hanicke W, Bomsdorf H, Kunz D, Tischler R (1986): MR imaging using stimulated echoes (STEAM). *Radiology* 160: 787–790.
8. Lahrech H, Briguet A, Graveron-Demilly D, Hiltbrand E, Moran PR (1987): Modified stimulated echo sequence for elimination of signals from stationary spins in MRI. *Magn Reson Med* 5:196–200.
9. Lahrech H, Briguet A, Hiltbrand E (1989): Self-referencing subtractive angiography by modified stimulated echo in magnetic resonance imaging. *Phys Med Biol* 34:1–4.
10. Matthaei D, Frahm J, Haase A, Merboldt KD, Hanicke W (1986): Multipurpose NMR imaging using stimulated echoes. *Magn Reson Med* 3:554–561.
11. Matthaei D, Haase A, Frahm J, Bomsdorf H, Vollmann W (1986): Multiple chemical shift selective (CHESS) MR imaging using stimulated echoes. *Radiology* 160:791–794.
12. Merboldt KD, Hanicke W, Frahm J (1986): Flow NMR imaging using stimulated echoes. *J Magn Reson* 67:336–341.
13. Mills P, Chew W, Litt L, Moseley M (1987): Localized imaging using stimulated echoes. *Magn Reson Med* 5:384–389.
14. Prasad PV, Nalcioglu O (1991): A modified pulse sequence for in vivo diffusion imaging with reduced motion artifacts. *Magn Reson Med* 18:116–131.
15. Thomsen C, Jensen KE, Jensen M, Olsen ER, Henriksen O (1990): MR pulse sequences for selective relaxation time measurements: a phantom study. *Magn Reson Imag* 8:43–50.
16. Turner R, von Kienlin M, Moonen CTW, van Zijl PCM (1990): Single shot localized echo-planar imaging (STEAM-EPI) at 4.7 Tesla. *Magn Reson Med* 14:401–408.

40

Short Tau (TI) Inversion Recovery (STIR)

BASIC PRINCIPLES

As the name suggests, the STIR sequence is a modified inversion recovery (IR) sequence in which the inversion time (the time interval between the 180° inverting pulse and the following 90° pulse, TI) has been greatly reduced to less than 200 msec.

The use of STIR in clinical MRI was designed primarily to avoid signals from the hydrogen protons embedded in fatty tissue so that fat-related motion could be reduced. There are two possible ways in which this goal is accomplished using an IR sequence.

1. Adjust the pulse repetition time ($-90° - 180° -$) such that the signal from fat remains saturated while the other tissues recover. However, this approach would be feasible only if the T1 of fat were longer than that of the other tissues. Unfortunately, of all known biological tissues, fat has one of the lowest T1 values (Table 40.1). Therefore, the TR value that would suppress the signal from the fat would also suppress the signal from most other tissues.
2. Adjust the TI value ($-180° - 90° -$) such that the inverted longitudinal magnetization of fat passes through the time axis before that of any other tissue (Fig. 40.1). The rate at which this null point is reached is determined by the T1 time constant. As different tissues have different T1 values, and most of these values are higher than that of fat, they lag the fat signal along the T1 recovery path. At this axis crossover point, there is no excitable magnetization for fat; therefore, no signal is obtained from fat by the following 90° pulse (Fig. 40.2).

In general, in about ln 2 × T1 time, this null point is reached (only if

TABLE 40.1.

Tissue	T1 (msec)[a]	T2 (msec)[a]
Gray matter	453 ± 77	101 ± 13
White matter	353 ± 60	92 ± 22
Liver	206 ± 45	43 ± 14
Spleen	364 ± 69	62 ± 37
Kidney	368 ± 99	58 ± 24
Cardiac muscle	377 ± 60	57 ± 16
Skeletal muscle	330 ± 59	47 ± 13
Fat	173 ± 49	84 ± 36

[a] At 0.15 T.

Modified, with permission, from Bottomley et al [3].

TR ≥ 5 T1) [4]. For the T1 value of fat given in Table 40.1, this suggests that if TI of the IR sequence is kept in the range of 121 ± 34 msec, the signal from fat would be suppressed. The subset of IR sequences in which the TI is less than 200 msec is called the short tau (TI) inversion recovery (STIR). To find a more accurate TI value, the graphic relationship between TI/T1 and TR/T1 may be used (Fig. 40.3) [14]. This approach is particularly useful when short TR values are used for rapid imaging and the condition TR ≥ 5 T1 is not met.

As we saw above, the degree of fat suppression is sensitive to the TI value, and the choice of the latter is influenced by the T1 value. In view of the fact that fat T1 varies from person to person (due to different composition) and from region to region even in the same person, it is of paramount importance to determine the T1 value of fat in the region of interest before beginning the actual examination to achieve optimum suppression of the signal. Shuman et al [19,20] have proposed that the

FIG. 40.1 Fat has a very short T1 value; therefore, its magnetization crosses the time axis (null point) earlier (upper curve) than the tissue with a longer T1 value (lower curve).

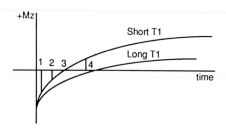

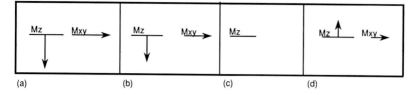

(a)   (b)   (c)   (d)

FIG. 40.2 Recovering longitudinal magnetization (Mz) is captured at four different time points along its recovery curve (see upper curve of Fig. 40.1). At (1) and (2) time points, there is considerable negative Mz that can be brought into the transverse plane (Mxy) for echo collection **(a)** and **(b)**. However, at time point (3), there is no magnetization (in reality, all spin vectors are randomly oriented) and, therefore, no signal can be elicited **(c)**. By time point (4), sufficient spin vectors have made the transition from the negative to the positive side, so that true positive signal is elicited **(d)**.

TI value should be tuned before choosing the final value. Many MR scanners have the ability to display the intensity of water and fat signals separately (the central frequency spectral display) from the selected region during the preimaging procedure. Therefore, it is simply a matter of varying the TI and observing the relative peak amplitudes. The TI value chosen should be such that it would give a minimum fat signal.

Variants   Even though the standard STIR pulse repetition time (about 1000 to 1500 msec) is lower than the typical TR value for a T2-weighted SE sequence, the image acquisition times are still on the order of 5 to 7

FIG. 40.3 For a tissue with known T1 value, the exact TI value that will null the signal (for a given TR value) can be determined from this graphical representation. (Modified, with permission, from Patrizio et al [14].)

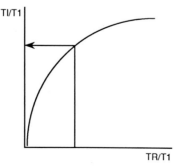

minutes. Therefore, an imaging scheme, fast short tau inversion recovery (FASTIR), has been proposed to reduce the imaging times [8].

(A) In FASTIR, a reduction in the total image acquisition time is accomplished by:

1. reducing further the TR to about 250 msec;
2. limiting the number of excitations; and
3. employing half-Fourier imaging (see UNSAD).

When decreasing TR, TI also has to be proportionally decreased to suppress the signal from the same tissues as in the case of longer TR. While all these steps lead to a considerable reduction in image acquisition times (50% to 60%), a reduction in TR also decreases the number of slices in a multislice examination. Note that, in general, these steps will decrease the image acquisition times for any pulse sequence. The choice of a particular step is influenced by the clinical problem at hand. For example, if long TR is desired for lesion sensitivity, then only step 2 or step 3 may be used; if excellent resolution is desired, step 2 may not be used.

(B) Unwanted tissue signal suppression (UTSS) uses short TR/TE SE sequence back-to-back with a STIR sequence (Fig. 40.4) [10,13]. A similar sequence has been used by Pykett et al for T1 measurement [15]. While the purpose of STIR is to null the signal from normal hepatic tissue, the SE sequence provides a superior lesion/tissue contrast-to-noise ratio [23]. Thus, an additive effect is obtained by combining them in one pulse sequence. Moreover, the phase angle between the SE and STIR magnetization vectors helps to determine the sign of the latter [14]. Thus, phase-corrected artifact-free IR images can be obtained along with T1-weighted SE images. Redpath et al [17] have used a similar approach (saturation recovery/IR instead of SE/IR) to phase correct IR images.

UTSS differs from STIR in that the signal from normal tissue is suppressed, rather than the pathology [14]. According to Patrizio et al [14],

FIG. 40.4 A short TE SE sequence is followed by a short TI STIR sequence. It is important to note that the effective repetition time for the SE sequence is determined by the duration of the STIR sequence; the effective repetition time for the STIR sequence is determined by the duration of the SE sequence. (Modified, with permission, from Lehmann et al [13].)

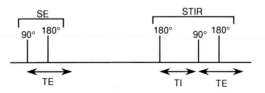

this approach reduces partial volume effects and thicker slices may be employed to increase the signal-to-noise ratio.

(C) Bakker et al [26] have recently proposed a combination of short TI with reduced (less than 90°) excitation flip angle pulse sequence. This approach has benefits of reduced RF-power deposition and more signal acquisitions per unit time; however, the signal-to-noise ratio is somewhat degraded when compared to the standard STIR images.

See also: IR.

CLINICAL APPLICATIONS
TISSUE CONTRAST

In addition to TR and TE, the value of TI considerably controls the final image contrast. While TR and TE determine the T2 weighting, TI determines the T1 weighting. Usually, long TR and TE (for T2 contrast) and short TI (for T1 contrast) are employed simultaneously. Due to this synergism, an increase in either T1 or T2 or both results in increased signal intensity. The brain and the CSF (very long T1) appear isointense, but the distinction between the gray matter (long T1) and white matter (short T1) is made more conspicuous [22]. Solid tumors usually give a strong signal (appear bright), with the surrounding tissue appearing as a low resolution dark region with loss of anatomic detail [7]. However, cysts containing lipid-rich fluid give a very weak signal, and thus appear dark, as do retrobulbar and subcutaneous fat. Bertino et al [2] have reported that STIR images (TR = 1400 msec) provide better differentiation between epidural abscesses and the CSF compared to spin echo imaging.

THE BRAIN

STIR has been particularly useful in differentiating brain lesions in the pediatric age group. Intracranial tumors have been better visualized by applying the STIR technique at relatively low field strengths of less than 0.1 T. For example, midline intracranial neoplasms, such as craniopharyngioma, pinealoma, and chordoma of the brainstem, are better highlighted on STIR (TI = 140 msec) sequences [22]. However, as the signal from CSF is not suppressed, periventricular lesions may be missed if the STIR sequence is employed alone. In such cases, TR or TI can be further reduced (or DIR, a variant of IR, may be used) to decrease the CSF signal.

THE ORBIT

As STIR suppresses the signal from retrobulbar fat, the contrast-to-noise ratio for the optic nerve is increased and is easily visualized [12]. This may benefit the diagnoses of pathologies such as optic neuritis, optic neuroma, and demyelinating diseases. However, the CSF in the peroptic subarachnoid space also appears bright; this may decrease the contrast-to-noise ratio for the CSF/lesion [1]. Therefore, Atlas et al [1] conclude that spin echo imaging should be the method of choice for orbital MR.

FIG. 40.5 (a) FASTIR (TR = 1500 msec; TE = 30 msec; TI = 100 msec) abdominal image acquired with half-Fourier imaging in one minute. To achieve better fat suppression, two different TI values were tried **(b)** and **(c)** before acquiring the time-consuming high resolution image **(d)**. Note the absence of motion artifacts on these images. (Courtesy of J.L. Fleckenstein; reproduced, with permission, from Fleckenstein et al [8].)

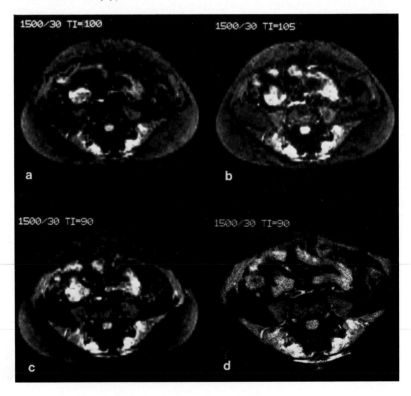

THE ABDOMEN

In comparison to T1- and T2-weighted SE sequences, the dual spin echo STIR (TI = 80 msec) sequence has been found to yield the highest contrast-to-noise ratio in identifying primary and metastatic tumors of the liver by suppressing the signal from normal liver tissue [6]. As the signal from fat is suppressed, a reduction in fat-related motion artifacts also is achieved [5]. However, artifacts due to breathing and splenic and bowel motion may be enhanced due to relatively long TR. The usefulness of FASTIR in abdominal imaging is shown in Fig. 40.5.

THE MUSCULOSKELETAL SYSTEM

STIR images clearly depict various pathologies, such as neoplasms and avascular necrosis associated with the intraosseous compartment of the bone. While the healthy (yellow) marrow appears dark, the pathologic marrow (eg, marrow infiltrated by metastases) appears bright because

1. the neoplastic tissue usually has longer T1 and T2 relaxation times;
2. the absence of the normal hemopoietic process in the diseased marrow further reduces local susceptibility artifacts and thereby decreases the loss of signal; and
3. normal fat is replaced by the diseased marrow with longer T1 time.

FIG. 40.6 Intramarrow edema from biopsy-proven stress fracture (arrows) of the left medial tibia was identified on coronal STIR (TR = 2 sec; TE = 120 msec; TI = 40 msec) image **(a)**, but was not seen on axial T2-weighted (TR = 2 sec; TE = 80 msec) image **(b)**. (Courtesy of M. Patten; reproduced, with permission, from Shuman et al [21].

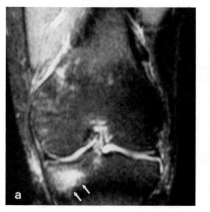
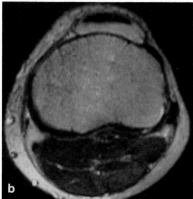

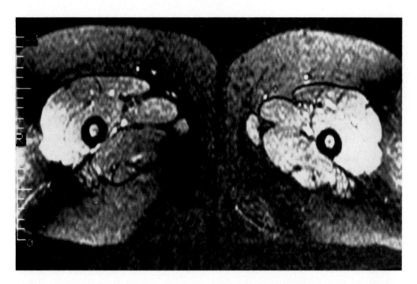

FIG. 40.7 Axial STIR images showing high signal intensities in the lateral parts of the thigh muscles in a patient with acute dermatomyositis. (Courtesy of D. Fraser; reproduced, with permission, from Fraser et al [9].)

A difficulty may arise, however, if the pathology lies in the red marrow, which also appears bright [24].

Generally, STIR has been found superior to T2-weighted SE images in demonstrating bone marrow pathologies (Fig. 40.6) [21]. However, as both the tumor and surrounding edema appear bright, the precise assessment of the boundaries of the tumor becomes rather difficult [11]. In this situation, Gd-DTPA contrast-enhanced T1-weighted SE images may provide better anatomic delineation of the pathology.

The STIR sequence has been found valuable in detecting dermatomyositis in the leg muscles (Fig. 40.7) [9]. Using FASTIR with the half-Fourier imaging approach, Fleckenstein et al [8] have successfully demonstrated the postexercise muscle necrosis (Fig. 40.8).

THE BLOOD AND THE ANGIOGRAPHY

Intravenous clots show clearer demarcation from the surrounding fatty tissue [16] than do T1- or T2-weighted SE images, and it is possible to quantify accurately the size of the clots.

Recently, a projective angiographic method built around the STIR sequence was proposed [25]. Initially, a STIR sequence is applied in order to suppress the signal from bone marrow and subcutaneous fat. To

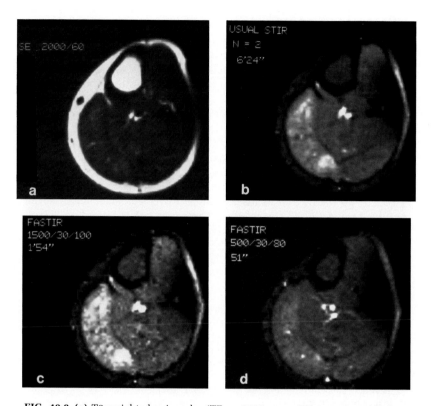

FIG. 40.8 (a) T2-weighted spin echo (TR = 2000 msec; TE = 60 msec) fails to highlight the pathology. **(b)** STIR (TR = 1500 msec; TE = 30 msec; TI = 100 msec) acquired in 6.4 min with 14 sections. **(c)** Half-Fourier FASTIR acquired in 1.9 min with 14 sections. **(d)** Short TR FASTIR (TR = 500 msec) acquired in 51 sec with four sections. FASTIR images (c and d) adequately show the lesion in lesser time than the time-consuming STIR image (b). (Courtesy of J.L. Fleckenstein; reproduced, with permission, from Fleckenstein et al [8].)

achieve complete suppression of the fat signal, the 90° RF pulse is made water-selective. After a fairly long TE (about 200 msec, to suppress the muscle signal), a series of echoes is acquired by applying 180° refocusing pulses. Under these conditions, the signal is obtained primarily from the flowing blood.

Note that any fluid (with long T1 and T2), such as CSF and urine, appears bright using this approach. Thus, its implementation in such regions as the head, neck, thorax, abdomen, and pelvis is not desirable. Even though the synovial fluid appears bright, the projection angiograms of the extremities are not severely degraded by the interfering artifacts.

ADVANTAGES AND DISADVANTAGES

At the cost of somewhat reduced spatial resolution, STIR provides a better contrast-to-noise ratio. Due to additive effects of both T1 and T2 contrast, the STIR sequence produces maximal lesion contrast and can be used as a screening method where the exact nature of the lesion is not known in advance. Near complete fat suppression by STIR makes it very attractive in such regions as the abdomen, orbit, breast [17], spine, and lymph nodes.

Moreover, it is possible to shorten TR to a value less than that employed in a standard T2-weighted SE sequence and still maintain the contrast characteristics of a T2-weighted sequence. This results in considerable savings in total image acquisition time. A STIR sequence with TR 1600 msec, TE 36 msec, TI 100 msec, and two averages takes about seven minutes for a set of 14 slices. When compared to STIR, the FASTIR sequence decreases total data acquisition time from 6 to 7 minutes to less than two minutes (for comparable values of TR, TE, and TI). However, it also results in some signal loss. The latter may be balanced by using a larger pixel size and a smaller coil size, each with its own limitations.

REFERENCES

1. Atlas SW, Grossman RI, Hackney DB, Goldberg HI, Bilaniuk LT, Zimmerman RA (1988): STIR MR imaging of the orbit. *Am J Roentgen* 151:1025–1030.

2. Bertino RE, Porter BA, Stimac GK, Tepper SJ (1988): Imaging spinal osteomyelitis and epidural abscess with short TI inversion recovery (STIR). *Am J Neuroradiol* 9:563–564.

3. Bottomley PA, Foster TH, Argsinger RE, Pfeifer LM (1984): A review of normal tissue hydrogen NMR relaxation time and relaxation mechanisms from 1-100 MHz: dependence on tissue type, NMR frequency, temperature, species, exercise and age. *Med Phys* 11:425–448.

4. Bydder G, Young I (1985): MR Imaging: Clinical use of the inversion recovery sequence. *J Comput Assist Tomogr* 9:659–675.

5. Bydder GM, Pennock JM, Steiner RE, Khenia S, Payne JA, Young IR (1985): The short TI inversion recovery sequence—an approach to MR imaging of the abdomen. *Magn Reson Imag* 3:251–254.

6. Dousset M, Weissleder R, Hendrick RE, Stark DD, Fretz CJ, Elizondo G, Hahn PF, Saini S, Ferrucci JT (1989): Short TI inversion-recovery imaging of the liver: pulse-sequence optimization and comparison with spin-echo imaging. *Radiology* 171:327–333.

7. Dwyer AJ, Frank JA, Sank VJ, Reinig JW, Hickey AM, Doppman JL (1988): Short-TI inversion-recovery pulse sequence: analysis and initial experience in cancer imaging. *Radiology* 168:827–836.

8. Fleckenstein JL, Archer BT, Barker BA, Vaughan JT, Parkey RW, Peshock RM (1991): Fast short-tau inversion-recovery MR imaging. *Radiology* 179:499–504.

9. Fraser DD, Frank JA, Dalakas M (1991): Inflammatory myopathies: MR imaging and spectroscopy. *Radiology* 179:341–344.

10. Gigli F, Mengozzi E, Lehman B, Burzi M, Gervasio M, Sartoni GS (1990): Short TR–short TE and UTSS sequences compared in an NMR study of focal neoplastic pathology in the liver. *Radiologia Medica* 79:321–330.

11. Golfieri R, Baddeley H, Pringle JS, Souhami R (1990): The role of the STIR sequence in magnetic resonance imaging examination of bone tumors. *Br J Radiol* 63:251–256.

12. Johnson G, Miller DH, MacManus D, Tofts PS, Barnes D, du Bouley EP, McDonald WI (1987): STIR sequences in NMR imaging of the optic nerve. *Neuroradiology* 29:238–245.

13. Lehmann B, Fanucci E, Gigli F, Uhlenbrock D, Bartolozzi C (1989): Signal suppression of normal liver tissue by phase corrected inversion recovery: a screening technique. *J Comput Assist Tomogr* 13:650–655.

14. Patrizio G, Pavone P, Testa A, Marsili L, Tettamanti E, Passariello R (1990): MR characterization of hepatic lesions by t-null inversion recovery sequence. *J Comput Assist Tomogr* 14:96–101.

15. Pykett K, Rosen BR, Buonanno FS, Brady TJ (1983): Measurement of spin-lattice relaxation times in nuclear magnetic resonance imaging. *Phys Med Biol* 28:723–729.

16. Rapoport S, Sostman HD, Pope C, Camputaro CM, Holcomb W, Gore JC (1987): Venous clots: evaluation with MR imaging. *Radiology* 162:527–530.

17. Redpath TW, Smith FW, Hutchison JMS (1988): Magnetic resonance image synthesis from an interleaved saturation recovery/inversion recovery sequence. *Br J Radiol* 61:619–624.

18. Schnapf DJ, Dabb RW, Tiruchelvam V, Wilson D, Livaditis S, Smeltzer M (1989): MRI of the post-mastectomy reconstructed breast: evaluation of the short TI. *Magn Reson Imag* 7:S122.

19. Shuman WP, Baron RL, Peters MJ, Tazioli PK (1989): Comparison of STIR and spin-echo MR imaging at 1.5 T in 90 lesions of the chest, liver and abdomen. *Am J Roentgen* 152:853–859.

20. Shuman WP, Lambert DT, Patten RM, Baron RL, Tazioli PK (1991): Improved fat suppression in STIR MR imaging: selecting inversion time through spectral display. *Radiology* 178:885–887.

21. Shuman WP, Patten RM, Baron RL, Liddell RM, Conrad EU, Richardson ML (1991): Comparison of STIR and spin-echo MR imaging at 1.5 T in 45 suspected extremity tumors: lesion conspicuity and extent. *Radiology* 179:247–252.

22. Smith FW (1987): Magnetic resonance imaging of midline brain tumors using inversion recovery sequences at 0.08 T (3.4 MHz). *Magn Reson Med* 5:118–128.

23. Stark DD, Wittenberg J, Edelman RR, Middleton MS, Saini S, Butch RJ, Brady TJ, Ferrucci JT (1986): Detection of hepatic metastases: analysis of pulse sequence performance in MR imaging. *Radiology* 159:365–370.

24. Vogler JB, Murphy WA (1988): Bone marrow imaging. *Radiology* 168:679–693.

25. Wright GA, Nishimura DG, Macovski A (1991): Flow-independent magnetic resonance projection angiography. *Magn Reson Med* 17:126–140.

26. Bakker CJG, Witkamp TD, Janssen WM (1991): Short TI short TR inversion recovery imaging using reduced flip angles. *Magn Reson Imag* 9:323–330.

41

Time of Flight Angiography (TOF)

BASIC PRINCIPLES

When an aqueous material flows under the influence of a magnetic gradient field, loss of the signal occurs due to two principle mechanisms. (1) the gradient-induced rapid dephasing of the moving spins, and (2) washing out of the magnetized spins. Both of these factors result in decreased signal amplitude. Based upon this realization, two varieties of MR angiography technique exist: (1) methods that depend primarily on the signal amplitude of the flowing spins, and (2) methods that depend primarily on the phase information of the flowing spins. The latter techniques are called phase contrast angiographic (PBANG) methods, of which FLAG and FEER pulse sequences are two examples.

The angiographic techniques that exploit the signal amplitude of flowing spins for showing the vasculature are classified as time of flight techniques. There are two basic time of flight effects in MR imaging [18,26]:

1. signal loss due to out-flow of the magnetized spins from the excited region before data acquisition (also called the high velocity signal loss)
2. signal enhancement due to in-flow of the unmagnetized spins (also called flow-related paradoxical enhancement, Fig. 41.1) [2].

Depending on the blood velocity and status of the cardiac cycle, either the first or the second TOF effect will predominate and the blood vessels may appear either dark (the first TOF effect) or bright (the second TOF effect).

Note that, without any kind of triggering or controlling mechanism, the appearance of blood vessels on conventional spin echo MR images is unpredictable. To achieve some control over the blood flow signal, var-

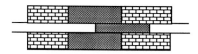

FIG. 41.1 Flow-related paradoxical signal enhancement. The incoming unsaturated spins replace the partially saturated spins (shaded area within the vessel lumen). As the stationary spins remain saturated (shaded areas outside the vessel) for a longer period of time, the flow signal is easily identified. The degree of signal enhancement is proportional to the flow velocity up to a certain limit. This signal enhancement has been termed paradoxical because, conventionally, the flow has been associated with signal loss and the resulting decrease in signal amplitude. However, this is true only for high velocity or turbulent flow conditions.

ious schemes may be used to tag the blood and then identify this tag once it is within the field of view. The tagging technique can be either inversion (depletion) of the longitudinal magnetization of the incoming spins [5,16] or the presaturation of the stationary spins in the volume being imaged [8,24] (Fig. 41.2).

Variants   (A) A novel MR angiographic technique has been proposed by Kwiat et al [10], in which the excited slice does not remain stationary, but moves in the direction of flow with the same velocity as the flow (Fig. 41.3).

Note that, like any other angiographic method, the goal of this technique is to image only the flowing spins. Let us understand how the technique works. As in sequential one-pass multislice imaging, multiple slices perpendicular to the flow direction are excited at a predetermined rate by a series of RF pulses of constant angle. As shown in Fig. 41.3, when slice number 1 is excited by this pulse, all spins, stationary as well as flowing, are flipped by an angle equal to the excitation angle. Next, slice number 2 is excited by an RF pulse of the same angle. Note that if the flowing spins have arrived into the region of the second slice by the time it is excited, they will flip by an angle equal to the RF pulse angle, but their net accumulated flip angle will be larger than the RF pulse angle, provided that the time interval between the excitation of successive slices is short compared to the T1 and T2 values of blood (Fig. 41.4). It is easy to see that if a sufficient number of slices is excited, the flowing spins eventually will possess a flip angle of 90°. At this time, if a 180° RF pulse is applied, an echo is collected that primarily consists of the contributions only from the flowing spins. It is important to note that the excitation rate of the slices determines which flow component will be visualized on the image. Moreover, slice thickness and slice interval regulate the amount of spins entering the slice and, thus, influence the intensity of the images.

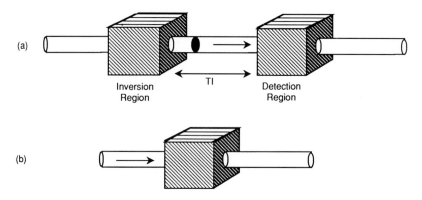

FIG. 41.2 (a) Longitudinal magnetization of the flowing spins is inverted in the inversion region. After time interval TI, it enters the detection region, where its signal intensity is proportional to the signal loss caused by T1 relaxation during TI. **(b)** In this scheme, the region of interest is repeatedly excited so that the magnetization of the stationary spins saturates, but that of the flowing spins is constantly being replaced by the incoming unsaturated spins.

(B) *Direct bolus imaging (DBI):* If we know how much distance (d) an object has traveled in what time (t), then the velocity of the object during the time period t can be derived simply by dividing d by t. Direct bolus imaging uses this rather naive equation for calculating blood velocity. Various investigators have proposed different approaches for this type of angiography [1,4,6,13,20,23].

Figure 41.5 illustrates an imaging technique in which direct bolus imaging has been implemented. Here, the blood is excited in the direction perpendicular to flow and a projection of the spins is obtained on a plane parallel to the direction of flow. The flowing spins appear as a single mass (bolus) whose shape varies with flow velocity. In order to calculate the velocity, a minimum of two images are obtained at different times showing the displacement of the bolus (Fig. 41.6).

In the approach proposed by Shimizu et al [23], the excitation is performed perpendicular to the flow (just as described above). However, to detect the position of the bolus, a three-dimensional acquisition is performed by phase encoding the data in two directions. This approach is particularly useful if there are many overlapping vessels in the region.

While the above approaches depict the moving bolus as a bright object against the dark background, the technique of Edelman et al [4] depicts the bolus as a dark object surrounded on either side by bright blood. Their technique works in the following way: first, the flowing spins in a plane

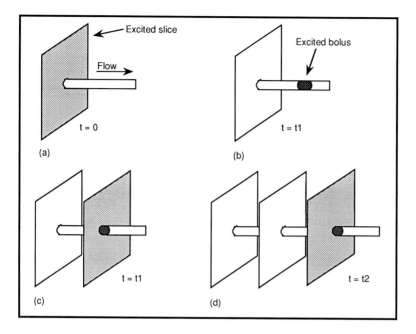

FIG. 41.3 The principle of time of flight angiography by the moving slice excitation. **(a)** At t = 0, one slice is excited. The excited bolus then moves a certain distance, depending on the velocity and the time interval t1. At this time, some TOF methods obtain a projection of this bolus **(b)**, and some other TOF methods locate this bolus by exciting a second slice, perpendicular to the flow direction **(c)**. If this latter approach is extended for several slices as shown in **(d)**, it becomes readily apparent that slice excitation is moving, and if the speed of slice excitation is same as the flow velocity, the same bolus will be excited multiple times. In the proposed technique, the excitation RF pulses are such that the bolus magnetization progressively flips towards 90° and, at that time, a readout pulse samples the flowing spins. The stationary spins do not experience this cumulative effect of the RF pulses; therefore, their magnetization does not contribute considerably to the final signal. (See also Fig. 41.4.)

perpendicular to the flow are saturated by a 90° pulse and their coherent transverse magnetization is destroyed by a spoiler pulse. Thus, they are stripped of their magnetization. Second, they are imaged in a plane parallel to the flow direction. While saturated spins show up as an area of signal loss, unsaturated flowing spins appear bright. The velocity is calculated as above.

Unlike the above approaches in which only one bolus is tagged at any

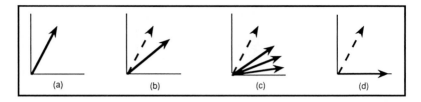

FIG. 41.4 The first RF pulse flips the magnetization of the stationary as well as the flowing spins by a certain degree **(a)**. **(b)** If the excited flowing spins have arrived into the second slice by the time the second RF pulse is applied, they experience additional excitation (b, the solid arrow) but the stationary spins of that slice do not experience this cumulative effect of the RF pulse (b, the broken arrow). If this process is continued for several RF cycles **(c)**, it can be seen that the flowing spins eventually will accumulate 90° excitation **(d)**. At this time, the readout RF pulse generates a spin echo mainly from the flowing magnetization that has been excited at a predetermined rate by a series of RF pulses.

instance of time, the technique of Saloner and Anderson [21] gives multiple boli of alternate intensities. Figue 41.7 schematically explains how their technique works.

(C) In conventional two-dimensional TOF angiography, all the phase encoding steps comprising a slice are carried out before advancing to the next slice (sequential sampling). In what is called the suppressed tissue with refreshment angiography method (STREAM) [3], the parallel k-space sampling strategy is employed as in conventional multislice SE imaging. In parallel k-space sampling, at every phase encoding step, all the desired slices are sampled before advancing to the next phase level (Fig. 41.8). However, this results in the prolonging of TR with the disadvantage that longitudinal magnetization of the stationary spins is not fully suppressed. Therefore, to minimize the signal contribution from stationary tissue, all

FIG. 41.5 Flow is excited in the plane perpendicular to the flow direction, and a projection of the excited bolus is obtained in a plane parallel to the flow direction.

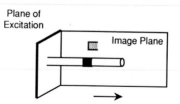

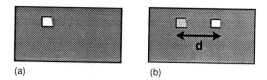

(a)   (b)

FIG. 41.6 Snapshot of the bolus at t = t1 **(a)**, and t = t2 **(b)**. The flow velocity is simply d/(t2-t1).

slices distal to the selected slice are presaturated every time data acquisition from the selected slice is carried out (Fig. 41.9).

Recently, STREAM has been implemented in a projective mode by eliminating the phase encode gradient [14]. This has resulted in very short examination times (four seconds for a 64-line angiogram).

(D) The three-dimensional approach for angiography has the advantage that the signal-to-noise ratio is enhanced due to inherent signal averaging. However, it is difficult to visualize small vessels against the vast background. While the use of thinner slices gives a better visualization of the small vessels, such images have a degraded signal-to-noise ratio, depending on the slice thinness. Parker et al [19] have combined the signal-to-noise ratio advantage of three-dimensional angiography with the better visualization advantage of the thin slices in their technique, multiple overlapping thin slab acquisition (MOTSA).

FIG. 41.7 Some flowing spins (indicated by the left diagonal area) in the excitation region receive more than one RF pulse before they exit. Therefore, their magnetization is more saturated than the spins that receive fewer RF pulses before they exit from the excitation region (right shaded area). As a result, given proper imaging conditions (and the flow velocity), the flow bolus has alternating black and white stripes.

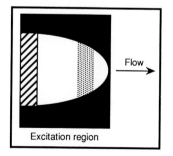

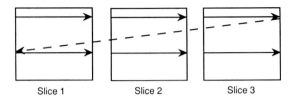

Slice 1   Slice 2   Slice 3

FIG. 41.8 In parallel k-space sampling, for each slice, a phase encode step is performed before advancing to the next phase encode step in the same slice.

As the name suggests, the volume of interest is divided into several overlapping slabs of fixed width; within each slab, multiple thin slices are excited (Fig. 41.10). After data acquisition, the slices falling in overlapping regions are discarded and the remaining slices are stacked together. An algorithm that projects the maximum intensity regions of a slice onto the subsequent slices (maximum intensity projection, or MIP) is then used to map the vessels in the volume of interest. To minimize the signal loss from the small vessels, Parker et al have used a combination of an asymmetric RF pulse and an asymmetric echo readout (Fig. 41.11). By bringing the RF pulse and the echo closer, this approach minimizes TE. However, the partial loss of echo results in a somewhat decreased signal-to-noise ratio.

(E) Kim and Cho [9] have proposed a three-dimensional TOF angiography in which both arteries and veins are displayed simultaneously (simultaneous data acquisition of arteries and veins, SAAV). In this technique, three RF excitation pulses are used to excite three different regions, as shown in Fig. 41.12. Several such sampled planes are then stacked together to reconstruct the three-dimensional volume data set.

FIG. 41.9 Before acquiring data from the first slice, slices 2 through 4 are excited (shaded areas). Next, before acquiring data from the second slice, slices 3 and 4 are excited. In this manner, the slices distal to the slice of interest receive multiple excitations, which saturate their magnetizations.

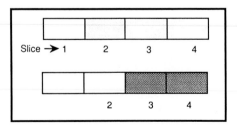

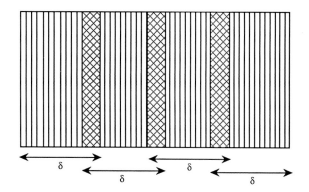

FIG. 41.10 The entire imaging volume is subdivided into several slabs of equal width δ, each containing equal number of partitions (vertical lines). In order to adequately cover the region occurring near the borders of the slabs, the slab widths are made to overlap (cross-hatched regions).

FIG. 41.11 **(a)** Symmetric RF excitation and echo sampling. The echo time is defined as the time interval between the center of the excitatory RF pulse and the sampled echo. To decrease the echo time and, thereby, reduce the intraview spin dephasing, the excitatory RF pulse and the echo are brought closer by making the RF excitation asymmetric around the center and by more data sampling during the rising part of the echo (off-centered echo) **(b)**.

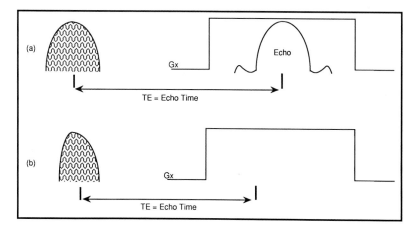

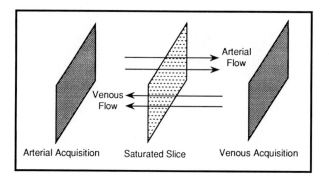

FIG. 41.12 In the SAAV technique of angiography, three sequential RF excitations excite three different slices during each pulse repetition cycle. The first RF excitation saturates a slice between the arterial and venous slices, which are excited thereafter. When the arterial slice is excited, the venous blood entering it already has been saturated once; therefore, it does not contribute significantly to the arterial slice. Similarly, when the venous slice is acquired, the arterial blood entering it already has been excited twice; therefore, it does not contribute significantly to the venous acquisition. The individual slices are then stacked together to create a three-dimensional data set.

(F) Most TOF angiographic methods detect the signal amplitude of the flowing spins. If the saturated flowing spins can be relaxed sooner, their longitudinal magnetization can be made available for the next excitation early, and thus an enhanced signal can be obtained from them. Moseley et al [17] have used gadolinium to shorten the T1 of blood and obtain brighter angiograms. The decreased T1 value also allows the use of a shorter TR and, therefore, data acquistion can be performed rapidly.

See also: FANG, LISA, PBANG, SIR.

CLINICAL APPLICATIONS
TISSUE CONTRAST

Based upon the type of TOF technique used, blood vessels may appear either dark or bright. In general, the intensity of the signal is determined by the flow velocity. The signal intensity increases with increasing velocity; but, for very high flow velocities, it actually may decrease due to rapid washing out of the excited spins and the presence of higher derivatives of motion. If desired, the signal from flowing blood may be further increased by suppressing stationary spins using very short pulse repetition time and gradient recalled data acquisition [25]. Along with the

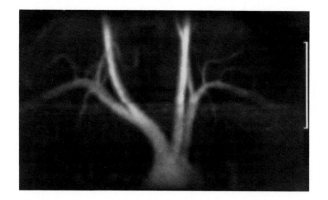

FIG. 41.13 This angiogram of the aortic arch and associated arteries was obtained using three-dimensional FISP (20° excitation; TR = 22 msec; asymmetric echo collection with TE = 5.6 msec). To cover the anatomic region shown here, two 75 mm thick (64 partitions) acquisitions, each obtained in 6.5 min, were combined. A line artifact appears due to misregistration of the overlapping regions because of the motion between the scans. (Courtesy of J.S. Lewin; reproduced, with permission, from Lewin et al [11].)

FIG. 41.14 Anterioposterior **(a)** and oblique **(b)** views of the abdominal aorta along with the iliac bifurcation and renal arteries. This angiogram has been produced by combining three image slabs (each slab is 100 mm thick with 64 partitions and is acquired in 8 min) with the three-dimensional FISP imaging parameters of pulse flip angle 20°; TR = 29 msec; TE = 5.6 msec. (Courtesy of J.S. Lewin; reproduced, with permission, from Lewin et al [11].)

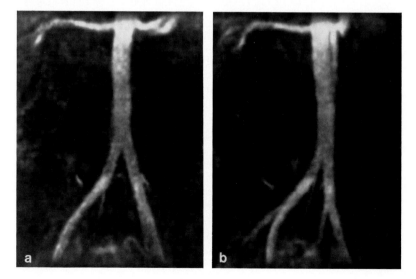

use of presaturation of the stationary spins, this approach yields an increased contrast-to-noise ratio.

CEREBROSPINAL FLUID

In TOF flow techniques, the signal amplitude of the flowing spins directly depends on the velocity; the flow velocity of CSF is on the order of only a few millimeters per second. Thus, the time of flight effect based imaging techniques do not effectively demonstrate CSF flow.

THE ANGIOGRAPHY

A variety of vascular structures, such as the cerebral vessels [15,22], carotid areries [12], aortic arch (Fig. 41.13) [11], and abdominal arteries (Fig. 41.14) [11] have been studied using TOF methods. Usually, the qualitative assessment of the vessel is far superior to the quantitative assessment of the blood flow, and a good degree of correlation exists between the contrast-based x-ray angiography and the TOF-based MR angiography.

ADVANTAGES AND DISADVANTAGES

Overall, TOF angiograms furnished excellent morphological information regarding the geometry and patency of a blood vessel. Unlike phase-based angiography, TOF-based angiographic methods depict all directional components of the flow in a single acquisition (if the slice thickness is wide enough). For comparable imaging parameters, TOF methods generally are 30% to 40% faster than the phase-based methods.

Blood flow pulsatality and peristalsis related artifacts are absent from STREAM angiograms because their periodicity is effectively destroyed by employing the parallel k-space sampling strategy (Fig. 41.15) [3]. In addition, as STREAM has a higher TR, ECG triggering may be incorporated in the study without any additional time penalty. The ECG-triggered acquisition has its own advantages and disadvantages (see Gating).

The disadvantage of relying only upon the signal amplitude for obtaining dynamic information is that, in addition to the velocity, the signal amplitude also is affected by proton density. Thus, accurate determination of flow velocity is not possible with TOF techniques, and only semiquantitative information is obtained by using these methods. However, Matsuda et al [13] have found a fairly acceptable correlation between their TOF method of velocity measurement and Doppler ultrasound.

As the signal intensity is directly dependent upon the bulk blood flow,

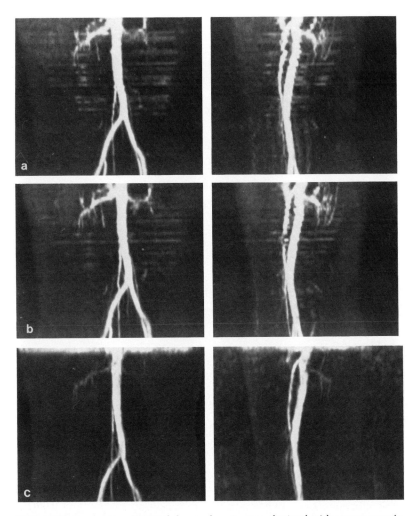

FIG. 41.15 Conventional TOF abdominal angiogram obtained with one average in 7 min **(a)** and with two averages in 14 min **(b)**. The right column of images represents lateral views of the images in the left column. Notice the high degree of motion artifacts in both sets of images. The STREAM angiogram **(c)** of the same section (obtained with TR = 3.9 sec; TE = 15 − 17 msec; one average in 8.3 min) shows near complete elimination of the artifacts. (Courtesy of M. Doyle; reproduced, with permission, from Doyle et al [3].)

vessels with slower flow velocity or smaller diameter vessels (such as the capillaries) with reduced blood volume give less intense signals and thus are often difficult to visualize and quantify.[1]

The TOF angiographic techniques are easier to implement because, in general, they do not require complicated pulse sequences or hardware modifications.

REFERENCES

1. Axel L, Shimakawa A, MacFall J (1986): A time-of-flight method of measuring flow velocity by magnetic resonance imaging. *Magn Reson Imag* 4:199–205.

2. Bradley WG, Waluch V (1985): Blood flow: magnetic resonance imaging. *Radiology* 154:443–450.

3. Doyle M, Matsuda T, Pohost GM (1991): A new acquisition mode for 2D inflow refreshment angiography. *Magn Reson Med* 18:51–62.

4. Edelman RR, Mattle HP, Kleefield J, Silver MS (1989): Quantification of blood flow with dynamic MR imaging and presaturation bolus tracking. *Radiology* 171:551–556.

5. Felmlee JP, Ehman RL (1987): Saptial presaturation: a method for suppressing flow artifacts and improving depiction of vascular anatomy in MR imaging. *Radiology* 164:559–564.

6. Foo TK, Perman WH, Poon CS, Cusma JT, Sandstrom JC (1989): Projection flow imaging by bolus tracking using stimulated echoes. *Magn Reson Med* 9:203–218.

7. Gore JC, Majumdar S (1990): Measurement of tissue blood flow using intravascular relaxation agents and magnetic resonance imaging. *Magn Reson Med* 14:242–248.

8. Hennig J, Mueri M, Friedburg H, Brunner P (1987): MR imaging of flow using the steady state selective saturation method. *J Comput Assist Tomogr* 11:872–877.

9. Kim JH, Cho ZH (1990): 3-D MR angiography with scanning 2-D images— simultaneous data acquisition of arteries and veins (SAAV). *Magn Reson Med* 14:554–561.

---

[1] A unique approach has been proposed by Gore and Majumdar [7] for quantifying tissue blood flow at the capillary level. In their scheme, a tracer (such as a paramagnetic contrast agent) is infused in the vessel at time = 0. For the next two minutes, the MR signal intensity is measured from each pixel with a very high temporal resolution (two samples per second). This sampling rate can be even higher by using the echo planar or turboFLASH imaging techniques. From the plot of the signal intensity versus the time, the mean transit time is calculated after integrating the area under the curve. The mean transit time is multiplied by the fraction of the tissue that is blood to obtain the tissue blood flow. However, there are two major difficulties: (1) as one of the axes displays the signal intensity, a way has to be found for deriving the tracer concentration from the signal intensity; and (2) the tissue fraction that is blood has to be estimated, which may involve drawing a blood sample, and this makes the procedure invasive.

10. Kwiat D, Einav S, Elad D (1990): A magnetic resonance imaging method of flow by successive excitation of a moving slice. *Med Phys* 17:258–263.

11. Lewin JS, Laub G, Hausmann R (1991): Three-dimensional time-of-flight MR angiography: applications in the abdomen and thorax. *Radiology* 179:261–264.

12. Masaryk TJ, Laub GA, Modic MT, Ross JS, Haacke EM (1990): Carotid-CNS MR flow imaging. *Magn Reson Med* 14:308–314.

13. Matsuda T, Shimizu K, Sakurai T, Fujita A, Ohara H, Okamura S, Hashimoto S, Tamaki S, Kawai C (1987): Measurement of aortic blood flow with MR imaging: comparative study with Doppler US. *Radiology* 162:857–861.

14. Matsuda T, Doyle M, Pohost GM (1991): Direct projective time-of-flight NMR angiography within 4 s. *Magn Reson Med* 18:395–404.

15. Mattle HP, Wentz KU, Edelman RR, Wallner B, Finn JP, Barnes P, Atkinson DJ, Kleefield J, Hoogewoud HM (1991): Cerebral venography with MR. *Radiology* 178:453–458.

16. Mayo JR, Culham JA, MacKay AL, Aikins DG (1989): Blood MR signal suppression by preexcitation with inverting pulses. *Radiology* 173:269–271.

17. Moseley ME, White DL, Wang SC, Wikstrom MG, Dupon JW, Gobbel G, Roth K, Brasch RC (1989): Vascular mapping using albumin (Gd-DTPA), an intravascular MR contrast agent, and projection MR imaging. *J Comput Assist Tomogr* 13:215–221.

18. Nishimura DG (1990): Time-of-flight MR angiography. *Magn Reson Med* 14:194–201.

19. Parker DL, Yuan C, Blatter DD (1991): MR angiography by multiple thin slab 3D acquisition. *Magn Reson Med* 17:434–451.

20. Saloner D, Hinson WH, Moran PR, Tsui BMW (1988): MR flow imaging in projection through a stationary surround. *J Comput Assist Tomogr* 12:122–129.

21. Saloner D, Anderson CM (1990): Flow velocity quantitation using inversion tagging. *Magn Reson Med* 16:269–279.

22. Sevick RJ, Tsuruda JS, Schmalbrock P (1990): Three-dimensional time-of-flight MR angiography in the evaluation of cerebral aneurysms. *J Comput Assist Tomogr* 14:874–881.

23. Shimizu K, Matsuda T, Sakurai T, Fujita A, Ohara H, Okamura S, Hashimoto S, Mano H, Kawai C, Kiri M (1986): Visualization of moving fluid: quantitative analysis of blood flow velocity using MR imaging. *Radiology* 159:195–199.

24. Wehrli FW, Shimakawa A, MacFall JR, Axel L, Perman W (1985): MR imaging of venous and arterial flow by a selective saturation-recovery spin echo (SSRSE) method. *J Comput Assist Tomogr* 9:537–545.

25. Wehrli FW, Shimakawa A, Gullberg GT, MacFall JR (1986): Time-of-flight MR flow imaging: selective saturation recovery with gradient refocusing. *Radiology* 160:781–785.

26. Wehrli FW (1990): Time-of-flight effects in MR imaging of flow. *Magn Reson Med* 14:187–193.

42

Ultra-Low Field MRI (ULF-MRI)

BASIC PRINCIPLES

The current generation of clinical MRI scanners require a powerful and highly homogeneous main magnetic field (Bo) to magnetize the protons. Three main types of magnets have been used in MR scanners to provide the required main magnetic field: resistive, permanent, and superconductive. The range of commercially available Bo is from 0.5 T to 2 T. Only the superconductive magnet is able to provide such high field strength homogeneous Bo within practical limitations (eg, the size and weight of the magnet).

The installation and maintenance of such a magnet poses immense technological and economic challenges. In addition, the cost of a fully operational MR system rises with increasing main magnetic field strength. However, the clinical utility of a field strength in excess of 0.5 T is questionable [14]. Even though image resolution and the signal-to-noise ratio at ultra-low field strengths (≤ 0.1 T) are inferior to higher field strength images, several studies have demonstrated the feasibility of such low field scanners in limited applications [1–3,11–13,15,17–19]. Thus, there always has been an incentive to develop innovative and inexpensive designs of the MR scanner [6,8].

The following features of the ULF-MRI should be noted.

1. The Larmor frequency (ω) at lower Bo field strengths is lower (as $\omega = \gamma Bo$). Therefore, as T1 is frequency dependent [5,9], it is also shortened (1/T1 is increased). (The T2 relaxation time usually is not affected by variations of the Larmor frequency in the range of 1 to 100 MHz [16].)

2. At lower field strengths, the amplitude of the equilibrium magneti-

zation is very low. Therefore, the signal-to-nose ratio generally is very low.

The signal-to-noise ratio is related to Bo field strength (M) by the following relationship:

SNR = M × n,

where n = 0.3 − 1.0. For M = 0.02, the signal-to-noise ratio of an image is approximately 1 [7]. However, as the T1 also is decreased, pulse repetition time (TR) may be reduced and, thus, more averages may be obtained to increase the signal-to-noise ratio.

Variants   (A) Recently, an experimental system capable of obtaining MR images using the earth's magnetic field has been proposed (magnetic resonance imaging in earth's field, MRIE) [4,21]. In brief, the sample is placed in the earth's magnetic field where it is most homogeneous and is magnetized with a primary coil for a time interval at least three times the T1 of the sample. During this prepolarization period, the low magnetic field induced by the coil determines the steady state value of the magnetization. The strength of this preparatory magnetic field is about 1000 times higher than the earth's magnetic field.

During this preparatory period, the attainment of equilibrium follows the standard equation

$$M(t) = Ms(1 - e^{(t/T1)}),$$

where Ms = steady state magnetization, and t = time. After the magnetization attains its near equilibrium (steady state) position, the external field is switched off. Now, the earth's magnetic field determines the frequency of free precession (Larmor frequency) of the magnetized spins. As the magnitude of the earth's magnetic field is very low (on the order of 10^{-5} T or 0.1 G), the Larmor frequency also is very low. A highly sensitive receiving coil is, therefore, needed to sense the induced electric flux (FID).

Transverse magnetization may be formed in two ways [4]:

1. if the external field is switched off at a rate faster than the Larmor frequency (nonadiabetically), the magnetization remains aligned along the external field, and an FID is directly observed without the need for RF pulses;
2. if the external field is switched off at a rate slower than the Larmor frequency (adiabatically), the precessing magnetization is aligned along the earth's magnetic field. RF pulse (for example, 90°) is then used to bring it into the transverse plane, and an FID is collected. Additional RF pulses may be used to refocus the echo.

Figure 42.1 shows a phantom image obtained using the technique of MRIE. Many of us who have seen the first NMR zeumatographic projection images of Lauterbar (Nature, 1973) may notice the similarity in the quality of those images and the phantom images of Fig. 42.1. Within a decade of that original publication, the image quality had improved so

FIG. 42.1 Early images obtained in the earth's magnetic field: **(a)** water-filled tubes; **(b)** an apple. (Courtesy of J. Stepisnik; reproduced, with permission, from Stepisnik et al [21].)

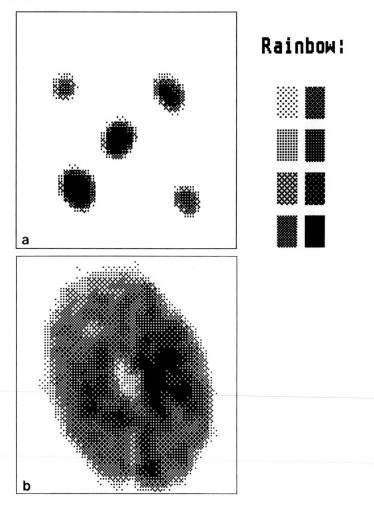

much that regularly scheduled clinical studies had begun at most centers. It may be too premature to expect that the same magnitude of improvement will be attained in the field of MRIE in the near future, as the momentum behind its development is not as great. However, any significant improvement in the science of ULF-MRI, in general, and that of MRIE, in particular, will prove beneficial for a variety of purposes, including economic incentives and defense issues (for example, these techniques may make MRI accessible at war fronts).

CLINICAL APPLICATIONS
TISSUE CONTRAST

Recall that, under the influence of BO, a net magnetization is induced in the sample, and the amplitude of this signal determines pixel intensity. Obviously, the acquired signal intensity is low at lower field strength. Therefore, the image quality of the low field MRI is poor due to an inferior signal-to-noise ratio.

CONTRAST ENHANCEMENT AND ULTRA LOW FIELD MRI

The paramagnetic ions decrease both the T1 and T2 relaxation times for a tissue. While the shortened T1 may increase tissue intensity, the shortened T2 usually decreases tissue intensity. Usually, a balance between these two opposite effects determines the contrast-to-noise ratio of the paramagnetic ion-enhanced images.

At lower field strengths, the relaxivity of the paramagnetic ion is increased [10]. This means that a lower concentration of paramagnetic ions is required to achieve the desired contrast effect. In addition, the tissue T1 relaxation rate (1/T1) also is shortened, and the T2 remains practically unchanged. The cumulative effect of all these factors offers an opportunity for enhancing the contrast-to-noise ratio.

THE BRAIN

In a limited number of brain pathologies, images obtained at 0.02 T have been found at least equivalent to x-ray CT images [17]. Compared to 0.17 T, IR images at 0.02 T showed acute intracranial and subdural hematomas more easily by increasing their signal intensity [18,20]. Recently, Sa-

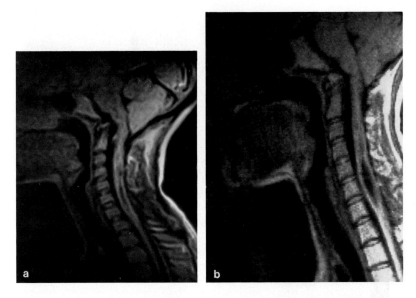

FIG. 42.2 (a) 0.02 T and **(b)** 0.5 T sagittal images showing chiari malformations and syrinx at C3-C6 level: (a) was obtained using the saturation recovery sequence (TR = 250 to 500 msec, TE = 40 msec; 12 min data acquisition time); (b) was obtained with the spin echo sequence (TR = 500 msec; E = 30 msec; 4.5 to 8.5 min data acquisition time). (Courtesy of L. Samuelsson; reproduced, with permission, from Samuelsson et al [15].)

muelsson et al [15] have evaluated the size and extent of the syrinx and the chiari malformations at 0.02, 0.04, and 0.5 T; they have reported excellent correlation between the values at different field strengths (Figs. 42.2 and 42.3). At 0.08 T, a variety of midline brain tumors have been examined by using the STIR sequence [20].

THE ABDOMEN

As early as 1982, the short T1 advantage of low field MRI was recognized and, in the studies performed at 0.04 T, Smith et al [19] were able to identify various types of pancreatic inflammation, cysts, and tumors. Since then, a variety of abdominal organs, such as the liver [2] and kidneys [11], have been examined at field strengths ranging from 0.02 T to 0.04 T.

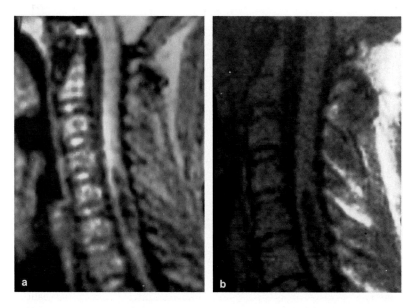

FIG. 42.3 (a) 0.04 T and (b) 0.5 T sagittal images showing herniated cerebellar tonsils and syrinx at C4-C6 level: (a) was obtained using the saturation recovery sequence (TR = 320 msec; TE = 40 msec; 19 min data acquisition time); (b) was obtained with the spin echo sequence (TR = 500 msec; TE = 30 msec; 4.5 to 8.5 min data acquisition time). (Courtesy of L. Samuelsson; reproduced, with permission, from Samuelsson et al [15].)

In a series by Lotz et al [11], it was possible to distinguish renal cysts from renal tumors at 0.02 T. Several other studies in the normal and hydronephrotic kidney seem to indicate that the efficacy of the paramagnetic contrast agents at low field strength (0.02 T) is similar to that observed at conventional BO field strength [10,11].

THE MUSCULOSKELETAL SYSTEM

Ekelund et al have examined lower extremity bone tumors at 0.02 T [1] and normal and abnormal knee joints [3] at 0.04 T. While their experience with the bone tumors at 0.02 T is not encouraging, they have demonstrated the ability of a 0.04 T scanner in identifying cruciate ligament tears (Fig. 42.4) in close agreement with the results obtained by arthroscopy.

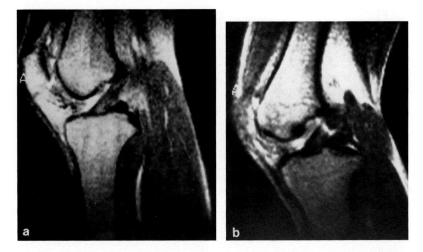

FIG. 42.4 These images of the knee joint obtained at 0.04 T show normal anterior cruciate ligament (ACL) **(a)** and ACL with a partial tear **(b)**. Both images were acquired using partial saturation technique (TR = 1000 msec; TE = 40 msec). The total data acquisition time was 15 to 17 min for 12 slices. However, the total examination time (including postprocessing of the data) was 45 to 60 min. (Courtesy of L. Ekelund; reproduced, with permission, from Ekelund et al [3].)

ADVANTAGES AND DISADVANTAGES

The single most expensive part of any MR scanner is the cost of the main magnet. This fixed cost liability can be reduced considerably by finding a less expensive source to generate the BO field. Alternative methods, such as those described herein, therefore, deliver the promise of reducing the cost of NMR imaging equipment.

As field homogeneity is proportional to the BO field strength, inhomogeneity effects are more pronounced in the ULF-MRI. Therefore, signal decay (T2*) in low magnetic fields is very fast, which makes imaging of the samples with very short relaxation times problematic.

The spatial resolution of low field images generally is low (sometimes, as high as one centimeter) compared to conventional MRI. Besides lower spatial resolution, the problem of external RF noise (in the case of MRIE) greatly hampers the sensitivity of this type of imaging method. Several modifications have been suggested to improve the signal-to-noise ratio of MRIE images [5] but more technological improvements are needed before such a system can be fully implemented in the clinical setting.

REFERENCES

1. Ekelund L, Toolanen G (1989): Low field (0.02 T) magnetic resonance imaging of bone and soft tissue tumors. *Skeletal Radiology* 18:585–590.

2. Ekelund L, Athlin L (1989): Low field magnetic resonance imaging of focal hepatic masses at 0.02 T. *Acta Radiologica* 30:591–595.

3. Ekelund L, Bjornebrink J, Elmquist LG (1991): Ultra-low field magnetic resonance imaging of acute cruciate ligament tears. *Magn Reson Imag* 9:179–185.

4. Favre B, Bonche JP, Mehier H, Peyrin JO (1990): Environmental optimization and shielding for NMR experiments and imaging in the earth's magnetic field. *Magn Reson Med* 13:299–304.

5. Fullerton GD, Cameron IL, Ord VA (1984): Frequency dependence of magnetic resonance spin-lattice relaxation of protons in biological materials. *Radiology* 151:135–138.

6. Gronemeyer DH, Kaufman L, Rothschild P, Seibel RM (1989): New possibilities and aspects of low-field magnetic resonance tomography. *Radiologia Diagnostica.* 30:519–527.

7. Hoult DI, Lauterbur PC (1979): The sensitivity of zeumatographic experiment involving human samples. *J Magn Reson* 34:425–433.

8. Kaufman L, Arakawa M, Hale J, Rothschild P, Carlson J, Hake K, Kramer D, Lu W, van Heteren J (1989): Accessible magnetic resonance imaging. *Magn Reson Quarterly* 5:283–297.

9. Koenig SH, Brown RD, Adams D, Emerson D, Harrison CG (1984): Magnetic field dependence of 1/T1 of protons in tissue. *Invest Radiol* 19:76–81.

10. Koenig SH, Spiller M, Brown RD, Wolf GL (1986): Magnetic field dependence (NMRD profile) of 1/T1 of rabbit kidney medulla and urine after intravenous injection of Gd(DTPA). *Invest Radiol* 21:697–704.

11. Lotz H, Ekelund L, Hietala SO, Wickman G (1988): Low field (0.02 T) MR imaging of the whole body. *J Comput Assist Tomogr* 12:1006–1013.

12. Metcalfe MJ, Jones RA, Redpath TW, Smith FW, Jennings K, Walton S (1989): Low-field cine magnetic resonance imaging in aortic valve disease. *Br J Radiol* 62:1063–1066.

13. Niemi P, Paajanen H, Maattanen H, Komu M, Erkintalo M, Alanen A, Dean PB, Kormano M (1988): Paramagnetic contrast enhancement at 0.02 T: an experimental study using Gd-DOTA in normal and hydronephrotic kidneys. *Magn Reson Med* 7:311–318.

14. Oldendorf W (1985): Low field strength magnetic scanners. *J Comput Assist Tomogr* 9:1153–1154.

15. Samuelsson L, Saaf J, Wahlund LO, Thuomas KA, Bergstrom K (1990): Evaluation of syringomyelia and chiari malformations using ultra-low magnetic resonance imaging. *Magn Reson Imag* 8:123–129.

16. Sepponen RE, Pohjonen JA, Sipponen JT, Tanttu JI (1985): A method for T1 rho imaging. *J Comput Assist Tomogr* 9:1007–1011.

17. Sepponen RE, Sipponen JT, Sivula A (1985): Low field (0.02 T) nuclear magnetic resonance imaging of the brain. *J Comput Assist Tomogr* 9:237–241.

18. Sipponen JT, Sepponen RE, Tanttu JI, Sivula A (1985): Intracranial hematomas studied by MR imaging at 0.17 and 0.02 T. *J Comput Assist Tomogr* 9:698–704.

19. Smith FW, Reid A, Hutchison JMS, Mallard JR (1982): Nuclear magnetic resonance imaging of the pancreas. *Radiology* 142:677–680.

20. Smith FW (1987): Magnetic resonance imaging of midline brain tumors using inversion recovery sequence at 0.08 T. (3.4 MHz) *Magn Reson Med* 5:118–128.

21. Stepisnik J, Erzen V, Kos M (1990): NMR imaging in the earth's magnetic field. *Magn Reson Med* 15:386–391.

43

Undersampling of Data (UNSAD)

BASIC PRINCIPLES

In the most commonly employed spin warp imaging technique, the phase encoding steps are sequentially applied (from K_{min} to k_{max}, or k_{max} to k_{min}) at a rate determined by the pulse repetition time (TR) (Fig. 43.1). Therefore, the time consumed by the entire process of phase encoding is $Np \times TR$ where Np is the total number of the phase encoding steps. For most imaging experiments (excluding those that may require preparatory phase or postprocessing of the data), this time is equivalent to the total experiment time. For example, for a single echo, T2-weighted spin echo image with TR = 2.5 sec, the process of phase encoding 256 steps means that the experiment will last for $256 \times 2.5 = 10.7$ min! And the perils of very long imaging times are well-known: primarily, the high number of motion artifacts and the low patient throughput.

Many fast imaging techniques have been proposed and a number of them are used widely in clinical studies. These techniques have been found to be successful in, among other things, reducing or eliminating motion artifacts. In general, fast imaging techniques achieve reduced data acquisition times by reducing the pulse repetition time. However, there is yet another avenue for achieving reduced imaging times—that is, by decreasing the amount of data (or phase encoding steps, Np) that are acquired. Most commonly, only about half the total phase encode steps are explicitly acquired, which translates directly into a 50% savings in the phase encoding time. Several techniques, as described below, exist for such undersampling of the data. They differ mainly in the manner in which the remaining data set (the k-space) is filled.

(A) In the frequently used technique of zero filling the data, the inner

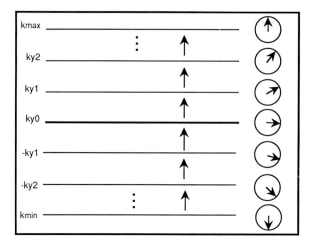

FIG. 43.1 The goal of any MR imaging technique is to acquire enough phase encoded echoes so that an image with acceptable spatial resolution can be reconstructed. In this illustration, the k-space representation of the most commonly employed spin warp imaging data acquisition is shown. Each horizontal line indicates a different phase encoding amplitude and, therefore, different positions of the transverse magnetization in the rotating frame (circles). Each phase encoded transverse magnetization (or, equivalently, the echo signal) is then frequency encoded along the horizontal axis of the k-space. Typically, this process of phase and frequency encoding is repeated at regular time intervals, determined by TR, before advancing to the next phase level.

k steps (lower valued) are explicitly acquired and the remaining outer steps (higher valued) are zero filled (Fig. 43.2). As the higher valued k-steps determine image resolution, the image resolution is degraded (in the phase encode direction) as a result of this data undersampling scheme. If, on the other hand, the outer k-steps are acquired and the inner k-steps zero filled, then a terrible loss in spatial information would occur.

(B) Alternatively, only every other phase encode step is explicitly acquired, and the missing steps are derived by interpolation (Fig. 43.3). With this scheme, the image resolution is undisturbed, as the highest-valued phase encode step is acquired. However, as the sampling interval is inadvertently increased, aliasing artifacts appear, which degrade the image quality. The following two approaches have been proposed to prevent such image degradation.

In the technique of the conjugate reconstruction by off-center undersampling (CROCUS), the phase encoding lines are slightly offset from the origin of the k-space by a certain percentage of the sampling interval (Fig.

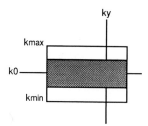

FIG. 43.2 The shaded area (the zero numbered phase step and the neighboring steps) represents the phase steps that are explicitly acquired (see Fig. 43.1).

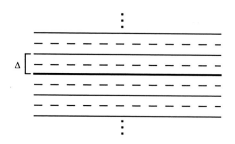

FIG. 43.3 The solid lines represent the phase steps that are explicitly acquired; the dashed lines represent the phase steps that are derived by interpolation. Note that the sampling interval (Δ) has doubled.

FIG. 43.4 The explicitly acquired phase steps (solid lines) are offset by a time delay δ from the origin. When δ = 25% of the sampling interval, the remaining steps (dashed lines) may be derived by using the principle of conjugate symmetry which, unlike interpolation, eliminates aliasing artifacts.

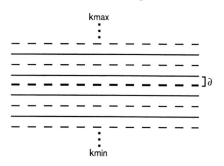

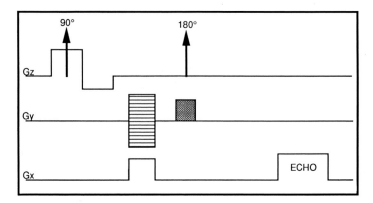

FIG. 43.5 In the strip scan method, the conventional two-dimensional Fourier transform spin warp pulse sequence is modified by applying a gradient pulse (shaded area on the Gy axis) at the same time the 180° readout pulse is being applied. This restricts the field of view in the Gy direction. However, the resolution along the frequency encode axis remains unaltered. As a result, the height of the final image is less than the width of the image (see Fig. 43.6).

FIG. 43.6 (a) Represents the case when the aliasing ghosts (shaded areas) try to encroach upon the actual image of the object due to undersampling of the data (see the original reference for the optical analogy). In order to prevent image degradation as a result of this aliasing, the field of view is limited in the phase encode direction as explained in Fig. 43.5. The resultant image **(b)** is elongated in the frequency encode direction, and so the name 'strip' scan technique. Similar aliasing artifacts also appear because of respiratory motion. See ROPE for the other means for removing aliasing artifacts.

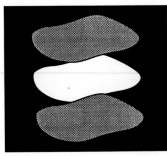

(a)

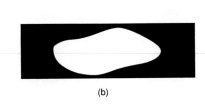

(b)

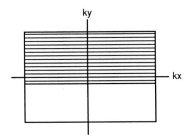

FIG. 43.7 In half-Fourier imaging, one contiguous half of the k-space is explicitly acquired (in this illustration, the upper half). In reality, a few additional phase steps are acquired, which are used to calculate the phase correction factor so that an artifact-free image can be reconstructed.

43.4) [1]. Ehrhardt et al [1] have demonstrated that this tends to remove aliasing artifacts that would have occurred due to the undersampling of data.

In the second alternative, the field of view (FOV) is decreased by applying a monopolar gradient pulse along the phase encode direction at the time of the 180° readout RF pulse (Fig. 43.5) (the strip scan method [7]). The decreased FOV effectively keeps artifacts away from degrading the region of interest (Fig. 43.6).

(C) In what is called the partial-Fourier imaging or half-Fourier imaging, one entire half of the k-space is explicitly acquired, and the other half is filled by the principle of conjugate symmetry. The conjugate symmetry of the Fourier transform dictates that if all the image data are real, then one-half of the image data can be derived by taking the complex conjugate of the corresponding other half of the image data. In practical terms, this means that if the phase encoding steps are carried out only from the origin to either end of the ky axis, the remaining phase values may be obtained by using conjugate symmetry (Fig. 43.7) [2,6].

The undersampling of data, as discussed above, is mainly used for the phase encoding process. However, the half-Fourier technique also may be used along the frequency encode direction. This decreases the minimum echo time and the intraview motion-related artifacts.

CLINICAL APPLICATIONS
TISSUE CONTRAST

In general, the amount of noise increases in proportion to the number of data steps that are explicitly not acquired. The image contrast-to-noise ratio (CNR), as a result, also decreases. However, such a decrease in the

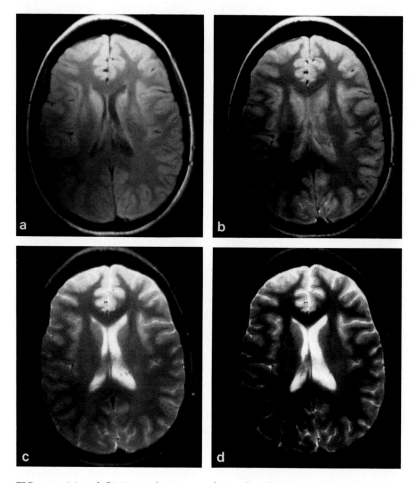

FIG. 43.8 (a) and **(b)** First echo images obtained with TE = 15 msec and TR = 2.5 msec (conventional) and TR = 5 sec (half-Fourier), respectively. **(c)** and **(d)** Second echo images obtained with TE = 90 msec and TR = 2.5 msec (conventional) and TR = 5 sec (half-Fourier), respectively. Notice the improved contrast-to-noise ratio for the half-Fourier images, which were obtained in similar acquisition times as the conventional full Fourier images. (Courtesy of E.M. Haacke; reproduced, with permission, from Haacke et al [4].

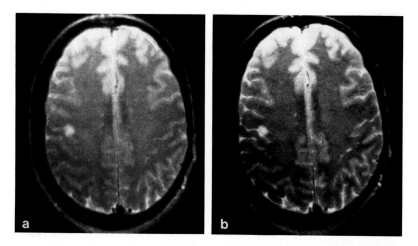

FIG. 43.9 **(a)** Conventional second echo image with TR = 2.5 sec; **(b)** half-Fourier second echo image with TR = 4 sec. Although data acquisition times for these images were similar, (b) shows the lesion in the right cerebral hemisphere more conspicuously than (a) because of the improved contrast-to-noise ratio. (Courtesy of E.M. Haacke; reproduced, with permission, from Haacke et al [4].)

contrast-to-noise ratio may be offset by employing a longer TR or taking multiple averages (Fig. 43.8). In such circumstances, the advantage of the speed is, of course, no longer retained. But image contrast may be modulated without unduly increasing the imaging time. Haacke et al [4] have recently analyzed the contrast behavior of full-Fourier and half-Fourier images of the brain. They have shown that the half-Fourier imaging can be used effectively for increasing the contrast-to-noise ratio of T2-weighted spin echo images (and thus enhance their diagnostic value) (Fig. 43.9), and also for vascular imaging.

ADVANTAGES AND DISADVANTAGES

The elimination of explicit phase encoding may give rise to aliasing artifacts, especially if the first or second schemes of the data undersampling are used (see above).

In addition, conjugate symmetry works only if all the sources of phase change other than gradients are removed. However, this is not true in real-life situations because of main field inhomogeneities and flow effects. Therefore, phase errors creep into the final image and make it blurry. To account for phase errors that may exist due to imperfect imaging conditions, several phase correction schemes have been proposed

[3,5]. Commonly, a few phase values are collected in addition to the usual 50% phase values. An estimate of the system phase errors is, then, derived from these extra phase values and a correction factor is applied while subjecting the image data to the conjugate symmetry principle.

REFERENCES

1. Ehrhardt JC, Tian ZC, Chang W (1988): Reduced MR acquisition time with the CROCUS technique. *J Comput Assist Tomogr* 12:468–473.
2. Feinberg DA, Hale JD, Watts JC, Kaufman L, Mark A (1986): Halving MR imaging time by conjugation: demonstration at 3.5 kg. *Radiology* 161:527–531.
3. Feinberg DA, Turner R, Jakab PD, Von Kienlin M (1990): Echo planar imaging with asymmetric gradient modulation and inner-volume excitation. *Magn Reson Med* 13:162–169.
4. Haacke EM, Mitchell J, Lee D (1990): Improved contrast at 1.5 Tesla using half-Fourier imaging: application to spin-echo and angiographic imaging. *Magn Reson Imag* 8:79–90.
5. MacFall JR, Pelc NJ, Vavrek RM (1988): Correction of spatially dependent phase shifts for partial Fourier imaging. *Magn Reson Imag* 6:143–155.
6. Margosian P, Schmitt F, Purdy P (1986): Faster MR imaging: imaging with half the data. *Health Care Instr* 1:195–197.
7. Mezrich RS, Axel L, Dougherty L, Kressel HY (1986): Strip scan: a method for faster MR imaging. *Radiographics* 6:833–845.
8. Runge VM, Wood ML (1990): Half-Fourier MR imaging of CNS disease. *Am J Neuroradiol* 11:77–82.

Index

Echo rephasing, field even, 49–54. *See also* Field even echo rephasing
Echo scan hybrid, mosaic, 5
Edema, brain, inversion recovery imaging of, 130
End diastolic phases, 93
End systolic phases, 93
EPI. *See* Echo planar imaging
Equilibrium magnetization, in ultra-low field MRI, 314–315
Even echo rephasing. *See also* Field even echo rephasing
 artifacts due to, 109
 field even, 49–54
 principle of, 51
Excitation-readout time lapse artifacts, 194
Excited spins, flow, 260
 in flow adjustable gradient echo, 64
Extracerebral arteries, phase-based angiography of, 218
Extradural pathologies
 fast low angle shot imaging of, 80
 gradient acquisition in steady state imaging of, 113

F
FADE. *See* Fast acquisition double echo
FANG. *See* Fourier angiography
FAST. *See* Fast acquisition in steady state
Fast acquisition double echo (FADE)
 advantages and disadvantages, 34
 basic principles, 30–32
 clinical applications, 34, 35f
Fast acquisition in steady state (FAST)
 advantages and disadvantages, 45–48
 basic principles, 43–45
 clinical applications, 45
 compared to resonant offset averaging in the steady state, 240
Fast field echoes (FFE)
 fast action double echo comparisons with, 34
 generation of, 111
 techniques
  basic principles, 87
  fast low angle shot, 76–84
  in steady state free precession, 275

Fast imaging techniques, 323. *See also* specific technique
 Fourier based, 273–274
 reasons for, 87
 in respiratory ordered phase encoding, 247–248
Fast imaging with steady state precession (FISP), 32, 43, 239, 240, 247
 advantages and disadvantages, 60, 62
 basic principles, 56
  variants, 56–57
 clinical applications, 57–60, 309f
Fast low angle excitation echo planar technique (FLEET), 23
 advantages of, 26–27
Fast low angle multiecho (FLAME), 70
Fast low angle rapid acquisition relaxation enhanced imaging (FLARE), 228
 clinical applications, 228, 230
 variant of, 228
Fast low angle shot (FLASH), 30, 31f, 87, 139, 189. *See also* Inversion recovery—fast low angle shot imaging; Snapshot FLASH imaging
 advantages and disadvantages, 83–84
 basic principles, 76–78
  variants, 78–79
 cine-FLASH, 83, 257
 clinical applications, 32, 60, 79, 83f
 compared to fast imaging with steady state precession, 60
 compared to fast low angle spin echo, 74
 inversion recovery imaging, 134–138
 phase encoding gradient in, 43
 refocused, 43, 77, 274
 snapshot, 254–258
 spoiled, 274
 transverse magnetization in, destruction of, 56
 turboFLASH, 83, 97, 211, 254, 312
Fast low angle spin echo (FLASE), 234
 advantages and disadvantages, 74
 basic principles, 69–70
  variants, 70–72
 clinical applications, 72–74

values, in respiratory ordered phase encoding, 248, 249
Phase encoding gradient
   direction of, changing of, 248
   in fast low angle shot, 78
   in line scan angiography, 139
Phase errors, in undersampling of data, 329–330
Phase information
   in double phase encoding, 18
   in field even echo rephasing, 53
Phase map
   creation of, 218
   pixel intensity in, 51, 52f, 221
Phase offset multiplanar imaging (POMP), 187
Phase shift, 212, 213, 214
   factors contributing to, 213
   in field even echo rephasing, 49
   of flowing spins, 220
Phase shift artifacts, suppression of, 149
Phase values, in undersampling of data, 330
Pi-EPI (π-EPI), 23
POMP. See Phase offset multiplanar imaging
POPE. See Projection ordered phase encoding
Portal venous system, fast low angle shot imaging of, 81–82
Postgadolinium fast low angle shot images, 80
Poststenotic flow, field even echo rephasing imaging of, 53
Pregnancy
   echo planar imaging in, 26
      blipped, 7
   rapid acquisition relaxation enhanced imaging in, 232
Preinversion pulses, in noninvasive image tagging, 198
PREP. See Projection-reconstruction echo planar imaging
Projection ordered phase encoding (POPE), 251, 252
Projection-reconstruction echo planar imaging (PREP), 23–24
Projective Fourier angiography (PFA), 36–37, 41
Prostate, fast low angle spin echo imaging of, 74
Prosthesis, metallic, 179

Proton images
   in gradient recalled echo and spin echo, 121
   rapid acquisition of, 79
Proton spectroscopy, of brain, 287
Pseudo cine-GRASS, 115
Pseudodynamic cine-FLASH, 82
Pseudogating, 94

Q
Quick T1 (QT1), 161, 162

R
RAPID. See Rapid acquisition of proton images using DIGGER
Rapid acquisition of proton images using DIGGER (RAPID), 79
Rapid acquisition relaxation enhanced imaging (RARE), 16
   advantages and disadvantages, 232
   basic principles, 224–225
      variants, 225–228
   clinical applications, 228–232
Rapid gradient echo, magnetization-prepared, 171–175. See also Magnetization-prepared rapid gradient echo
Rapid relaxation with repeated echoes. See Rapid acquisition relaxation enhanced imaging
Rapid sequential excitation (RSE) approach, 67
Rapid spin echo (RASE)
   advantages and disadvantages, 237–238
   basic principles, 234–235
   clinical applications, 235–237
Rapid spin echo excitation (RASEE), 70, 74
RARE. See Rapid acquisition relaxation enhanced imaging
RARE ROAST. See Refocused acquisition in the readout direction
RASE. See Rapid spin echo
RASEE. See Rapid spin echo excitation
Recovery delay (Te)
   defined, 134
   in inversion recovery—fast low angle shot imaging, 134–138

Striped tags (STAG), 200, 201, 203f
advantages and disadvantages, 206
Subarachnoid cyst, double phase
    encoding images of, 17f, 18
Subject motion, 89
Subtraction angiography, advantages
    and disadvantages of, 220–221
Suppressed tissue with refreshment
    angiography method
    (STREAM), 304–305, 306f
SURGE. See Spin echo using repeated
    gradient echoes
Symmetry, conjugate, 327, 327f,
    329–330
Syncopated periodic excitation
    (SPEX), 177f, 178
Synovial fluid, in short tau inversion
    recovery imaging, 297
Synthetic imaging
    advantages of, 167
    principle of, 165–166
Syrinx malformations, ultra-low field
    MRI of, 318, 318f, 319f

T

T1 calculation, in echo planar
    imaging, 26
T1 contrast
    in fast imaging with steady state
        precession, 56, 58
    in fast low angle shot imaging, 138
    in inversion recovery, 131, 138
        short tau, 298
    in rapid acquisition relaxation
        enhanced imaging, 225
T1 relaxation
    in fast acquisition double echo, 30
    in fast low angle shot, 77
    in inversion recovery, 126, 128
    inverted spins and, 260
    stimulated echo acquisition mode
        and, 287
T1 relaxation curve, in inversion
    recovery—fast low angle shot
    imaging, 138
T1 relaxation time
    in gradient recalled echo and spin
        echo, 119
    measurement of, 157, 158t, 158–162
        advantages and disadvantages,
        166–167
        brain, 158t, 166

simultaneous with T2, 164–165
    stimulated echo acquisition mode
        for, 282
T1 values
    in inversion recovery, 128
        selective, 263
        short tau, 293
    in steady state free precession, 277
    in time of flight techniques, 301,
        304f
T1 weighted images, 157
    in fast acquisition in steady state,
        45
    in fast imaging with steady state
        precession, 60
    in inversion recovery—fast low
        angle shot imaging, 134
    motion artifact suppression
        technique and, 146
    in multislice imaging, 183
    in rapid spin echo, 235
    in short tau inversion recovery, 293
    spin echo
        fast low angle, 74, 81
        in gradient acquisition in steady
            state, 113
        of joints, 82
T1/T2 ratio, in fast imaging with
    steady state precession, 57
T2 contrast
    motion artifact suppression
        technique and, 146
    in short tau inversion recovery
        imaging, 298
T2 decay, 287
    stimulated echo acquisition mode
        and, 287
T2 relaxation
    in fast acquisition double echo, 30
    in fast low angle shot, 77
    in gradient recalled echo and spin
        echo, 119
    in inversion recovery, 126
T2 relaxation time
    measurement of, 157, 158t,
        162–163, 167
        simultaneous with T1, 164–165
    in rapid acquisition relaxation
        enhanced imaging, 228
T2 values
    in short tau inversion recovery, 293
    in steady state free precession, 277
    in time of flight techniques, 301,
        304f